Review of
Medical Microbiology

Review of Medical Microbiology

Patrick R. Murray, PhD

Chief, Microbiology Service
Department of Laboratory Medicine
National Institutes of Health
Bethesda, Maryland

Ken S. Rosenthal, PhD

Professor
Department of Microbiology and Immunology
Northeastern Ohio Universities College of Medicine
Rootstown, Ohio

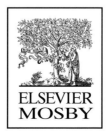

ELSEVIER
MOSBY

**ELSEVIER
MOSBY**

1600 John F. Kennedy Boulevard, Suite 1800
Philadelphia, Pennsylvania 19103-2899

Review of Medical Microbiology   ISBN: 0-323-03325-3

Patrick R. Murray's role as author of this book was carried out in his private capacity, and his contribution does not reflect official support or endorsement by the National Institutes of Health or the Department of Health and Human Services.

International Standard Book Number: 0-323-03325-3

Acquisitions Editor: William Schmitt
Developmental Editor: Katie Miller
Publishing Services Manager: Joan Sinclair
Project Manager: Cecelia Bayruns

Printed in China.

Last digit is the print number: 9 8 7 6 5 4 3 2 1

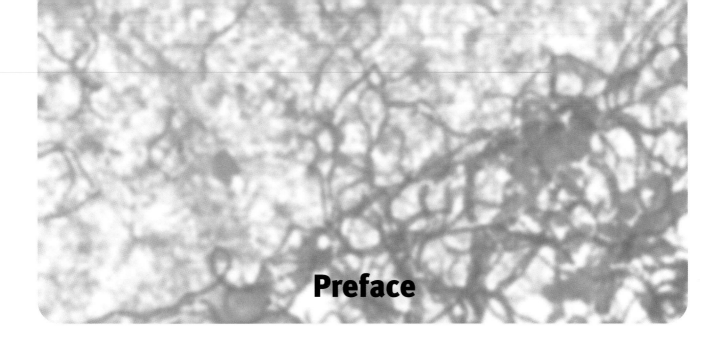

Preface

The difficulty all students have is "separating the wheat from the chaff"; that is, distinguishing what is important from what is "interesting and nice to know." In our textbook, *Medical Microbiology*, we attempted to reduce the complex fields of microbiology and infectious diseases to a manageable but comprehensive body of information. We supplemented the text with clinical illustrations, diagrams, and summary tables and provided clinical scenarios to help students understand disease from the perspective of their knowledge of basic microbial biology.

Review of Medical Microbiology was prepared as another tool for students to help them assess their understanding of microbiology and—incidentally—perform well on related exams. The *Review* consists of 550 USMLE-type questions covering the four major microbial pathogen groups: bacteria, viruses, fungi, and parasites. Most questions are framed in reference to the clinical presentation of the patient and deal with subject matter that we think should be mastered by a student. Students can also learn from the discussion of the correct and incorrect answers that is provided for each question. In this case, a student can even learn from his or her mistakes. We hope students will find this a useful tool not only for successfully passing their examinations, but also for building upon their foundation of knowledge in microbiology.

Patrick R. Murray, PhD
Ken S. Rosenthal, PhD

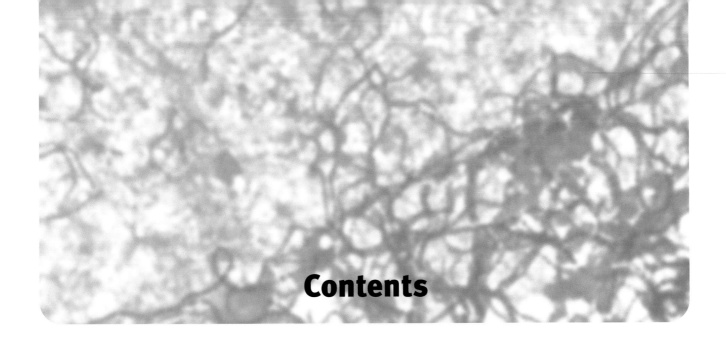

Contents

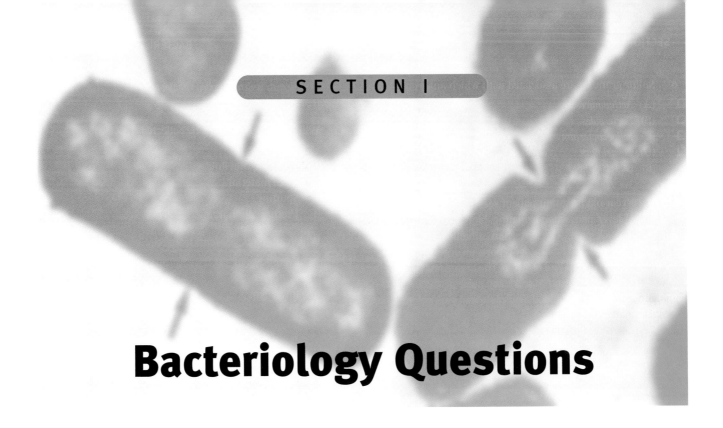

Bacteriology Questions

1 A 6-year-old boy arrives with his mother to the pediatric emergency room complaining of pain in his right hand where a stray cat had bit him the previous day. The mother had washed the wound with soap and water but noticed the area around the wound was red by that evening. The next morning, the boy awoke crying and complaining of pain in his hand. The physical exam reveals that he has an oral temperature of 39°C. The skin over the wound is erythematous. A serosanguineous drop is expressed from the puncture wound and submitted for a culture and Gram stain. The microbiology laboratory reports abundant growth of gram-negative coccobacilli. The organisms were facultatively anaerobic but failed to grow on MacConkey agar. Which organism is most likely responsible for this infection?

- ☐ (A) *Capnocytophaga*
- ☐ (B) *Eikenella*
- ☐ (C) *Escherichia*
- ☐ (D) *Fusobacterium*
- ☐ (E) *Pasteurella*

2 A mother brings her 3-month-old baby to her pediatrician because he has been progressively more listless for 3 days. The baby has been constipated and has refused to nurse or take a bottle. Upon physical examination, the physician notes that the baby has a sluggish papillary reaction to light, a weak gag reflex, and poor anal sphincter control. The physician tentatively diagnosis this 3-month-old with infant botulism. Which test would be the most reliable for confirming this diagnosis?

- ☐ (A) Culture of the baby's blood
- ☐ (B) Culture of the baby's stool
- ☐ (C) Detection of toxin in food products
- ☐ (D) Detection of toxin in the baby's serum
- ☐ (E) Detection of antitoxin antibodies in the baby's serum

3 Which bacterial species is most commonly associated with septicemia?

- ☐ (A) *Campylobacter coli*
- ☐ (B) *Campylobacter fetus*
- ☐ (C) *Campylobacter jejuni*
- ☐ (D) *Campylobacter upsaliensis*
- ☐ (E) *Helicobacter pylori*

4 Which property is responsible for the survival and replication of *Mycobacterium tuberculosis* in an infected patient?

- ☐ (A) Production of phospholipase C that degrades cellular membranes
- ☐ (B) Production of proteases that degrade IgM and IgG
- ☐ (C) Phagocytized bacteria inhibit phagosome lysosome fusion
- ☐ (D) Phagocytized bacteria inactivate lysosomal enzymes
- ☐ (E) Presence of a capsule that inhibits phagocytosis

5 Which test is most reliable for diagnosing *Clostridium difficile* disease?

- ☐ (A) Gram stain of the stool
- ☐ (B) Culture of the stool
- ☐ (C) Assay of stool filtrates for toxin
- ☐ (D) Assay of blood for toxin
- ☐ (E) Nucleic acid amplification (NAA) for specific bacteria in stool

6 Sulfur granules are associated with which anaerobe?

❑ (A) *Actinomyces*

❑ (B) *Bacteroides*

❑ (C) *Bifidobacterium*

❑ (D) *Clostridium*

❑ (E) *Lactobacillus*

7 A 28-year-old pregnant patient sees her obstetrician and complains of fever, pain when urinating, blood in her urine, and severe lower back pain. The physician submits her urine for culture; the next day, the laboratory reports an organism growth count of greater than 10^5/ml of urine. The organisms grew well on both the blood agar and MacConkey agar, producing beta-hemolytic colonies on the blood agar plate and pink colonies on the MacConkey agar. Which of the following is the most likely causal organism?

❑ (A) *Candida albicans*

❑ (B) *Enterococcus faecalis*

❑ (C) *Escherichia coli*

❑ (D) *Proteus mirabilis*

❑ (E) *Staphylococcus aureus*

8 Rifampin acts in a bactericidal manner by which mechanism?

❑ (A) Blocks peptide elongation by inhibiting peptidyl-transferase

❑ (B) Inhibits cross-linking of cell wall peptidoglycan

❑ (C) Inhibits DNA topoisomerases

❑ (D) Inhibits initiation of RNA synthesis

❑ (E) Initiates premature release of peptide chains from ribosome

9 *Streptococcus pneumoniae* can escape phagocytic clearance by which mechanism?

❑ (A) Capsule-mediated inhibition of phagocytosis

❑ (B) Inhibition of phagosome/lysosome fusion

❑ (C) Inhibition of opsonization mediated by protein A

❑ (D) Lysis of phagosome and replication in cytoplasm

❑ (E) Replication in fused phagosome/lysosome

10 A 14-day-old baby is admitted to the hospital with a fever, hyperactivity, and a stiff neck. At the time of giving birth to the baby, the mother complained of flu-like symptoms. Blood and cerebrospinal fluid (CSF) were collected for culture. No organisms were seen in the Gram stain of the CSF; however, the culture of blood and CSF became positive after 48 h of incubation. Colonies appeared weakly beta-hemolytic, and the Gram stain was interpreted as gram-positive cocci or coccobacilli arranged in single cells and pairs. Which organism is most likely responsible for this baby's infection?

❑ (A) *Escherichia coli*

❑ (B) *Listeria monocytogenes*

❑ (C) *Neisseria meningitidis*

❑ (D) Group B *Streptococcus agalactiae*

❑ (E) *Streptococcus pneumoniae*

11 Which specimen should be collected on a swab?

❑ (A) Blood

❑ (B) Cerebrospinal fluid

❑ (C) Fecal material

❑ (D) Sputum

❑ (E) Urethral discharge

12 Which antibiotic prevents transcription of DNA into RNA?

❑ (A) Ciprofloxacin

❑ (B) Erythromycin

❑ (C) Imipenem

❑ (D) Rifampin

❑ (E) Tetracycline

13 A 56-year-old man undergoes coronary bypass surgery. He receives cefazolin prophylactically and at a dosage that is continued for 2 days postoperatively. On the 10th postoperative day, he develops a fever of 40°C with a heart rate of 110 beats per minute (bpm) and a blood pressure of 100/70 mm Hg. His white blood cell (WBC) count is 14,000/mm^3, and a urinalysis reveals many white blood cells per high power field. Cultures of blood, urine, and the surgical wound are then obtained. The urine and wound cultures are positive with gram-negative rods. The organism is oxidase-positive and unable to ferment glucose. Large, spreading, beta-hemolytic colonies are seen on sheep blood agar, and colorless colonies are noted on MacConkey agar. Antimicrobial susceptibility testing reveals the organism is susceptible to imipenem and piperacillin-tazobactam, but it is resistant to trimethoprim/sulfamethoxazole. These results are characteristic of which organism?

❑ (A) *Acinetobacter haemolyticus*

❑ (B) *Burkholderia cepacia*

❑ (C) *Moraxella catarrhalis*

❑ (D) *Pseudomonas aeruginosa*

❑ (E) *Stenotrophomonas maltophilia*

14 A 16-year-old boy is taken to his family physician with a 1-week history of rhinitis and pharyngitis, as well as a low-grade fever, malaise, and headache. The boy has no history of a rash. He has a nonproductive cough and is short of breath upon exertion. Chest radiograph reveals a density in the lower lobes. Gram stain of induced sputum shows inflammatory cells, a few squamous epithelial cells, and no predominant organism. No respiratory pathogens are recovered in culture on routine media. A rapid group A *Streptococcus* test is negative; a heterophil test is also negative; the VDRL test is weakly positive; and serum cold agglutinins are positive. Which organism is most likely responsible for this patient's infection?

❑ (A) *Chlamydophila (Chlamydia) pneumoniae*

❑ (B) *Legionella pneumophila*

❑ (C) *Mycoplasma pneumoniae*

❑ (D) *Streptococcus pneumoniae*

❑ (E) *Treponema pallidum*

15 When waking her 6-year-old son for school, a mother observes that the boy is limping. She notices that his left knee is swollen, red, warm to the touch, and movement is painful. He states he fell on the knee 2 days ago while playing with friends. The mother brings her son to see their pediatrician, who removes 15 ml of cloudy fluid from the knee. A Gram stain and culture of the fluid shows gram-positive cocci arranged in clusters (see figure). Which organism is most likely the cause of the boy's symptoms?

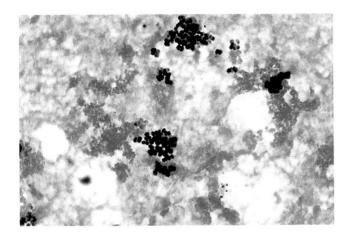

- ❑ (A) *Bacillus cereus*
- ❑ (B) *Enterococcus faecalis*
- ❑ (C) *Neisseria gonorrhoeae*
- ❑ (D) *Staphylococcus aureus*
- ❑ (E) *Streptococcus pyogenes*

16 A physician working in a rural community in Russia sees a number of local residents with signs and symptoms suggestive of diphtheria. Which antibiotic should be used to treat these patients?

- ❑ (A) Chloramphenicol
- ❑ (B) Ciprofloxacin
- ❑ (C) Doxycycline
- ❑ (D) Metronidazole
- ❑ (E) Penicillin

17 Which statement about *Staphylococcus aureus* is correct?

- ❑ (A) Resistance to ampicillin/sulbactam is mediated by beta-lactamases.
- ❑ (B) Resistance to dicloxacillin is mediated by beta-lactamases.
- ❑ (C) Resistance to oxacillin is mediated by beta-lactamases.
- ❑ (D) Resistance to penicillin is mediated by beta-lactamases.
- ❑ (E) Resistance to vancomycin is mediated by beta-lactamases.

18 Which test is most commonly used to detect *Tropheryma whipplei*?

- ❑ (A) Culture
- ❑ (B) Enzyme immunoassay
- ❑ (C) Gram stain
- ❑ (D) Nucleic acid-based tests
- ❑ (E) Silver stain

19 *Bartonella quintana* is the etiologic agent of trench fever or "5-day" fever. This disease is characterized by severe headaches, fever (recurring at 5-day intervals), weakness, and pain in the long bones. Which arthropod is a vector of this disease?

- ❑ (A) Fleas
- ❑ (B) Lice
- ❑ (C) Mosquitoes
- ❑ (D) Sand flies
- ❑ (E) Ticks

20 After an automobile accident, a 23-year-old woman requires an emergency splenectomy. Her subsequent recovery is uneventful. However, 4 weeks after the surgery, she is brought to the emergency department unconscious and nonresponsive. The emergency department physicians are unable to stabilize her, and she expires 1 h after she arrived. Blood is collected for culture, chemistry tests, and hematology tests. The technologist examining the peripheral blood smear observes abundant bacteria. Within 6 h, the blood culture is also reported to be positive with gram-positive cocci (see figure). Which organism is most likely responsible for this overwhelming infection?

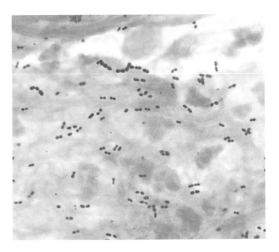

- ❑ (A) *Enterococcus faecium*
- ❑ (B) *Peptostreptococcus anaerobius*
- ❑ (C) *Staphylococcus aureus*
- ❑ (D) *Streptococcus pneumoniae*
- ❑ (E) *Streptococcus pyogenes*

21 A 46-year-old man had a bone marrow transplant in July to manage his hematologic malignancy. In November, his family notices that he seems confused and disoriented, and they bring him to see his oncologist. The physician notes that the man is unable to stand without assistance and cannot state his location or the day of the week. A computerized tomographic (CT) scan of his brain reveals multiple lesions. He is taken to surgery, and purulent material is drained from one of the accessible lesions. This sample is submitted to the microbiology laboratory for a Gram stain and culture. Gram-positive cocci and long, thin gram-negative rods are seen on Gram stain. After 2 days, no growth is observed on blood, chocolate, or MacConkey agars. Which organisms are most likely responsible for this man's infection?

- ❏ (A) *Peptostreptococcus* and *Bacteroides*
- ❏ (B) *Peptostreptococcus* and *Fusobacterium*
- ❏ (C) *Peptostreptococcus* and *Prevotella*
- ❏ (D) *Staphylococcus* and *Haemophilus*
- ❏ (E) Viridans group *Streptococcus* and *Haemophilus*

22 Which statement is correct?

- ❏ (A) *Bacteroides fragilis* is a gram-positive, non–spore-forming rod.
- ❏ (B) *Propionibacterium* is found on the skin's surface.
- ❏ (C) *Lactobacillus* is a common pathogen that colonizes the genitourinary tract and causes urinary tract infections.
- ❏ (D) Most anaerobic infections are exogenous infections.
- ❏ (E) Most anaerobic infections are monomicrobic.

23 A family of two adults and three children develop gastroenteritis while vacationing in New York. The onset is abrupt with abdominal cramps and watery diarrhea. None of the family members has a fever or nausea; nobody experiences vomiting. Within 24 h, the symptoms have resolved. The family notes that the condition developed 10 h after they had eaten a buffet dinner in a roadside café. When they report the disease to the public health office, an investigator is assigned to investigate the restaurant. The investigation reveals that one of the food products eaten by the family was contaminated with a high concentration of type A *Clostridium perfringens*. Which food is the most likely source of this infection?

- ❏ (A) Beef stew
- ❏ (B) Chicken
- ❏ (C) Custard
- ❏ (D) Milk shake
- ❏ (E) Salad

24 *Campylobacter* infections are associated most commonly with which of the following foods?

- ❏ (A) Apple pie
- ❏ (B) Chicken
- ❏ (C) Hamburgers
- ❏ (D) Rice
- ❏ (E) Shrimp

25 *Bacteroides fragilis* is the most common cause of which condition or disease?

- ❏ (A) Intraabdominal abscesses
- ❏ (B) Gas gangrene
- ❏ (C) Brain abscesses
- ❏ (D) Pelvic inflammatory disease
- ❏ (E) Pseudomembranous colitis

26 A 59-year-old man punctures his hand while clearing brush on his property. He develops signs and symptoms consistent with tetanus 4 days after the accident. The toxin produced by this organism acts by which mechanism?

- ❏ (A) Catalyzes hydrolysis of membrane phospholipids
- ❏ (B) Integrates into cell membranes, leading to pore formation with cell lysis
- ❏ (C) Stimulates macrophages to release proinflammatory cytokines
- ❏ (D) Blocks release of the neurotransmitter acetylcholine
- ❏ (E) Blocks release of neurotransmitters for inhibitory synapses

27 Which association is correct?

- ❏ (A) *Lactobacillus* frequently causes opportunistic infections in patients with prosthetic devices, such as intravascular catheters.
- ❏ (B) *Clostridium difficile* can survive in an environment (e.g., hospital floors, medical instruments) for a prolonged period.
- ❏ (C) Tetanus toxin binds irreversibly to its receptor and stimulates a vigorous antibody response.
- ❏ (D) Important virulence factors produced by *Bacteroides fragilis* include enterotoxin and exfoliative toxin.
- ❏ (E) *Bacteroides fragilis* is typically susceptible to metronidazole, penicillin, and broad-spectrum cephalosporins.

28 Which respiratory pathogen can be detected in clinical specimens by Gram stain?

- ❏ (A) *Chlamydophila (Chlamydia) pneumoniae*
- ❏ (B) *Legionella pneumophila*
- ❏ (C) *Mycobacterium tuberculosis*
- ❏ (D) *Mycoplasma pneumoniae*
- ❏ (E) *Nocardia asteroides*

29 Approximately 4 h after eating a meal in a neighborhood restaurant, three members of a family develop a sudden onset of nausea, vomiting, and severe abdominal cramps. Nobody is febrile, and only one family member has diarrhea. Within 24 h, the symptoms have resolved with no subsequent recurrences. Which organism is most likely responsible for this outbreak?

❑ (A) *Bacillus cereus*
❑ (B) *Campylobacter jejuni*
❑ (C) *Salmonella enterica*
❑ (D) *Shigella sonnei*
❑ (E) *Yersinia enterocolitica*

30 Which test can be used to identify *Streptococcus pneumoniae?*

❑ (A) Bacitracin susceptibility
❑ (B) Bile solubility
❑ (C) Catalase
❑ (D) Coagulase
❑ (E) Oxidase

31 A 35-year-old man with AIDS presents to his physician with a 2-month history of fever, drenching night sweats, and weight loss. At the time of presentation, his CD4 cell count is 15/mm³. Hepatomegaly and a palpable spleen are noted during the physical examination. Specimens of blood, sputum, and stool are collected for microbiology testing. Acid-fast rods are seen upon examination of the sputum specimen, and these organisms are recovered from all specimens submitted to the laboratory. Colonies of the organism are nonpigmented, niacin-negative, and nitrate reductase-negative. Which antibiotic would be most effective against this organism?

❑ (A) Ciprofloxacin
❑ (B) Clarithromycin
❑ (C) Ethambutol
❑ (D) Isoniazid
❑ (E) Rifampin

32 Which antibiotic inhibits peptidoglycan synthesis?

❑ (A) Ciprofloxacin
❑ (B) Erythromycin
❑ (C) Imipenem
❑ (D) Rifampin
❑ (E) Tetracycline

33 A 32-year-old woman sees her gynecologist with complaints of a low-grade fever, weight loss, abdominal pain, and vaginal bleeding. She has noticed these symptoms for more than 4 weeks. She reports that she had an IUD inserted 5 years previously but has been sexually inactive for more than 1 year. Pelvic examination and palpation reveal a firm mass, so the woman is taken to surgery. The IUD is found to be associated with fibrosis and a collection of pus. The IUD and mass are removed, and the mass is submitted to pathology for histological examination and cultures. Thin, branching gram-positive rods are observed, and this organism is then isolated in culture after incubation for 5 days. Which organism is most likely responsible for this woman's infection?

❑ (A) *Actinomyces*
❑ (B) *Lactobacillus*
❑ (C) *Mobiluncus*
❑ (D) *Nocardia*
❑ (E) *Propionibacterium*

34 A 43-year-old woman sees her family physician with complaints of a dull persistent pain surrounding her nose and the feeling of paranasal fullness. These symptoms developed after a viral respiratory infection that she had 3 weeks prior to this visit. A CT scan of the head shows opacity in the paranasal sinuses (see figure) and confirms the clinical diagnosis of chronic sinusitis. Which organism is most likely responsible for this infection?

From Cohen J, Powderly WG: *Infectious diseases*, ed 2, St Louis, 2004, Mosby.

❑ (A) *Haemophilus influenzae*, type b
❑ (B) *Neisseria meningitides*
❑ (C) *Staphylococcus aureus*
❑ (D) *Streptococcus pneumoniae*
❑ (E) *Streptococcus pyogenes*

35 Which antibiotic can be used to treat infections caused by *Mycoplasma pneumoniae?*

❑ (A) Ampicillin-sulbactam
❑ (B) Ceftazidime
❑ (C) Erythromycin
❑ (D) Imipenem
❑ (E) Vancomycin

36 Which arthropod is the most important vector of tularemia?

❑ (A) Deer fly
❑ (B) Flea
❑ (C) Lice
❑ (D) Mosquito
❑ (E) Tick

37 During a routine physical examination, a 48-year-old man complains to his physician of chronic, persistent gastric pain. The pain is a burning sensation that is relieved by meals or milk but reoccurs within a few hours after eating. The physician suspects the patient has a duodenal ulcer. Because the patient has denied use of aspirin and nonsteroidal anti-inflammatory drugs, the physician also suspects the ulcer has an infectious etiology. Which important virulence factor for the organism is most likely responsible for this patient's disease?

- ❑ (A) Capsule
- ❑ (B) Endotoxin
- ❑ (C) Enterotoxin
- ❑ (D) Phospholipase C
- ❑ (E) Urease

38 A 7-year-old girl sees her pediatrician for a cutaneous pustule on her right arm at the site where her kitten had scratched her 1 week prior to the appointment. Her mother has also noticed an enlargement of the right axillary lymph nodes. The girl has a low-grade fever and complains of feeling tired. The pediatrician collects cultures of the pustule, lymph node, and blood, but all results are negative after incubation for 1 week. Which organism is most likely responsible for this infection?

- ❑ (A) *Bartonella henselae*
- ❑ (B) *Klebsiella (Calymmatobacterium) granulomatis*
- ❑ (C) *Capnocytophaga ochracea*
- ❑ (D) *Eikenella corrodens*
- ❑ (E) *Pasteurella multocida*

39 Which arthropod is the vector of Lyme disease?

- ❑ (A) Flea
- ❑ (B) Tick
- ❑ (C) Lice
- ❑ (D) Mite
- ❑ (E) Mosquito

40 A 52-year-old man develops peritonitis after rupture of his appendix. After surgery for repair of the rupture, the man is treated with clindamycin and ceftazidime. Approximately 5 days later, the patient develops profuse diarrhea, abdominal cramps, and a fever of 38.5°C. During an additional 5 days, the diarrhea worsens, with gross blood present in the stools and white plaques observed over the colonic mucosa (see figure). Which organism is most likely responsible for this patient's symptoms?

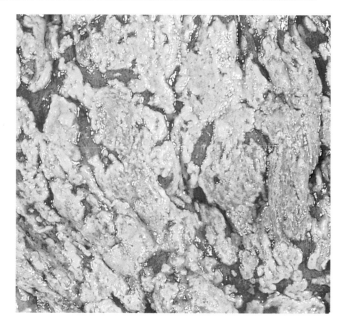

- ❑ (A) *Bacillus cereus*
- ❑ (B) *Clostridium difficile*
- ❑ (C) *Escherichia coli* O517
- ❑ (D) *Shigella sonnei*
- ❑ (E) *Staphylococcus aureus*

41 Which microscopic staining methods should be used to detect the *Mycobacterium avium* complex?

- ❑ (A) Calcofluor white stain
- ❑ (B) Gram stain
- ❑ (C) Kinyoun stain
- ❑ (D) Trichrome stain
- ❑ (E) Giemsa stain

42 A 54-year-old woman, with a previous history of rheumatic heart disease, has developed mild fevers and night sweats. During the next 4 weeks, the fevers and sweats become more frequent, and she experiences a loss of appetite with a corresponding 10-lb weight loss. When she goes to her physician, he notices a new heart murmur. Upon questioning, the woman mentions that she had her teeth cleaned 2 months previously and did not receive prophylactic antibiotics at the time of the procedure. Three sets of blood cultures are collected, and empiric therapy for subacute bacterial endocarditis is initiated. After incubation for 5 days, all three sets of blood cultures are positive with gram-negative rods. It is noted that colonies of the organism are observed sticking to the surface of the blood culture bottles. Which organism is most likely responsible for this infection?

- ❑ (A) *Actinobacillus actinomycetemcomitans*
- ❑ (B) *Eikenella corrodens*
- ❑ (C) *Kingella kingii*
- ❑ (D) *Staphylococcus epidermidis*
- ❑ (E) *Streptococcus mutans*

43 Infection with *Neisseria gonorrhoeae* is characterized by intracellular growth of the bacteria and stimulation of a vigorous inflammatory response. Which virulence factor is responsible for the inflammatory response?

- ❑ (A) Capsule
- ❑ (B) Lipooligosaccharide (LOS)
- ❑ (C) Opacity (Opa) protein
- ❑ (D) Reduction-modifiable (RMP) protein
- ❑ (E) Teichoic acid

44 After 2 days of increasing pain during urination, a 20-year-old female college student goes to the student health center. Upon examination, she complains of left flank tenderness and low-grade fevers. Her urine is cloudy and shows microscopic evidence of erythrocytes, pyuria, and abundant gram-positive bacteria. Her relevant past medical history is significant for no previous urinary tract infections, and she admits to being sexually active. Which organism is most likely responsible for this woman's infection?

- ❑ (A) *Candida albicans*
- ❑ (B) *Enterococcus faecalis*
- ❑ (C) *Escherichia coli*
- ❑ (D) *Neisseria gonorrhoeae*
- ❑ (E) *Staphylococcus saprophyticus*

45 Which susceptibility pattern would be considered accurate for an oxacillin-resistant *Staphylococcus aureus?*

- ❑ (A) Resistant to penicillin; susceptible to ampicillin-sulbactam, cephalothin, ceftazidime, imipenem, and vancomycin
- ❑ (B) Resistant to penicillin, ampicillin-sulbactam, and cephalothin; susceptible to ceftazidime, imipenem, and vancomycin
- ❑ (C) Resistant to penicillin, ampicillin-sulbactam, cephalothin, and imipenem; susceptible to ceftazidime and vancomycin
- ❑ (D) Resistant to all beta-lactam antibiotics; susceptible to vancomycin
- ❑ (E) Resistant to all beta-lactam and vancomycin

46 A 35-year-old woman with a long-standing but clinically stable history of systemic lupus erythematosus presents to her physician with a 1-week history of low-grade fevers, nausea, vomiting, and fatigue. Her medications at the time of presentation are prednisone, hydrochloroquine, and coumadine. Her physical examination is unremarkable, and her chest radiograph is normal. She has a Hickman catheter, and no erythema or purulence is present at the site. Her laboratory values are stable. Two blood cultures are drawn, and the patient is discharged for further follow-up. The laboratory calls her 2 days later and says that both blood cultures are positive with a poorly staining gram-positive rod. The laboratory explains that an acid-fast stain was performed and was positive. The organism grew 2 days after the blood culture bottles were subcultured to blood and chocolate

agars. Acid-fast staining of the colonies showed uniform staining acid-fast rods, with no branching apparent. Upon further questioning, the patient admits that she had expressed pus from the insertion site of the catheter. Additional cultures collected from this site grow the same organism. Which organism is most likely responsible for this woman's infection?

- ❑ (A) *Mycobacterium fortuitum*
- ❑ (B) *Mycobacterium haemophilum*
- ❑ (C) *Nocardia asteroides*
- ❑ (D) *Nocardia brasiliensis*
- ❑ (E) *Rhodococcus equi*

47 A 23-year-old man presents to the emergency department of a local hospital with a swollen hand that has lacerations on its dorsal surface. Erythema and some purulent exudate are present. The patient stated that he injured the hand in a fistfight when he hit a man in the mouth. Radiograph studies show bones broken in two fingers and the presence of soft tissue swelling. The exudate is collected for aerobic and anaerobic bacterial culture. After 2 days, the laboratory reports that both the aerobic and anaerobic cultures are positive. Among the mixture of bacteria growing in culture is a small gram-negative rod that grew in both the aerobic and anaerobic atmospheres. In the aerobic atmosphere, it grew slowly on both blood and chocolate agars, but it did not grow on MacConkey agar. The laboratory also notes that the organism had a bleach-like odor and pitted the blood agar. Which antibiotic would be considered the drug of choice for treating infections caused by this organism?

- ❑ (A) Cephalothin
- ❑ (B) Clindamycin
- ❑ (C) Erythromycin
- ❑ (D) Oxacillin
- ❑ (E) Penicillin

48 Antibiotic therapy is contraindicated for management of infection with which organism?

- ❑ (A) *Campylobacter jejuni*
- ❑ (B) *Clostridium difficile*
- ❑ (C) *Escherichia coli* O157
- ❑ (D) *Helicobacter pylori*
- ❑ (E) *Shigella sonnei*

49 Approximately 4 weeks after a bone marrow transplant, a 42-year-old man returns to his physician with complaints of fevers and a productive sputum. The symptoms have developed during the preceding 5 days. A chest x-ray is obtained, and a cavitary lesion is observed in the upper right lobe. While the patient is in the radiology department, he has a seizure. A CT scan of his head shows a mass in the right parietal area of the brain. Cultures of the brain and lung are performed, and, after 4 days of growth, gram-positive filamentous rods are observed (see figure). The organism stains poorly with the Gram stain and is weakly acid-fast. Which pathogen is the most likely the cause of this man's condition?

- ❑ (A) *Actinomyces israelii*
- ❑ (B) *Corynebacterium jeikeium*
- ❑ (C) *Mycobacterium tuberculosis*
- ❑ (D) *Nocardia asteroides*
- ❑ (E) *Rhodococcus equi*

50 *Salmonella* can escape phagocytic clearance by which mechanism?

- ❑ (A) Capsule-mediated inhibition of phagocytosis
- ❑ (B) Inhibition of phagosome/lysosome fusion
- ❑ (C) Inhibition of opsonization mediated by protein A
- ❑ (D) Lysis of phagosome and replication in cytoplasm
- ❑ (E) Replication in fused phagosome/lysosome

51 Which bacteria can stain weakly acid-fast when detected in clinical specimens?

- ❑ (A) *Actinomyces israelii*
- ❑ (B) *Bartonella bacilliformis*
- ❑ (C) *Corynebacterium jeikeium*
- ❑ (D) *Legionella micdadei*
- ❑ (E) *Propionibacterium propionicus*

52 *Coxiella burnetii* can escape phagocytic clearance by which mechanism?

- ❑ (A) Capsule-mediated inhibition of phagocytosis
- ❑ (B) Inhibition of phagosome/lysosome fusion
- ❑ (C) Inhibition of opsonization mediated by protein A
- ❑ (D) Lysis of phagosome and replication in cytoplasm
- ❑ (E) Replication in fused phagosome/lysosome

53 Which statement about *Erysipelothrix rhusiopathiae* is accurate?

- ❑ (A) This organism is typically susceptible to penicillin.
- ❑ (B) This organism is catalase-negative and can be mistaken for *Streptococcus*.
- ❑ (C) Infection with this organism is associated with human bites.

- ❑ (D) The primary virulence factor associated with organism is endotoxin.
- ❑ (E) This organism is a strict anaerobe.

54 A 54-year-old man sees his physician because he has been feeling ill for 2 months. His illness is nonspecific, with complaints of fatigue, muscle aches, low-grade fevers, and a loss of appetite. Physical examination reveals he is underweight and has poor oral hygiene, a temperature of 38°C, a palpable spleen, and a heart murmur. Three blood cultures are collected, and, after incubation for 7 days, the microbiology laboratory reports the blood cultures are positive for a pleomorphic gram-negative rod. The blood culture broths are subcultured, and growth is detected on blood and chocolate agars after incubation for 4 days. No growth is detected on MacConkey agar. The results of the preliminary biochemical tests are catalase-negative, oxidase-positive, and indole-weakly positive. Which organism is most likely responsible for this man's infection?

- ❑ (A) *Acinetobacter baumanni*
- ❑ (B) *Cardiobacterium hominis*
- ❑ (C) *Capnocytophaga ochracea*
- ❑ (D) *Eikenella corrodens*
- ❑ (E) *Haemophilus parainfluenzae*

55 A 54-year-old man goes to his family physician with complaints of a persistent nonproductive cough with severe chest pain that have lasted 1 week. His physician hears rales bilaterally, and chest radiographs demonstrate a diffuse bilateral infiltrates with no signs of consolidation or abscess formation. The man has a low-grade fever, heart rate of 110 bpm, respiratory rate of 25/min (breaths per minute), and blood pressure of 130/80 mm Hg. Sputum is induced for microscopy and culture, and blood is collected for culture. No organisms are observed on a Gram stain of the sputum specimen, and no organisms grow in the blood cultures. Growth of a gram-negative rod is observed on buffered charcoal-yeast extract (BCYE) agar inoculated with sputum after 4 days of incubation. Which organism is most likely responsible for this man's infection?

- ❑ (A) *Chlamydophila (Chlamydia) pneumoniae*
- ❑ (B) *Klebsiella pneumoniae*
- ❑ (C) *Legionella pneumophila*
- ❑ (D) *Mycoplasma pneumoniae*
- ❑ (E) *Streptococcus pneumoniae*

56 Which antibiotic is consistently active against anaerobic gram-negative rods?

- ❑ (A) Carbenicillin
- ❑ (B) Clindamycin
- ❑ (C) Imipenem
- ❑ (D) Metronidazole
- ❑ (E) Penicillin

57 *Francisella tularensis* can escape phagocytic clearance by which mechanism?

- ❑ (A) Capsule-mediated inhibition of phagocytosis
- ❑ (B) Inhibition of phagosome/lysosome fusion
- ❑ (C) Inhibition of opsonization mediated by protein A
- ❑ (D) Lysis of phagosome and replication in cytoplasm
- ❑ (E) Replication in fused phagosome/lysosome

58 A 34-year-old woman visits her family physician complaining of pain when urinating, lower back pain, and low-grade fevers. A urine specimen is collected for culture and Gram stain. Abundant gram-positive rods are observed by microscopy, and small colonies are detected on the culture medium after 48 h of incubation. Which organism is most likely responsible for this urinary tract infection?

- ❑ (A) *Clostridium perfringens*
- ❑ (B) *Corynebacterium urealyticum*
- ❑ (C) *Enterococcus faecium*
- ❑ (D) *Escherichia coli*
- ❑ (E) *Lactobacillus acidophilus*

59 Which feature is unique to gram-positive bacteria?

- ❑ (A) Cytoplasmic membrane
- ❑ (B) Endotoxin
- ❑ (C) Outer membrane
- ❑ (D) Peptidoglycan
- ❑ (E) Spore formation

60 An 8-year-old boy falls while playing and abrades the skin over his thigh and hip. The injury does not appear serious, and no effort is made to clean the wound or apply topical antibiotic creams. The wound over the hip worsens after 3 days, with inflammation and a small amount of purulence. That evening, the child develops a high-grade fever (40°C), headache, and a diffuse rash. By the time the child arrives at the hospital, he is hypotensive, complains of severe myalgias, and has diarrhea. After 1 more day, his skin desquamates (including over the palms and soles), and he develops renal and hepatic abnormalities. Which toxin is most likely responsible for this illness?

- ❑ (A) Alpha-toxin
- ❑ (B) Enterotoxin A
- ❑ (C) Exfoliative toxins
- ❑ (D) Leukocidin
- ❑ (E) Toxic shock syndrome toxin-1

61 Which factor is primarily responsible for the tissue damage seen in syphilis?

- ❑ (A) Production of bacterial hyaluronidase
- ❑ (B) Outer membrane proteins facilitating adherence to host cells
- ❑ (C) Fibronectin coat protecting the bacteria from phagocytosis

- ❑ (D) Release of endotoxin
- ❑ (E) Host immune response to bacteria

62 A gastroenterologist in a small community hospital notices that five of his patients have developed a diarrheal disease 2 to 4 days after they underwent colonoscopies. The only other common factor among the patients is that they are being treated with empiric clindamycin. The physician feels that in this setting, these patients were most likely infected with *Clostridium difficile*. Which test should be performed with a collected stool specimen to confirm this diagnosis?

- ❑ (A) Culture on blood agar
- ❑ (B) Culture on MacConkey agar
- ❑ (C) Culture on sorbitol/MacConkey agar
- ❑ (D) Culture on selective agar incubated in a micro-aerophilic atmosphere
- ❑ (E) Immunoassay for toxins

63 A 23-year-old man with HIV goes to a hospital emergency department with complaints of body aches, headaches, and low-grade fevers. He states that he has felt ill and has had fevers for more than 10 days. He previously had been treated for a pneumocystis infection but did not maintain his antiretroviral antibiotics. Blood cultures are collected for bacteria, fungi, and mycobacteria. After incubation for 2 weeks, the fungal and mycobacterial cultures remain negative, but the bacterial blood cultures are positive with short gram-negative rods. The positive blood culture broth is subcultured, and growth on agar media is observed after incubation for more than 1 week in an atmosphere of enriched carbon dioxide and high humidity. The organism is small, is slightly curved, and has negative catalase and oxidase reactions. Which organism is most likely responsible for this infection?

- ❑ (A) *Bartonella*
- ❑ (B) *Capnocytophaga*
- ❑ (C) *Eikenella*
- ❑ (D) *Prevotella*
- ❑ (E) *Vibrio*

64 A 54-year-old man living in Juarez, Mexico, arrives in a Dallas, Texas hospital with a grossly enlarged foot that is covered with multiple draining sinus tracts. The man states that the lesions on his foot developed over the period of months. They are not painful, but he has difficulty walking. The foot has localized subcutaneous swellings and suppuration. Radiographic studies demonstrate swelling in the underlying tissues and evidence of osteomyelitis. Tissue samples and drainage from one of the sinus tracts are collected. The specimens are cultured on blood agar, chocolate agar, MacConkey agar, and buffered charcoal yeast extract (BCYE) agar. These media are incubated in an air incubator supplemented with 5% carbon dioxide. After 3 days, growth on blood and chocolate agars as well as on BCYE agar are observed (see figure). Which organism is most likely responsible for this infection?

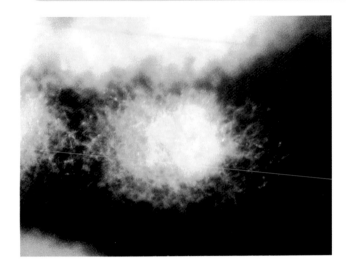

- ❏ (A) *Actinomyces israelii*
- ❏ (B) *Mycobacterium avium*
- ❏ (C) *Nocardia brasiliensis*
- ❏ (D) *Sporothrix schenckii*
- ❏ (E) *Vibrio vulnificus*

65 *Staphylococcus aureus* can escape phagocytic clearance by which mechanism?

- ❏ (A) Capsule-mediated inhibition of phagocytosis
- ❏ (B) Inhibition of phagosome/lysosome fusion
- ❏ (C) Inhibition of opsonization mediated by protein A
- ❏ (D) Lysis of phagosome and replication in cytoplasm
- ❏ (E) Replication in fused phagosome/lysosome

66 Which food is most commonly associated with *Listeria monocytogenes* infections?

- ❏ (A) Chicken
- ❏ (B) Ice cream
- ❏ (C) Carrots
- ❏ (D) Rice
- ❏ (E) Soft cheese

67 The lethal toxin produced by *Bacillus anthracis* works by which mechanism?

- ❏ (A) Blocks release of acetylcholine
- ❏ (B) Blocks release of gamma-aminobutyric acid
- ❏ (C) Inactivates elongation factor-2 (EF-2) and prevents protein synthesis
- ❏ (D) Stimulates increased adenylate cyclase activity
- ❏ (E) Stimulates release of proinflammatory cytokines

68 A 35-year-old man develops a persistent nonproductive cough with malaise and a headache for a 10-day period. A chest radiograph shows a patchy infiltrate in the left lower lobe, with no evidence of consolidation or pleural effusions. Gram stain and culture of induced sputum and routine blood cultures are negative; however, growth of bacteria is observed in monolayers of Hep-2 cell cultures. Which organism is most likely the cause of these results?

- ❏ (A) *Chlamydophila (Chlamydia) pneumoniae*
- ❏ (B) *Klebsiella pneumoniae*
- ❏ (C) *Legionella pneumophila*
- ❏ (D) *Mycoplasma pneumoniae*
- ❏ (E) *Streptococcus pneumoniae*

69 Which organism is associated with exogenous infections?

- ❏ (A) *Actinomyces*
- ❏ (B) *Clostridium*
- ❏ (C) *Eubacterium*
- ❏ (D) *Peptostreptococcus*
- ❏ (E) *Prevotella*

70 A 34-year-old man tells his wife that for the last 3 days he has been feeling progressively worse. His illness began with a headache, mild fever, and sweats. Over time, the symptoms have become more prominent, and his wife takes him to his physician. The physician notes that the man has a temperature of 39°C, blood pressure of 137/85 mm Hg, heart rate of 82 bpm, and respiratory rate of 25/min. This patient was previously in good health and returned from a trip to Mexico 3 weeks prior to this visit. While in Mexico, the man ate only in high quality restaurants although he did consume unpasteurized goat cheese. The physician orders blood cultures for his patient, and 3 days later the cultures are found to be positive. Very small gram-negative coccobacilli were observed when the culture broths were Gram stained. Which antibiotic would be considered the drug of choice for treating the organism responsible for this infection?

- ❏ (A) Ampicillin
- ❏ (B) Clindamycin
- ❏ (C) Doxycycline
- ❏ (D) Ceftazidime
- ❏ (E) Erythromycin

71 A 58-year-old man who is hospitalized with a glioblastoma develops a fever spike of 40°C. Three blood cultures are collected during a period of 12 h through an intravenous catheter port. All cultures are positive after 48 h of incubation and show small rods that are club-shaped and gram-positive; these are arranged in pairs and short parallel clusters. The organism grows slowly on subculture, is catalase-positive, and is resistant to most antibiotics tested, with the exception of vancomycin. Which organism is most likely responsible for this infection?

- ❏ (A) *Arcanobacterium haemolyticum*
- ❏ (B) *Corynebacterium jeikeium*
- ❏ (C) *Lactobacillus casei*
- ❏ (D) *Listeria monocytogenes*
- ❏ (E) *Propionibacterium acnes*

72 Which statement about *Treponema pallidum* is correct?

- ❑ (A) The bacteria are 2 to 4 µm wide and 6 to 20 µm long.
- ❑ (B) The bacteria grow best on blood agar or chocolate agar.
- ❑ (C) A syphilic patient's immune response may lead to tissue damage.
- ❑ (D) Late syphilis is characterized by the appearance of genital ulcers and a disseminated rash.
- ❑ (E) Penicillin resistance has become common for patients with syphilis.

73 Which test is most appropriate for confirming the diagnosis of sinusitis?

- ❑ (A) Blood culture
- ❑ (B) Nasopharyngeal culture
- ❑ (C) Sinus aspirate
- ❑ (D) Sputum culture
- ❑ (E) Throat culture

74 What is the optimum volume of blood that should be collected from an adult patient for a single blood culture?

- ❑ (A) <1 ml
- ❑ (B) 1-5 ml
- ❑ (C) 10 ml
- ❑ (D) 15 ml
- ❑ (E) 20 ml

75 Which intracellular pathogen is transmitted by the human body louse?

- ❑ (A) *Coxiella burnetii*
- ❑ (B) *Ehrlichia chaffeensis*
- ❑ (C) *Rickettsia prowazekii*
- ❑ (D) *Rickettsia rickettsii*
- ❑ (E) *Rickettsia typhi*

76 Which property is characteristic of *Chlamydophila (Chlamydia) pneumoniae?*

- ❑ (A) Important virulence factors and resistance genes are encoded on plasmid DNA.
- ❑ (B) The disease is infectious for many mammals, including humans.
- ❑ (C) Intracellular inclusions contain iodine-staining glycogen.
- ❑ (D) Only one serotype has been identified.
- ❑ (E) The organism is susceptible to trimethoprim/sulfamethoxazole.

77 Disease caused by *Corynebacterium diphtheriae* is mediated by an A-B type toxin. Which answer best describes the effect of this toxin?

- ❑ (A) Interferes with phagocytosis
- ❑ (B) Interferes with DNA replication
- ❑ (C) Interferes with protein synthesis

- ❑ (D) Stimulates macrophages to release the tumor necrosis factor
- ❑ (E) Stimulates lysis of erythrocytes, leukocytes, and platelets

78 A 64-year-old man undergoes intraabdominal surgery for colonic cancer. Five days after the surgery, the patient develops peritonitis for which he is treated with ceftazidime, gentamicin, and metronidazole. Although he initially responds to this therapeutic regimen, on the third night of treatment he develops spiking fevers and abdominal tenderness. He is taken to surgery that night, and 50 cc of purulent material is drained from his abdominal cavity. The material is submitted for Gram stain and culture. The Gram stain is positive (see figure), and both aerobic and anaerobic cultures are positive within 24 h. Which organism is most likely responsible for this infection?

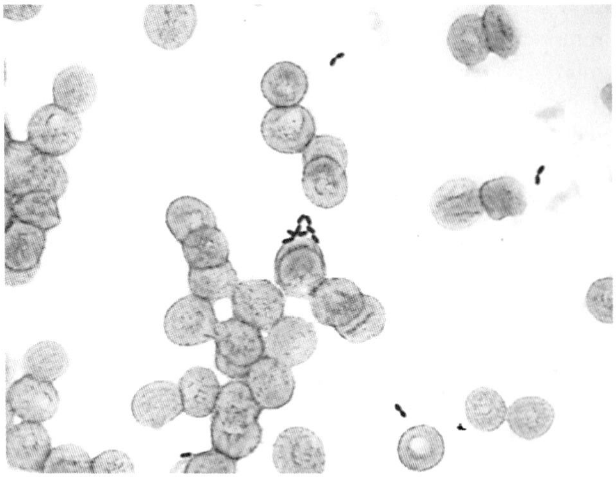

- ❑ (A) *Candida albicans*
- ❑ (B) *Enterococcus faecalis*
- ❑ (C) *Peptostreptococcus anaerobius*
- ❑ (D) *Staphylococcus aureus*
- ❑ (E) *Streptococcus pyogenes*

79 Which anaerobe is associated with gas gangrene?

- ❑ (A) *Actinomyces*
- ❑ (B) *Bifidobacterium*
- ❑ (C) *Clostridium*
- ❑ (D) *Fusobacterium*
- ❑ (E) *Lactobacillus*

80 Which mycobacteria is photochromogenic?

- ❑ (A) *Mycobacterium avium*
- ❑ (B) *Mycobacterium fortuitum*
- ❑ (C) *Mycobacterium haemophilum*
- ❑ (D) *Mycobacterium kansasii*
- ❑ (E) *Mycobacterium tuberculosis*

81 Which organism is uniformly susceptible to vancomycin?

- ❑ (A) *Enterococcus*
- ❑ (B) *Escherichia*
- ❑ (C) *Leuconostoc*
- ❑ (D) *Pediococcus*
- ❑ (E) *Streptococcus*

82 Which association is correct?

- ❑ (A) Strict anaerobic gram-positive cocci: *Enterococcus*
- ❑ (B) Strict anaerobic gram-positive rod: *Chlamydia*
- ❑ (C) Strict anaerobic gram-negative cocci: *Peptostreptococcus*
- ❑ (D) Strict anaerobic gram-negative rod: *Bacteroides*
- ❑ (E) Strict anaerobic gram-negative rod: *Clostridium*

83 A 54-year-old man develops an infection at his surgical incision site 2 days after cardiac surgery. The site is characterized by swelling, erythema, and purulent drainage around the sutures. Culture of the drainage is performed, and beta-hemolytic colonies grow on aerobic blood agar plates after 24 h of incubation. Which enzyme is an important virulence factor and diagnostic marker for this organism?

- ❑ (A) Catalase
- ❑ (B) Coagulase
- ❑ (C) Endotoxin
- ❑ (D) Exotoxin A
- ❑ (E) Lecithinase

84 During a routine physical, a man complains to his physician that he has had upper gastric burning pains and has had a problem with burping following his meals for the past week. The patient denies use of nonsteroidal anti-inflammatory drugs or alcohol. The physician suspects this man's symptoms are related to a bacterial infection. A test for which bacterial product would confirm this diagnosis?

- ❑ (A) Coagulase
- ❑ (B) Cytotoxin (also called toxin B)
- ❑ (C) Emetic enterotoxin
- ❑ (D) Endotoxin
- ❑ (E) Urease

85 *Shigella sonnei* can escape phagocytic clearance by which mechanism?

- ❑ (A) Capsule-mediated inhibition of phagocytosis
- ❑ (B) Inhibition of phagosome/lysosome fusion
- ❑ (C) Inhibition of opsonization mediated by protein A
- ❑ (D) Lysis of phagosome and replication in cytoplasm
- ❑ (E) Replication in fused phagosome/lysosome

86 Approximately 36 h after a neighborhood picnic, 14 people develop diarrhea, with the majority complaining of abdominal cramps. Most have low-grade temperatures and 8 to 10 bowel movements a day. Bloody stools affect two people. Although symptoms resolve for most of these people within 1 week, two children and one adult have to be hospitalized. For these patients, leukocytes are observed on a stool exam but with no predominant organism. Cultures are performed, and after 2 days of incubation, an organism grows on selective media at 42°C but does not grow on MacConkey agar. The organism is a thin, gram-negative rod (see figure). Which organism is most likely responsible for these infections?

- ❑ (A) *Campylobacter*
- ❑ (B) *Escherichia*
- ❑ (C) *Salmonella*
- ❑ (D) *Shigella*
- ❑ (E) *Yersinia*

87 A 63-year-old man sees his physician with complaints of a fever, dry cough, muscle aches, nausea, anorexia, and headache. The symptoms developed during the preceding 3 days. Chest radiograph shows consolidation in both his left and right lung fields. His past medical history contains significant relevant information of a 30-year history of smoking and consumption of 6 to 10 beers daily. He is admitted to the hospital, and therapy with ceftriaxone is initiated. During the next 5 days, he fails to show improvement. Sputum is collected at the time of admission into the hospital. A Gram stain, fungal stains, and acid-fast stains show no organisms. Routine bacterial, fungal, and mycobacterial cultures are negative; however, after 5 days, small colonies of weakly staining gram-negative rods grow on BCYE agar. Which organism is most likely responsible for this man's infection?

- ❑ (A) *Chlamydophila (Chlamydia) pneumoniae*
- ❑ (B) *Klebsiella pneumoniae*
- ❑ (C) *Legionella pneumophila*
- ❑ (D) *Mycoplasma pneumoniae*
- ❑ (E) *Streptococcus pneumoniae*

88 Which antibiotic is active against *Mycoplasma pneumoniae?*

- ❑ (A) Ampicillin-sulbactam
- ❑ (B) Azithromycin
- ❑ (C) Imipenem
- ❑ (D) Penicillin
- ❑ (E) Vancomycin

89 A variety of vaccines have been developed against *Neisseria meningitidis*. Which serogroup polysaccharide is a weak immunogen and does not elicit antibodies?

❑ (A) Serogroup A
❑ (B) Serogroup B
❑ (C) Serogroup C
❑ (D) Serogroup Y
❑ (E) Serogroup W135

90 A 10-year-old boy develops a sore throat, fever, and headache. After 3 days of these symptoms, he develops a diffuse erythematous rash on his chest that spreads to his extremities. His pediatrician makes the tentative diagnosis of streptococcal scarlet fever. A throat swab is tested by a "rapid strep test" but is reported to be negative. A second throat swab is cultured on blood and chocolate agars. After 48 h of incubation, the culture is reported to be negative for group A *Streptococcus* (*S. pyogenes*) but positive for a beta-hemolytic gram-positive rod. Which organism is most likely responsible for this infection?

❑ (A) *Arcanobacterium haemolyticum*
❑ (B) *Corynebacterium diphtheriae*
❑ (C) *Listeria monocytogenes*
❑ (D) *Staphylococcus aureus*
❑ (E) *Streptococcus dysgalactiae*

91 A 36-year-old woman in her last trimester of pregnancy goes to the local hospital complaining of an acute illness characterized by fevers, headaches, myalgias, and arthralgias. Two blood cultures are collected, and small gram-positive rods are detected after 48 h of incubation. The blood culture broths are subcultured to blood agar plates, and small, beta-hemolytic colonies are observed after overnight incubation. The bacteria are catalase-positive and motility-positive; they also hydrolyzed esculin. Which statement is correct for the organism responsible for this woman's infection?

❑ (A) Patients with defects in humoral immunity are at increased risk of disease.
❑ (B) The bacteria grow in phagolysosomes of macrophages.
❑ (C) Infection is associated with consumption of soft cheeses and undercooked meats.
❑ (D) The bacteria grow in a narrow range of temperature and pH.
❑ (E) Mortality for patients with this disease approaches 100%.

92 The exotoxin produced by *Clostridium botulinum* works by which mechanism?

❑ (A) Blocks release of acetylcholine
❑ (B) Blocks release of gamma-aminobutyric acid
❑ (C) Inactivates EF-2 and prevents protein synthesis
❑ (D) Stimulates increased adenylate cyclase activity
❑ (E) Stimulates release of proinflammatory cytokines

93 A 74-year-old man is admitted to the hospital because of a 3-day history of high fever, myalgia, and chills accompanied by back pain and elimination of dark urine during the previous 12 h. His temperature is 38.5°C, blood pressure is 120/70 mm Hg, and respiratory rate is 30/min. Laboratory results include hemoglobin 131 g/l, hematocrit 0.41, serum urea 71 mg/dl, total bilirubin 4.1 mg/dl, lactic dehydrogenase 1250 U/L, and potassium 6.5 mEq/L. A urinalysis shows the presence of blood, but less than five WBCs per high-power field are seen. Blood cultures are collected, and antibiotic treatment is initiated. Approximately 6 h after admission, however, the patient goes into cardiac arrest and expires. When the blood cultures are analyzed 6 h after they were collected, gas is observed in the culture bottles, and bacteria were seen on Gram stain. Postmortem examination of tissues reveals microabscesses in the liver and gall bladder. Which organism is responsible for this man's fatal infection?

❑ (A) *Bacteroides fragilis*
❑ (B) *Clostridium perfringens*
❑ (C) *Escherichia coli*
❑ (D) *Pseudomonas aeruginosa*
❑ (E) *Staphylococcus aureus*

94 During a military conflict in Somalia, several soldiers develop a febrile illness characterized by the abrupt onset of fever with rigors, severe headaches, myalgias, arthralgias, lethargy, photophobia, and coughing. Observed are conjunctival suffusion and a petechial rash that develop 4 days into the illness and then fade after 1 to 2 days at the time the symptoms wane. Splenomegaly and hepatomegaly are also characteristically present. After 1 week to 10 days, the symptoms recur. The tentative diagnosis of this disease is relapsing fever. Which diagnostic tests should be performed?

❑ (A) Blood culture
❑ (B) Skin rash culture
❑ (C) Enzyme immunoassay
❑ (D) Giemsa stain of blood
❑ (E) Proteus OXK agglutinin titer

95 A 55-year-old man is admitted to the hospital with complaints of chest pain and production of blood-tinged sputum. A chest radiograph confirms consolidation in the left upper lung field, and *Klebsiella pneumoniae* is isolated from blood cultures and sputum. Therapy with ceftazidime is initiated. After 10 days of treatment, the man develops profuse, watery diarrhea. During the next 2 days, the diarrhea becomes more frequent, and blood is present in stool samples. White plaques over the colonic mucosa are observed by coloscopy. Which toxin is most likely responsible for this patient's colitis?

❑ (A) *Bacillus cereus* enterotoxin
❑ (B) *Clostridium difficile* cytotoxin
❑ (C) *Escherichia coli* verotoxin
❑ (D) *Shigella dysenteriae* toxin
❑ (E) *Staphylococcus aureus* enterotoxin

96 Which enteric pathogen has been associated with hemolytic uremic syndrome?

- ❑ (A) *Bacillus cereus*
- ❑ (B) *Clostridium difficile*
- ❑ (C) *Salmonella enterica*
- ❑ (D) *Shigella dysenteriae*
- ❑ (E) *Yersinia enterocolitica*

97 Which diagnostic test is most commonly used for leptospirosis?

- ❑ (A) Giemsa stain
- ❑ (B) Gram stain
- ❑ (C) Culture on blood and chocolate agars
- ❑ (D) Serologic detection of specific antibodies
- ❑ (E) PCR amplification of bacterial DNA

98 A 54-year-old woman is diagnosed with acute lymphocytic leukemia and is hospitalized for 3 weeks for management of her disease. During the second week of hospitalization, she develops high fevers and hypotension. *Staphylococcus aureus,* susceptible to oxacillin, is isolated from multiple blood cultures and an intravenous catheter. Treatment with oxacillin is initiated, and the catheter is then removed. During the next week, she experiences defervescence and improves clinically. However, after 7 days of antibiotic treatment, she develops high spiking fevers. Blood cultures are positive for a gram-positive rod (see figure) resistant to all antibiotics tested except vancomycin. Which bacterial species is most likely responsible for this infection?

- ❑ (A) *Corynebacterium diphtheriae*
- ❑ (B) *Corynebacterium jeikeium*
- ❑ (C) *Corynebacterium macginleyi*
- ❑ (D) *Corynebacterium pseudotuberculosis*
- ❑ (E) *Corynebacterium ulcerans*

99 A live, attenuated vaccine is used to prevent infections caused by which bacterial species?

- ❑ (A) *Bordetella pertussis*
- ❑ (B) *Coxiella burnetii*
- ❑ (C) *Haemophilus influenzae*
- ❑ (D) *Mycobacterium tuberculosis*
- ❑ (E) *Streptococcus pneumoniae*

100 Which bacterium can contaminate foods and grow at refrigerator temperatures (e.g., 4° to 8°C)?

- ❑ (A) *Bacillus cereus*
- ❑ (B) *Campylobacter jejuni*
- ❑ (C) *Escherichia coli*
- ❑ (D) *Shigella sonnei*
- ❑ (E) *Yersinia enterocolitica*

101 A 7-year-old boy develops acute diarrhea and abdominal cramps. During an examination, the boy's pediatrician notes that he has a low-grade fever; a stool specimen indicates that the boy also has bloody stools. Upon questioning, the boy's mother remembers that he had eaten an undercooked hamburger 2 days earlier at a local fast food restaurant. The pediatrician is concerned that the boy is infected with *Escherichia coli* O157. Which tests should be performed with the collected stool specimen to confirm this diagnosis?

- ❑ (A) Culture on blood agar
- ❑ (B) Culture on MacConkey agar
- ❑ (C) Culture on sorbitol/MacConkey agar
- ❑ (D) Culture on selective agar incubated in a micro-aerophilic atmosphere
- ❑ (E) Immunoassay for toxins A and B

102 *Listeria monocytogenes* can escape phagocytic clearance by which mechanism?

- ❑ (A) Capsule-mediated inhibition of phagocytosis
- ❑ (B) Inhibition of phagosome/lysosome fusion
- ❑ (C) Inhibition of opsonization mediated by protein A
- ❑ (D) Lysis of phagosome and replication in cytoplasm
- ❑ (E) Replication in fused phagosome/lysosome

103 Which test is the most sensitive method for diagnosing endocarditis caused by *Coxiella burnetii?*

- ❑ (A) Culture of blood
- ❑ (B) Detection of specific antibodies
- ❑ (C) Detection of *Coxiella* antigens in urine
- ❑ (D) Gram stain of infected heart valve
- ❑ (E) Skin test

104 Which test can be used for the identification of genus *Enterococcus* members?

- ❑ (A) Bile solubility
- ❑ (B) Coagulase
- ❑ (C) Germ tube formation
- ❑ (D) L-pyrrolidonyl arylamidase (PYR) test
- ❑ (E) Bacitracin susceptibility

105 Which disease is the most common vector-borne disease in the United States?

- ❑ (A) Babesiosis
- ❑ (B) Ehrlichiosis
- ❑ (C) Legionnaire's disease
- ❑ (D) Lyme disease
- ❑ (E) Plague

106 Which organism is commonly associated with meningitis in a 1-week-old infant?

- ❑ (A) *Haemophilus influenzae*
- ❑ (B) *Neisseria meningitidis*
- ❑ (C) *Salmonella enteritidis*
- ❑ (D) *Streptococcus agalactiae* Group B
- ❑ (E) *Streptococcus pneumoniae*

107 The pathology of Rocky Mountain spotted fever is associated with infection of which cells?

- ❑ (A) Endothelial cells
- ❑ (B) Erythrocytes
- ❑ (C) Monocytes
- ❑ (D) Neutrophils
- ❑ (E) Squamous epithelial cells

108 A 47-year-old woman living in Ecuador is diagnosed with chronic myelocytic leukemia and is treated with a variety of antineoplastic drugs. A bone marrow biopsy 1 year later is consistent with acceleration of her disease. A month after the biopsy, she is scheduled to receive a stem cell transplant. However, she is noted to have profuse watery diarrhea 3 days before the transplant. Tests for *Clostridium difficile* are negative. A parasitology examination reveals *Strongyloides* and *Trichuris*. Bacterial cultures are also performed, and after 2 days of incubation, colorless colonies are observed on MacConkey agar; red colonies with a small black button are present on xylose-lysine-deoxycholate (XLD) agar. The colony is inoculated into a triple sugar iron (TSI) agar slant and urea agar slant. The following reactions are observed: alkaline over acid reaction with no gas formation and weak hydrogen sulfide production on TSI (see figure); the urease reaction is negative. Which organism is most likely responsible for this woman's infection?

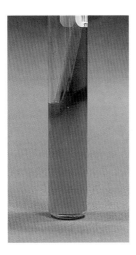

- ❑ (A) *Escherichia coli* O157
- ❑ (B) *Salmonella choleraesuis*
- ❑ (C) *Salmonella typhi*
- ❑ (D) *Shigella sonnei*
- ❑ (E) *Yersinia enterocolitica*

109 Quinupristin-dalfopristin is bacteriostatic by which mechanism?

- ❑ (A) Blocks peptide elongation by inhibiting peptidyl-transferase
- ❑ (B) Inhibits cross-linking of cell wall peptidoglycan
- ❑ (C) Inhibits DNA topoisomerase
- ❑ (D) Inhibits initiation of RNA synthesis
- ❑ (E) Initiates premature release of peptide chains from ribosome

110 A 36-year-old woman living in rural Illinois develops persistent nasal congestion, facial pain, and headache. Imaging studies of her sinuses demonstrate the presence of opacities. Repeated courses of antibiotics and anti-inflammatory drugs are unsuccessful, and the woman is taken to surgery to attempt to drain the sinuses. Fluids collected at the time of surgery are sent for Gram stain and culture. Small, gram-negative rods are observed on Gram stain and grow the next day on culture. Preliminary identification tests are consistent with the identification of *Haemophilus influenzae*. This organism, however, fails to agglutinate with typing sera. Which answer is the most likely explanation for this observation?

- ❑ (A) The agglutination test was performed incorrectly.
- ❑ (B) The organism is *Haemophilus parainfluenzae*.
- ❑ (C) The organism does not have a capsule.
- ❑ (D) The surface of the organism is covered with pili.
- ❑ (E) The organism produces an enzyme that degrades IgG.

111 A 6-year-old girl develops bloody diarrhea with severe abdominal cramps 4 days after eating an undercooked hamburger. During the next week, her condition progresses to acute renal failure, thrombocytopenia, and microangiopathic hemolytic anemia. The clinical diagnosis of hemolytic uremic syndrome (HUS) is made. Which property is characteristic of the toxin most likely responsible for this condition?

- ❑ (A) Binds to globotriaosylceramide (Gb_3) receptors
- ❑ (B) Chemotactic for neutrophils with release of cytokines
- ❑ (C) Facilitates uptake of bacterial proteins in colonic epithelium cells
- ❑ (D) Produces actin depolymerization with destruction of cytoskeleton
- ❑ (E) Stimulates increased cyclic adenosine monophosphate (cAMP) levels

112 Rheumatic fever is a complication of infection with selected strains of *Streptococcus pyogenes*. This disease is characterized by inflammatory changes of the heart, blood vessels, joints, and subcutaneous tissues. Which test would be most useful for the diagnosis of rheumatic fever?

❑ (A) Blood culture
❑ (B) Synovial (joint) fluid culture
❑ (C) Measurement of antistreptolysin O (ASO) antibodies
❑ (D) Measurement of antistreptokinase antibodies
❑ (E) Microscopic examination of subcutaneous skin nodules

113 A 34-year-old man goes to the emergency department complaining of pain when urinating and a urethral discharge. The urethral discharge is collected for Gram stain and culture. The Gram stain showed gram-negative diplococci with many polymorphonuclear leukocytes. After 1 day of incubation, growth is observed on a Thayer-Martin agar medium, and sheep blood agar and the Gram stain of the colony are consistent with the initial Gram stain. The following results are seen on biochemical testing: acid production in glucose and maltose broths, no acid in lactose or sucrose broth, and growth on nutrient agar. Which organism is most likely the cause of this man's condition?

❑ (A) *Moraxella catarrhalis*
❑ (B) *Neisseria gonorrhoeae*
❑ (C) *Neisseria lactamica*
❑ (D) *Neisseria meningitidis*
❑ (E) *Neisseria sicca*

114 A 24-year-old man sustains multiple injuries in a car accident and is hospitalized for more than 1 month. During the man's hospitalization, he develops peritonitis following his abdominal injuries and a postsurgical wound infection. The organisms responsible for these infections are *Escherichia coli*, *Bacteroides fragilis*, and *Enterococcus*. Antibiotic therapy includes imipenem, gentamicin, and metronidazole. The patient's abdominal infections eventually clear; however, evidence of pneumonia then develops. During a 1-week period, the patient has increased pulmonary secretions with a productive, blood-tinged sputum. Sputum and blood is collected for culture, and after 24 h of incubation, a gram-negative rod is isolated from both specimens. The organism appears lavender-green on blood agar plates and has an ammonia odor. Colonies on MacConkey agar are colorless. The organism is oxidase-negative and uses carbohydrate oxidatively but not fermentatively. The preliminary susceptibility tests demonstrate that the organism is susceptible to trimethoprim/sulfamethoxazole and ticarcillin/clavulanate but resistant to imipenem. Which organism is most likely responsible for this patient's pulmonary infection?

❑ (A) *Acinetobacter baumannii*
❑ (B) *Burkholderia pseudomallei*
❑ (C) *Legionella pneumophila*
❑ (D) *Pseudomonas aeruginosa*
❑ (E) *Stenotrophomonas maltophilia*

115 *Staphylococcus aureus* is associated with a variety of toxin-mediated and pyogenic infections. The range of infections caused by coagulase-negative staphylococci is more limited. Which condition is most commonly associated with the coagulase-negative staphylococci?

❑ (A) Brain abscess
❑ (B) Endocarditis of a prosthetic heart valve
❑ (C) Intraabdominal abscess
❑ (D) Osteomyelitis
❑ (E) Wound infection following trauma to the skin's surface

116 Approximately 1 week after orthopedic surgery for a fractured hip, an 84-year-old woman notices some purulent drainage and redness along the incision line. During the next 3 days, the drainage increases, the surgical incision becomes warm and tender to the touch, and she develops a low-grade fever. When she sees her physician, he is concerned that she has developed an infection at the operative site. Bacterial cultures are collected, and abundant gram-positive cocci grow within 24 h. Preliminary tests show that the organism is catalase-positive. Antimicrobial susceptibility tests are performed, and the organism is found to be resistant to oxacillin. Which drug should be used to treat this infection?

❑ (A) Ampicillin
❑ (B) Ceftazidime
❑ (C) Imipenem
❑ (D) Piperacillin-tazobactam
❑ (E) Vancomycin

117 Bacteria become resistant to chloramphenicol by which mechanism?

❑ (A) Acetylation of an antibiotic
❑ (B) Active efflux of an antibiotic out of the cell
❑ (C) Modification of penicillin-binding proteins (PBPs)
❑ (D) Modification of a pentapeptide side chain in cell wall peptidoglycan
❑ (E) Modification of a ribosomal binding site

118 Which bacterial species has been associated with the Guillain-Barré syndrome?

❑ (A) *Aeromonas hydrophila*
❑ (B) *Bartonella quintana*
❑ (C) *Campylobacter jejuni*
❑ (D) *Staphylococcus aureus*
❑ (E) *Yersinia enterocolitica*

119 *Bacillus cereus* is associated with diarrheal disease characterized by a rapid onset, short duration, and sudden onset of nausea, vomiting, and severe abdominal cramps. Which food is most commonly the source of these infections?

❑ (A) Chicken salad
❑ (B) Hamburger
❑ (C) Ice cream
❑ (D) Rice
❑ (E) Seafood

120 A 62-year-old woman is undergoing treatment for her leukemia when she develops a spiking temperature, chills, and hypotension. During the next 2 days, skin lesions develop. They first appear as small vesicles and progress to hemorrhage, necrosis, and finally ulceration. The skin surrounding the vesicles is erythematous. Aspiration of the fluid from the vesicles shows few inflammatory cells but abundant gram-negative rods. Culture of the fluid is positive after 24 h with gram-negative rods that grow on both blood agar and MacConkey agar plates. Growth on the blood agar plate appears as spreading beta-hemolytic colonies, with a distinct fruity odor. Growth on the MacConkey agar plate appears as a clear colony. Which virulence factor is responsible for the tissue destruction associated with this patient's skin lesions?

- ❑ (A) Alkaline protease
- ❑ (B) Elastase
- ❑ (C) Endotoxin
- ❑ (D) Exotoxin A
- ❑ (E) Pyocyanin

121 A 52-year-old woman is brought to the emergency department by her son, who found his mother unresponsive at home. By the time she arrives to the hospital, she has regained consciousness but is confused and cannot follow simple commands. A CT scan of her head shows numerous well-defined lesions, and multilobar infiltrates are seen in her chest radiograph (see radiograph figure). Her past medical history is notable for the diagnosis of multiple myeloma 2 years prior to this visit, with a subsequent bone marrow transplant performed. She has done well since the transplant and has resumed her normal activities that include gardening, hiking, and cooking. Because one of her brain lesions is at an accessible site, she is taken to surgery and an aspirate is collected. A bronchial alveolar lavage is also performed. Gram stain of the specimens demonstrates weakly staining, gram-positive rods arranged in filaments. The organisms are also weakly acid-fast (see stain figure). The same organism grows after 3 days on the following culture media: sheep blood agar, chocolate agar, BCYE agar, Sabouraud dextrose agar, and Lowenstein-Jensen agar. Which organism is most likely responsible for this infection?

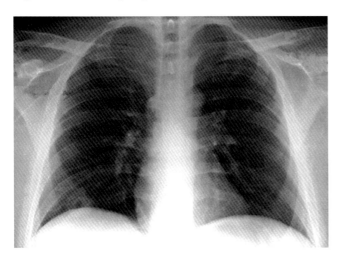

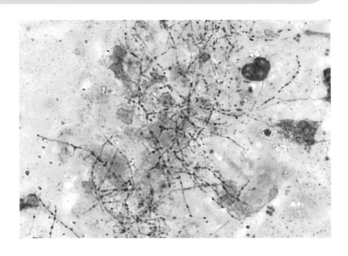

- ❑ (A) *Actinomyces israelii*
- ❑ (B) *Legionella micdadei*
- ❑ (C) *Mycobacterium chelonae*
- ❑ (D) *Nocardia asteroides*
- ❑ (E) *Rhodococcus equi*

122 Beta-lactam antibiotics bind to which bacterial cell wall structure?

- ❑ (A) Lipopolysaccharides
- ❑ (B) Pentaglycine bridge
- ❑ (C) Peptidoglycan
- ❑ (D) Teichoic acid
- ❑ (E) Transpeptidases

123 Which technique is considered the definitive method for defining a bacterial species?

- ❑ (A) Analysis of chromosomal DNA fragments by pulse field gel electrophoresis (PFGE)
- ❑ (B) Biochemical reactivity with selected substrates
- ❑ (C) Calculation of guanine to cytosine (G + C) ratio
- ❑ (D) DNA/DNA hybridization
- ❑ (E) Sequencing of 16S rRNA gene

124 Which mycobacteria is characterized by positive niacin and nitrate reductase tests?

- ❑ (A) *Mycobacterium avium*
- ❑ (B) *Mycobacterium chelonae*
- ❑ (C) *Mycobacterium fortuitum*
- ❑ (D) *Mycobacterium kansasii*
- ❑ (E) *Mycobacterium tuberculosis*

125 In September 2000, an outbreak of *Escherichia coli* gastroenteritis occurred in Pennsylvania. Most of the infected patients had visited a popular dairy farm, where they had contact with the animals and where lunch and snacks were served. Patients developed diarrhea (three or more loose stools in a period of 24 h) within 10 days of visiting the farm. Although the clinical presentation varied among the patients, the illness typically began with severe abdominal cramps and nonbloody diarrhea. Stools frequently became grossly bloody in day 2 or 3 of illness. Most patients became asymptomatic within 1 week; however, approximately 10% of the children with gastroenteritis developed acute renal failure, hypertension, and seizures. Which organism was most likely responsible for these infections?

- ☐ (A) Enteroaggregative *E. coli* (EAEC)
- ☐ (B) Enterohemorrhagic *E. coli* (EHEC)
- ☐ (C) Enteroinvasive *E. coli* (EIEC)
- ☐ (D) Enteropathogenic *E. coli* (EPEC)
- ☐ (E) Enterotoxigenic *E. coli* (ETEC)

126 In the twenty-first century, there has been a dramatic increase in community-acquired necrotizing pneumonia, particularly in pediatric patients; this type of pneumonia is typically caused by methicillin-resistant *Staphylococcus aureus*. A clonal relationship exists among the strains of bacteria. Which staphylococcal virulence factor has been implicated in this specific disease?

- ☐ (A) Alpha-toxin
- ☐ (B) Enterotoxin
- ☐ (C) Exfoliative toxin
- ☐ (D) Panton-Valentine (PV) leukocidin
- ☐ (E) TSST-1

127 A 65-year-old man is admitted to the hospital with exacerbation of his chronic pulmonary disease. Approximately 3 days after admission, his condition worsens, and he requires ventilatory assistance. After 7 days of treatment, his condition destabilizes. Chest radiograph show new infiltrates in both lung fields with cavitation in the left upper lobe. A bronchial alveolar lavage is performed, and gram-negative rods are observed on Gram stain and culture. Preliminary testing indicates that this organism is most likely *Pseudomonas aeruginosa.* Which scenario is the most likely source of this patient's infection?

- ☐ (A) Contact with nursing personnel
- ☐ (B) Contamination with an intravenous line
- ☐ (C) Ingestion of hospital food
- ☐ (D) Inhalation of airborne organism
- ☐ (E) Use of respiratory therapy equipment

128 Members of the family Chlamydiaceae are able to survive and replicate in humans by which mechanism?

- ☐ (A) A capsule inhibits phagocytosis.
- ☐ (B) Bacteria are phagocytosed, lyse the phagosome, and replicate in the cytoplasm.
- ☐ (C) Bacteria are phagocytosed but then prevent phagosome/lysosome fusion.
- ☐ (D) Bacteria are phagocytosed and fuse with lysosomes, but the bacteria are resistant to lysosomal enzymes.
- ☐ (E) Bacteria produce proteases that degrade IgG antibodies.

129 A 5-year-old boy complains to his mother that his throat hurts when he swallows his food. The mother notes that the boy's throat is red, and a whitish exudate has formed over his tonsils. The next day, a diffuse red rash develops on his chest. The mother takes the boy to his pediatrician, at which time the rash has spread over his neck, face, and limbs. The rash is most intense at folds of the skin. Which organism is most likely responsible for this infection?

- ☐ (A) *Bordetella pertussis*
- ☐ (B) *Haemophilus influenzae*
- ☐ (C) *Staphylococcus aureus*
- ☐ (D) *Streptococcus pneumoniae*
- ☐ (E) *Streptococcus pyogenes*

130 A 42-year-old man with septic shock is admitted to the hospital. His wife states that he is an alcoholic with hepatic cirrhosis. The other relevant history information is that the man may have cut his foot on a seashell while walking along the beach 3 days before his illness began. Blood cultures are collected, and after 12 h of incubation, a gram-negative rod is isolated. The organism ferments glucose and is oxidase positive. Which organism is most likely responsible for this man's infection?

- ☐ (A) *Acinetobacter baumannii*
- ☐ (B) *Burkholderia cepacia*
- ☐ (C) *Escherichia coli*
- ☐ (D) *Stenotrophomonas maltophilia*
- ☐ (E) *Vibrio vulnificus*

131 A 46-year-old woman presents to the emergency department with a 1-day history of high fevers and severe headaches. The emergency department physician notes a temperature of 39.5°C, palpable spleen and liver, and conjunctival ejection. The patient is hospitalized, and blood and urine specimens are submitted to the pathology laboratory for diagnostic tests. On the third hospital day, the patient develops a petechial rash over her body. On the fourth hospital day, the hematology laboratory reports seeing long, thin spirochetal organisms on the peripheral blood smear. The tentative diagnosis of endemic relapsing fever is made. Her fevers persist for 5 days, and then she suddenly experiences defervescence. Which arthropod is the most likely vector in this infection?

- ☐ (A) Flea
- ☐ (B) Soft tick
- ☐ (C) Louse
- ☐ (D) Mite
- ☐ (E) Mosquito

132 Which specimen would be appropriate to submit to the microbiology laboratory?

- ☐ (A) Midstream urine for anaerobic culture
- ☐ (B) A collection of sputum during a period of 24 h for mycobacterial culture
- ☐ (C) Blood specimen (1 ml) from a 10-year-old boy for routine bacterial culture
- ☐ (D) Urine refrigerated at 4° to 8°C after collection
- ☐ (E) Cerebrospinal fluid refrigerated at 4° to 8°C after collection

133 A 63-year-old man with chronic obstructive pulmonary disease (COPD) is hospitalized for 3 weeks because of deteriorating pulmonary function. Approximately 10 days into his hospitalization, he requires transfer into the respiratory intensive care unit and placement on a ventilator. His pulmonary function continues to deteriorate, and chest radiographs demonstrate multilobar infiltrates with cavitation. Sputum is collected for Gram stain and bacterial culture. The Gram stain shows gram-negative coccobacilli (see figure). The culture is positive after 24 h with growth on the blood, chocolate, and MacConkey agars. The organism is oxidase-negative, is nonfermentative, and fails to grow when subcultured onto anaerobic media. Susceptibility tests demonstrate susceptibility to imipenem, piperacillin-tazobactam, and trimethoprim/sulfamethoxazole. Which organism is most likely responsible for this infection?

- ❑ (A) *Acinetobacter baumannii*
- ❑ (B) *Burkholderia cepacia*
- ❑ (C) *Enterobacter cloacae*
- ❑ (D) *Pseudomonas aeruginosa*
- ❑ (E) *Stenotrophomonas maltophilia*

134 Bacteria become resistant to vancomycin by which mechanism?

- ❑ (A) Acetylation of the antibiotic
- ❑ (B) Active efflux of the antibiotic out of the cell
- ❑ (C) Modification of PBPs
- ❑ (D) Modification of a pentapeptide side chain in cell wall peptidoglycan
- ❑ (E) Modification of a ribosomal binding site

135 Resistance to vancomycin has not been reported for which species of *Enterococcus?*

- ❑ (A) *Enterococcus avium*
- ❑ (B) *Enterococcus casseliflavus*
- ❑ (C) *Enterococcus faecalis*
- ❑ (D) *Enterococcus faecium*
- ❑ (E) *Enterococcus gallinarum*

136 A 12-year-old girl with cystic fibrosis is admitted into the hospital with an exacerbation of her pulmonary disease. She has a productive cough with thick, tenacious secretions. A chest radiograph shows new infiltrates in both lung fields. Sputum is collected for Gram stain and culture. Gram-negative rods are observed in the Gram stain, and the organism is isolated after 48 h in culture. The following laboratory results are obtained for this organism: good growth on blood agar with dirt-like odor; slow growth on MacConkey agar with colorless colonies initially that progress to purple-red colonies after extended incubation; oxidase-positive; inability to ferment carbohydrates but ability to use glucose, lactose, and other carbohydrates oxidatively. Susceptibility tests show the organism is susceptible to trimethoprim/sulfamethoxazole, imipenem, and ceftazidime. Which organism is most likely responsible for this girl's infection?

- ❑ (A) *Acinetobacter baumannii*
- ❑ (B) *Burkholderia cepacia*
- ❑ (C) *Klebsiella pneumoniae*
- ❑ (D) *Pseudomonas aeruginosa*
- ❑ (E) *Stenotrophomonas maltophilia*

137 Which specimen is appropriate for diagnosing the indicated condition?

- ❑ (A) Abscess: pus
- ❑ (B) Epiglottitis: blood culture
- ❑ (C) Otitis media: ear swab
- ❑ (D) Sinusitis: nasopharyngeal washing
- ❑ (E) Urethritis: midstream urine

138 Which antibiotic is considered the drug of choice for treating infections with *Francisella tularensis?*

- ❑ (A) Ceftriaxone
- ❑ (B) Chloramphenicol
- ❑ (C) Penicillin
- ❑ (D) Streptomycin
- ❑ (E) Tetracycline

139 Which animal or insect is an important reservoir for *Francisella tularensis* in the United States?

- ❑ (A) Birds
- ❑ (B) Cattle
- ❑ (C) Deer
- ❑ (D) Fleas
- ❑ (E) Rabbits

140 Levofloxacin is bactericidal by which mechanism?

- ❑ (A) Blocks peptide elongation by inhibiting peptidyl-transferase
- ❑ (B) Inhibits cross-linking of cell wall peptidoglycan
- ❑ (C) Inhibits DNA topoisomerase
- ❑ (D) Inhibits initiation of RNA synthesis
- ❑ (E) Initiates premature release of peptide chains from ribosome

141 A 27-year-old man living in rural St. Louis goes to his physician with a 2-day history of progressive respiratory difficulties. He tells the physician that the onset of his disease was characterized by severe chest pain, drenching sweats, and a high-grade fever. During the next 2 days, he develops a productive cough with blood-tinged sputum. The physician orders a chest radiograph, which is abnormal with lobar consolidation (see figure). The relevant medical history for the patient includes HIV infection that was diagnosed 4 years previously, and a low CD4 count due to poor compliance with his anti-retroviral drug regimen. In addition, the patient explains that approximately 4 days before he became ill, he had mowed his lawn and accidentally run over a sick rabbit. Sputum is collected and cultures and stains are ordered for bacteria, fungi, and mycobacteria. The stains are all negative. After 3 days of incubation, pinpoint colonies are observed on chocolate agar and BCYE agar. Gram stain of the colonies shows very small gram-negative coccobacilli. Which organism is most likely responsible for this infection?

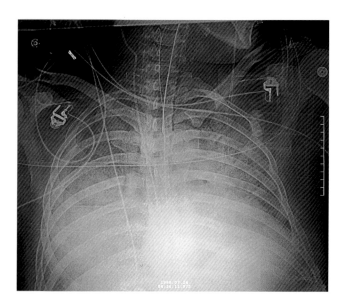

- ❏ (A) *Bordetella parapertussis*
- ❏ (B) *Francisella tularensis*
- ❏ (C) *Legionella pneumophila*
- ❏ (D) *Neisseria meningitidis*
- ❏ (E) *Pseudomonas aeruginosa*

142 Bacteria become resistant to clindamycin by which mechanism?

- ❏ (A) Acetylation of the antibiotic
- ❏ (B) Active efflux of the antibiotic out of the cell
- ❏ (C) Modification of PBPs
- ❏ (D) Modification of a pentapeptide side chain in cell wall peptidoglycan
- ❏ (E) Modification of a ribosomal binding site

143 *Brucella* is able to survive phagocytic killing by which factor?

- ❏ (A) Antiphagocytic capsule
- ❏ (B) Inhibition of phagosome/lysosome fusion
- ❏ (C) Inhibition of leukocyte chemotaxis
- ❏ (D) Lysis of phagosome followed by intracellular growth
- ❏ (E) Phospholipase C activity

144 Penicillin resistance has been reported most commonly for which *Streptococcus* species?

- ❏ (A) *S. agalactiae*
- ❏ (B) *S. anginosus*
- ❏ (C) *S. bovis*
- ❏ (D) *S. pneumoniae*
- ❏ (E) *S. pyogenes*

145 A conjugated, polysaccharide vaccine is used to prevent infections caused by which bacterial species?

- ❏ (A) *Bordetella pertussis*
- ❏ (B) *Haemophilus influenzae*
- ❏ (C) *Mycobacterium tuberculosis*
- ❏ (D) *Salmonella typhi*
- ❏ (E) *Yersinia pestis*

146 A sexually active 24-year-old homosexual man develops a tender papule with surrounding erythema on the foreskin of his penis. The papule expands, becomes pustular, and then ulcerates. The ulcer is extremely painful, and a bloody exudate is produced when the ulcer is manipulated. The man also develops tender inguinal lymphadenopathy. His physician swabs the ulcer and sends it for culture and Gram stain. Large numbers of gram-negative coccobacilli are seen on Gram stain. Which organism is responsible for this man's infection?

- ❏ (A) *Chlamydia trachomatis*
- ❏ (B) *Haemophilus ducreyi*
- ❏ (C) Herpes simplex virus
- ❏ (D) *Neisseria gonorrhoeae*
- ❏ (E) *Treponema pallidum*

147 A 6-year-old boy develops diarrhea with abdominal cramps. During the next 2 days, the diarrhea increases in frequency and is characterized by bloody stools. During this period, the patient has a low-grade fever. Cultures of the stool are positive for *Escherichia coli* O157. Which factor is responsible for this disease?

- ❏ (A) Autoagglutination of bacteria over intestinal epithelium with decreased fluid absorption
- ❏ (B) Heat-labile enterotoxin that increases cyclic adenosine monophosphate levels
- ❏ (C) Heat-stable enterotoxin that increases cyclic guanosine monophosphate levels
- ❏ (D) Plasmid-mediated invasion and destruction of colonic epithelium
- ❏ (E) Toxin-mediated disruption of protein synthesis with destruction of intestinal microvilli

148 A mother finds her 4-year-old son extremely agitated with a persistent cough. During the next 2 days, the child has coughing episodes that leave him gasping for air. After an episode that ends in the child vomiting, the mother takes her son to the local emergency department. The child is lethargic between coughing episodes, but his pulse rate and respiratory rate are elevated at the end of an episode. His white blood cell count is 15,000/mm³ with a predominance of lymphocytes. A nasopharyngeal aspirate is collected and sent to the lab for routine and special bacterial cultures. After 3 days, the lab reports small gram-negative rods that are growing on Bordet-Gengou medium. Which factor produced by the organism is most likely responsible for the clinical symptoms of this infection?

❑ (A) Cytotoxin that lyses polymorphonuclear leukocytes
❑ (B) Endotoxin that stimulates the release of cytokines
❑ (C) Exotoxin that causes unregulated cyclic adenosine monophosphate levels
❑ (D) Neuraminidase that alters host cell membrane glycolipids
❑ (E) Streptolysin O that lyses erythrocytes, leukocytes, and platelets

149 A 2-year-old boy is awakened from his sleep with acute pain in his left ear. During the previous 2 days, he developed an upper respiratory tract infection with nasal congestion. Because the pain persists for the next 24 h and is not relieved with warm compresses, the boy's mother takes him to the pediatrician. The physician finds the ear membrane swollen and red and makes the diagnosis of otitis media. What is the source of the organism that has infected this child?

❑ (A) Organism acquired by exposure to contaminated water
❑ (B) Organism acquired by inhalation of contaminated air
❑ (C) Organism normally found on the ear
❑ (D) Organism normally found in the oropharynx
❑ (E) Organism normally found on the skin surface

150 Which test is considered the most sensitive for detecting bacteria in the genus *Legionella?*

❑ (A) Direct fluorescent antibody stain
❑ (B) Dieterle silver stain
❑ (C) Culture on selective media
❑ (D) Detection of *Legionella* antigen in urine specimens
❑ (E) Detection of antibodies against *Legionella*

151 A 43-year-old woman in her sixth month of pregnancy goes to her regional hospital with malaise, muscle weakness, myalgias, and a low-grade temperature. She has been in good health and has maintained regular visits to her obstetrician throughout her pregnancy. No evidence of fetal distress is found. Her chest radiograph, differential, and routine chemistries are normal; however, two blood cultures collected at the time of admission become positive after 24 h of incubation. Gram-positive coccobacilli are observed on Gram stain, and weakly beta-hemolytic colonies on a sheep blood agar with a positive catalase reaction grow on subculture. The motility test for this isolate is positive. Which organism is most likely responsible for this woman's infection?

❑ (A) *Bacillus anthracis*
❑ (B) *Bacillus cereus*
❑ (C) *Corynebacterium ulcerans*
❑ (D) *Listeria monocytogenes*
❑ (E) *Streptococcus agalactiae*

152 Which enteric pathogen is able to invade and replicate in the M cells located in Peyer patches of the small intestine?

❑ (A) Enteroinvasive *Escherichia coli*
❑ (B) Enterohemorrhagic *Escherichia coli*
❑ (C) *Salmonella enteritidis*
❑ (D) *Shigella sonnei*
❑ (E) *Vibrio cholerae*

153 Which statement is correct?

❑ (A) Most patients with bacterial meningitis have small numbers of bacteria in their cerebrospinal fluid.
❑ (B) Most patients with cystitis have a bacteria count of more than 100,000/ml of urine.
❑ (C) Multiple blood cultures are generally required to diagnose subacute bacterial endocarditis.
❑ (D) Multiple stool cultures should be collected to diagnose bacterial gastroenteritis.
❑ (E) The most important factor for recovering bacteria in blood cultures is to collect a large volume of blood.

154 A 56-year-old woman is admitted to the hospital because she has had a 2-week history of pain and swelling in her right hand. Her hand has a 1-cm pustule with surrounding swelling and erythema. Epitroclear and axillary lymph nodes are also swollen and tender. Upon questioning by the emergency department physician, the woman cannot recall any injuries to her hand other than scratches she sustained while tending to her garden roses. Incision and drainage of the pustule is performed, and the collected material is sent to the laboratory for culture. After 3 days, small white colonies are observed on blood agar, chocolate agar, and BCYE agar. The organism is susceptible to trimethoprim/sulfamethoxazole, ciprofloxacin, and imipenem. Which organism is most likely responsible for this patient's infection?

❑ (A) *Erysipelothrix rhusiopathiae*
❑ (B) *Mycobacterium chelonae*
❑ (C) *Mycobacterium marinum*
❑ (D) *Nocardia brasiliensis*
❑ (E) *Sporothrix schenckii*

155 Which property is associated with *Enterococcus faecium* virulence?

❑ (A) Antibiotic resistance
❑ (B) Endotoxin production
❑ (C) Exfoliative toxin production
❑ (D) Exotoxin production
❑ (E) Phospholipase C production

156 A 9-month-old boy with persistent flu-like symptoms begins to suffer from coughing paroxysms that occur up to 50 times a day. Each paroxysm is so severe that the boy gasps for breath between coughs and sometimes vomits. Which answer describes the mechanism of two of the major toxins produced by the organism responsible for the disease?

❑ (A) Deregulation of adenylate cyclase in host cells
❑ (B) Disruption of cell membranes
❑ (C) Inhibition of acetylcholine release
❑ (D) Inhibition of protein synthesis
❑ (E) Stimulation of neurotransmitter release

157 A 23-year-old man is brought to the emergency department in a comatose state. He has a fever of 40°C, conjunctival petechiae, and embolic lesions on his palm. Blood and CSF are collected for culture and other laboratory tests. The CSF has a cell count of 1000/mm³ of predominantly leukocytes, an elevated protein, and decreased glucose. While in the emergency department, the patient has to be resuscitated before he is transferred to the medical intensive care unit (MICU). Approximately 12 h after admission to the unit, the patient expires. Early the next day, the microbiology laboratory contacts the emergency department and MICU to notify them that the blood and CSF cultures have grown gram-negative diplococci that are identified as *Neisseria meningitidis*. The hospital staff members who had direct and close contact with this patient should use which antibiotic as a prophylaxis?

❑ (A) Chloramphenicol
❑ (B)· Ciprofloxacin
❑ (C) Minocycline
❑ (D) Penicillin
❑ (E) Rifampin

158 Clindamycin is bacteriostatic by which mechanism?

❑ (A) Blocks peptide elongation by inhibiting peptidyl-transferase
❑ (B) Inhibits cross-linking of cell wall peptidoglycan
❑ (C) Inhibits DNA topoisomerase
❑ (D) Inhibits initiation of RNA synthesis
❑ (E) Initiates premature release of peptide chains from ribosome

159 A 42 year-old man undergoes an allogeneic bone marrow transplantation for treatment of chronic myelocytic leukemia. After engraftment, he develops severe graft versus host disease, for which he is treated with high doses of steroids. Approximately 2 weeks later, he develops a low-grade fever and a productive cough. Chest radiographs showed consolidation in the right upper lobe and evidence of cavitation. Expectorate sputa are collected; on Gram stain, abundant neutrophils, no squamous epithelial cells, and abundant filamentous and branching gram-positive rods are noted (see figure). A modified acid-fast stain is also positive. Which organism is most likely responsible for this man's infection?

❑ (A) *Actinomyces*
❑ (B) *Legionella*
❑ (C) *Mycobacterium*
❑ (D) *Nocardia*
❑ (E) *Rhodococcus*

160 The presence of squamous epithelial cells in expectorated sputum should be assessed for which culture?

❑ (A) Anaerobe culture
❑ (B) Fungal culture
❑ (C) Mycobacterial culture
❑ (D) Nocardia culture
❑ (E) Routine bacterial culture

161 When the wife of a 55-year-old man awakes one morning, she finds her husband extremely agitated and feverish. She takes him to the local emergency department, and upon arrival, her husband is nonresponsive with a temperature of 40°C, blood pressure of 100/60 mm Hg, heart rate of 80 bpm, and respiratory rate of 32/min. Past relevant history includes consumption of a pint of vodka each day, a splenectomy following an automobile accident 3 years previously, and a dog bite on his left leg 4 days before the onset of his illness. The bite wound is erythematous and has a serous sanguinous drainage. The drainage and blood are submitted for culture. Gram stain of the drainage shows thin, filamentous gram-negative rods, and the cultures of the drainage and blood are positive with the same organism after 3 days of incubation. The isolate is catalase-positive and oxidase-positive and requires a carbon dioxide–enriched atmosphere for growth. Which organism is most likely responsible for this infection?

❑   (A) *Capnocytophaga canimorsus*
❑   (B) *Eikenella corrodens*
❑   (C) *Pasteurella multocida*
❑   (D) *Spirillum minus*
❑   (E) *Vibrio vulnificus*

162   Which feature would be characteristic of lepromatous leprosy?

❑   (A) Absence of erythematous patches on the skin
❑   (B) Low infectivity
❑   (C) Normal immunoglobulin levels
❑   (D) Positive acid-fast stain
❑   (E) Positive skin test reaction

163   A toxoid vaccine is used to prevent infections caused by which bacteria?

❑   (A) *Corynebacterium diphtheriae*
❑   (B) *Neisseria meningitidis*
❑   (C) *Streptococcus pneumoniae*
❑   (D) *Vibrio cholerae*
❑   (E) *Yersinia pestis*

164   Approximately 12 h after a premature delivery, a baby girl is noted to be unresponsive, tachypnic, and cyanotic. Blood and CSF are collected for culture, and the baby is started on antibiotic therapy. The preliminary laboratory report of the Gram stain of the CSF indicates gram-positive cocci are present. Which organism is most likely responsible for this infection?

❑   (A) *Listeria monocytogenes*
❑   (B) *Neisseria meningitidis*
❑   (C) *Staphylococcus aureus*
❑   (D) Group B *Streptococcus agalactiae*
❑   (E) *Streptococcus pneumoniae*

165   An 18-month-old boy has a CSF shunt placed to alleviate hydrocephalus. The child becomes progressively more agitated 4 weeks after this procedure and is noted to be febrile (39°C). CSF is collected for Gram stain and culture, and gram-positive rods with abundant neutrophils are noted on the Gram stain. After 48 h of incubation, small gram-positive rods are seen on the anaerobic blood agar plate. Which organism is most likely responsible for this infection?

❑   (A) *Actinomyces*
❑   (B) *Bifidobacterium*
❑   (C) *Eubacterium*
❑   (D) *Lactobacillus*
❑   (E) *Propionibacterium*

166   Bacteria become resistant to oxacillin by which mechanism?

❑   (A) Acetylation of the antibiotic
❑   (B) Active efflux of the antibiotic out of the cell
❑   (C) Modification of PBPs

❑   (D) Modification of a pentapeptide side chain in cell wall peptidoglycan
❑   (E) Modification of a ribosomal binding site

167   Approximately 2 days after a church picnic, 13 children and adults develop a diarrheal disease characterized by 6 to 10 bowel movements per day, abdominal cramps, headaches, and fevers. Visible blood in stools affects three patients. The physician in the local hospital emergency department who sees these patients suspects an outbreak of *Campylobacter* or *Salmonella* food poisoning. Which test should be performed with the collected stool specimens to confirm the diagnosis of *Campylobacter jejuni* infection?

❑   (A) Culture on blood agar
❑   (B) Culture on MacConkey agar
❑   (C) Culture on sorbitol/MacConkey agar
❑   (D) Culture on selective agar incubated in a microaerophilic atmosphere
❑   (E) Immunoassay for toxin

168   Which association is correct?

❑   (A) *Clostridium perfringens*: antibiotic-associated colitis
❑   (B) *Clostridium botulinum*: blocked release of neurotransmitters from inhibitory synapses
❑   (C) *Clostridium tetani*: food-borne tetanus
❑   (D) *Clostridium perfringens*: food poisoning associated with meat products
❑   (E) *Clostridium difficile*: flaccid paralysis

169   A 42-year-old carpenter suffers a penetrating eye injury when a wooden splinter is deflected into his eye. Within 12 h of the injury, the eye is inflamed and painful. By the time the man goes to the emergency department, he has completely lost vision in the eye. Drainage from the eye is collected on a swab and submitted for Gram stain and culture. Abundant gram-positive rods are observed on Gram stain (see figure); within 12 h of incubation, large beta-hemolytic colonies are detected on the aerobic blood agar plates. Which organism is most likely responsible for this infection?

- ☐ (A) *Bacillus cereus*
- ☐ (B) *Clostridium perfringens*
- ☐ (C) *Corynebacterium jeikeium*
- ☐ (D) *Erysipelothrix rhusiopathiae*
- ☐ (E) *Pseudomonas aeruginosa*

170 The exotoxin produced by *Vibrio cholerae* works by which mechanism?

- ☐ (A) Blocks release of acetylcholine
- ☐ (B) Blocks release of GABA
- ☐ (C) Inactivates EF-2 and prevents protein synthesis
- ☐ (D) Stimulates increased adenylate cyclase activity
- ☐ (E) Stimulates release of proinflammatory cytokines

171 What is the most common source of *Shigella* infections?

- ☐ (A) Contaminated water
- ☐ (B) Person-to-person contact
- ☐ (C) Steamed rice
- ☐ (D) Undercooked chicken
- ☐ (E) Undercooked hamburger

172 A mother brings her 2-week-old baby girl to the emergency department. The baby was well until 1 day before presentation. During the past 24 h, the baby has become progressively more agitated, crying throughout the day and refusing to nurse. Perioral erythema (redness and inflammation around the mouth) and fever are noted at this first visit. During the next 2 days, a diffuse scarlatiniform rash and cutaneous blisters develop. Slight pressure displaces the skin, showing a bright red skin surface. The mother takes the baby back to the emergency room, and a Gram stain and culture of fluid aspirated from the bullae are performed; the results are negative. Which toxin is most likely responsible for this illness?

- ☐ (A) Alpha-toxin
- ☐ (B) Enterotoxin A
- ☐ (C) Exfoliative toxins A and B
- ☐ (D) Leukocidin
- ☐ (E) TSST-1

173 A 10-year-old girl develops a sore throat, erythema and exudates over the tonsils, cervical lymphadenopathy, and a fever. A pharyngeal swab is collected, and beta-hemolytic colonies of gram-positive cocci in chains grow the next day in culture. Which test can be used to identify this organism?

- ☐ (A) Catalase
- ☐ (B) Coagulase
- ☐ (C) Solubility in bile
- ☐ (D) Susceptibility to optochin
- ☐ (E) Susceptibility to bacitracin

174 Which disease is transmitted by mites?

- ☐ (A) African trypanosomiasis
- ☐ (B) Plague

- ☐ (C) Relapsing fever
- ☐ (D) Rickettsial pox
- ☐ (E) Tularemia

175 A 24-year-old man living in Kenya goes to his local physician with the complaint that a swelling in his groin enlarged to the point that it ruptured and drained cloudy fluid. After taking a careful history, the physician discovers that the sexually active man had initially developed a small blister that ulcerated and then rapidly healed. Approximately 1 week later, the lymph nodes that drained the area had become enlarged. The area surrounding the nodes became inflamed and the nodes were tender. It was these swollen nodes that enlarged to the point they ruptured through the skin and drained purulent material. At the time the nodes enlarged, the patient felt feverish and had a headache and muscle aches. The physician makes a diagnosis based on the isolation of the organism from the purulent exudate. Which organism is most likely responsible for this man's infection?

- ☐ (A) *Chlamydia trachomatis*
- ☐ (B) Herpes simplex virus
- ☐ (C) *Klebsiella (Calymmatobacterium) granulomatis*
- ☐ (D) *Neisseria gonorrhoeae*
- ☐ (E) *Treponema pallidum*

176 Which enteric pathogen produces disease by elaboration of toxin in food products (intoxication)?

- ☐ (A) *Clostridium difficile*
- ☐ (B) *Salmonella typhi*
- ☐ (C) *Shigella sonnei*
- ☐ (D) *Staphylococcus aureus*
- ☐ (E) *Yersinia enterocolitica*

177 A 22-year-old man develops pain when urinating and a urethral discharge 3 days after unprotected sex with a prostitute. Gram-negative diplococci are seen on Gram stain of the discharge (see figure). Which medium can be used for the selective isolation of this organism?

❑ (A) BCYE agar
❑ (B) Bordet-Gengou agar
❑ (C) Modified Thayer-Martin (MTM) agar
❑ (D) Mueller-Hinton agar
❑ (E) Nutrient agar

178 Recovery of which Mycobacterium species requires inoculation of chocolate agar and incubation at 30°C?

❑ (A) *Mycobacterium avium*
❑ (B) *Mycobacterium fortuitum*
❑ (C) *Mycobacterium haemophilum*
❑ (D) *Mycobacterium leprae*
❑ (E) *Mycobacterium marinum*

179 A 37-year-old woman is brought to the emergency department complaining of severe pain in her left eye. Examination of the eye reveals a corneal ulcer with surrounding edema. The patient wears an extended-wear contact lens and admits to not caring for the lens as recommended. A scraping of the involved cornea is performed for Gram stain and culture, and topical and intraocular antibiotics are started. Despite the prompt initiation of treatment, the condition of the eye worsens over the next 48 h, and she loses her vision in that eye. Abundant gram-negative rods are seen on Gram stain of the corneal scrapings, and the organism grows in culture the next day. Preliminary tests indicate this is a gram-negative, nonfermentative rod that is oxidase-positive and also able to produce a fluorescent pigment. Which toxin is responsible for this woman's destructive eye infection?

❑ (A) Alpha-toxin
❑ (B) Beta-toxin
❑ (C) Cereolysin
❑ (D) Endotoxin
❑ (E) Exotoxin A

180 During a period of 10 days, eight children in a first-grade class develop pharyngitis, characterized by a bright red throat with patchy white exudates over the tonsillar area. On the second day of the illness, a rash develops in three of the children. It is first observed on the upper chest and then spreads over the neck, trunk, and extremities but spares the palms, soles, and area around the mouth. Deep lines of red are noted along skin folds, and the rash blanches when pressure is applied. Which toxin is most likely responsible for this rash?

❑ (A) Endotoxin
❑ (B) Exfoliative toxin
❑ (C) Pertussis toxin
❑ (D) Pyrogenic exotoxin
❑ (E) Streptolysin O

181 The diagnosis of early localized Lyme disease is most commonly made by which of the following?

❑ (A) Detection of *Borrelia burgdorferi* by culture
❑ (B) Detection of *Borrelia burgdorferi* in Giemsa-stained blood

❑ (C) Detection of anti-*Borrelia burgdorferi* antibodies in the blood or CSF
❑ (D) History of tick exposure in endemic areas
❑ (E) Clinical diagnosis of erythema migrans

182 Which organism is a common cause of sinusitis?

❑ (A) *Bordetella pertussis*
❑ (B) *Corynebacterium diphtheriae*
❑ (C) *Moraxella catarrhalis*
❑ (D) *Mycoplasma pneumoniae*
❑ (E) *Neisseria gonorrhoeae*

183 Which organism is most numerous in the human colon?

❑ (A) *Bacteroides*
❑ (B) *Bifidobacterium*
❑ (C) *Enterococcus*
❑ (D) *Escherichia*
❑ (E) *Pseudomonas*

184 Which specimen is appropriate for the associated disease?

❑ (A) Cystitis: urethral swab
❑ (B) Ocular infection: corneal scraping
❑ (C) Pneumonia: oropharyngeal washing
❑ (D) Sinusitis: nasopharyngeal aspirate
❑ (E) Wound: swab of drainage

185 Which structural component of bacteria is unique to bacterial spores?

❑ (A) Dipicolinic acid
❑ (B) Lipid A
❑ (C) Lipoteichoic acid
❑ (D) O antigen
❑ (E) Peptidoglycan

186 A 20-year-old college student awakens in the middle of the night with a severe headache. During the next few hours, the headache worsens, and she is unable to think clearly. Her roommate becomes concerned that she is becoming more agitated and takes her to the student health care facility. When the 20-year-old arrives, the physician notes that she is in acute distress, has a stiff neck, and has conjunctival petechiae. The clinical diagnosis of meningitis is made, and samples of blood and cerebrospinal fluid are collected. A CSF cell count is 1200 cells/mm^3 with 95% PMNs, glucose 35 mg/dl, and protein 250 mg/dl. Gram stain of the CSF shows abundant gram-negative diplococci (see figure), and this organism is recovered in both blood and CSF the next day. Which property is responsible for the clinical manifestations of this disease?

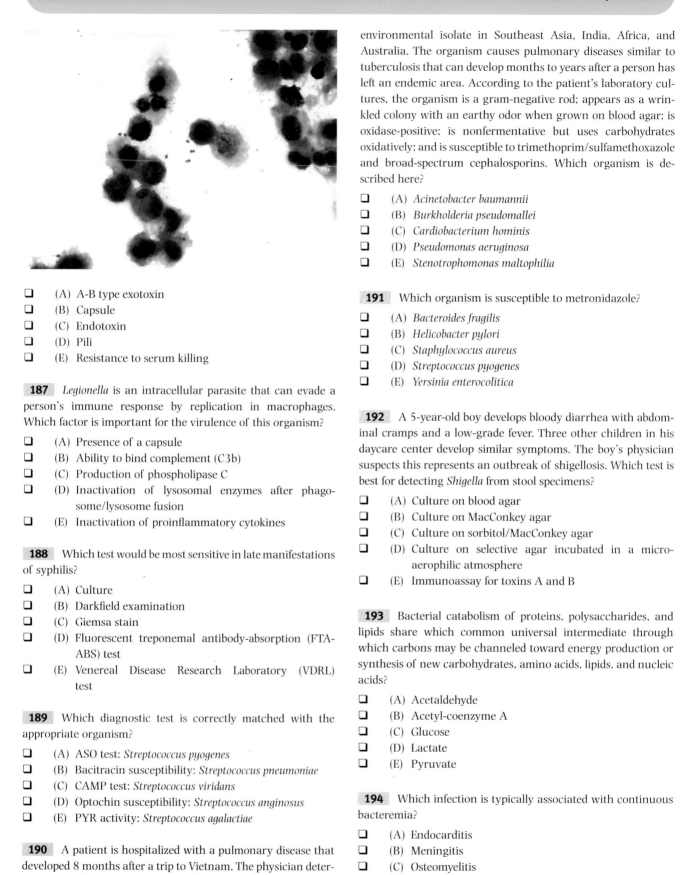

- ❑ (A) A-B type exotoxin
- ❑ (B) Capsule
- ❑ (C) Endotoxin
- ❑ (D) Pili
- ❑ (E) Resistance to serum killing

187 *Legionella* is an intracellular parasite that can evade a person's immune response by replication in macrophages. Which factor is important for the virulence of this organism?

- ❑ (A) Presence of a capsule
- ❑ (B) Ability to bind complement (C3b)
- ❑ (C) Production of phospholipase C
- ❑ (D) Inactivation of lysosomal enzymes after phagosome/lysosome fusion
- ❑ (E) Inactivation of proinflammatory cytokines

188 Which test would be most sensitive in late manifestations of syphilis?

- ❑ (A) Culture
- ❑ (B) Darkfield examination
- ❑ (C) Giemsa stain
- ❑ (D) Fluorescent treponemal antibody-absorption (FTA-ABS) test
- ❑ (E) Venereal Disease Research Laboratory (VDRL) test

189 Which diagnostic test is correctly matched with the appropriate organism?

- ❑ (A) ASO test: *Streptococcus pyogenes*
- ❑ (B) Bacitracin susceptibility: *Streptococcus pneumoniae*
- ❑ (C) CAMP test: *Streptococcus viridans*
- ❑ (D) Optochin susceptibility: *Streptococcus anginosus*
- ❑ (E) PYR activity: *Streptococcus agalactiae*

190 A patient is hospitalized with a pulmonary disease that developed 8 months after a trip to Vietnam. The physician determines that the organism responsible for this patient's illness is not commonly found in the United States, but it is a common environmental isolate in Southeast Asia, India, Africa, and Australia. The organism causes pulmonary diseases similar to tuberculosis that can develop months to years after a person has left an endemic area. According to the patient's laboratory cultures, the organism is a gram-negative rod; appears as a wrinkled colony with an earthy odor when grown on blood agar; is oxidase-positive; is nonfermentative but uses carbohydrates oxidatively; and is susceptible to trimethoprim/sulfamethoxazole and broad-spectrum cephalosporins. Which organism is described here?

- ❑ (A) *Acinetobacter baumannii*
- ❑ (B) *Burkholderia pseudomallei*
- ❑ (C) *Cardiobacterium hominis*
- ❑ (D) *Pseudomonas aeruginosa*
- ❑ (E) *Stenotrophomonas maltophilia*

191 Which organism is susceptible to metronidazole?

- ❑ (A) *Bacteroides fragilis*
- ❑ (B) *Helicobacter pylori*
- ❑ (C) *Staphylococcus aureus*
- ❑ (D) *Streptococcus pyogenes*
- ❑ (E) *Yersinia enterocolitica*

192 A 5-year-old boy develops bloody diarrhea with abdominal cramps and a low-grade fever. Three other children in his daycare center develop similar symptoms. The boy's physician suspects this represents an outbreak of shigellosis. Which test is best for detecting *Shigella* from stool specimens?

- ❑ (A) Culture on blood agar
- ❑ (B) Culture on MacConkey agar
- ❑ (C) Culture on sorbitol/MacConkey agar
- ❑ (D) Culture on selective agar incubated in a microaerophilic atmosphere
- ❑ (E) Immunoassay for toxins A and B

193 Bacterial catabolism of proteins, polysaccharides, and lipids share which common universal intermediate through which carbons may be channeled toward energy production or synthesis of new carbohydrates, amino acids, lipids, and nucleic acids?

- ❑ (A) Acetaldehyde
- ❑ (B) Acetyl-coenzyme A
- ❑ (C) Glucose
- ❑ (D) Lactate
- ❑ (E) Pyruvate

194 Which infection is typically associated with continuous bacteremia?

- ❑ (A) Endocarditis
- ❑ (B) Meningitis
- ❑ (C) Osteomyelitis
- ❑ (D) Peritonitis
- ❑ (E) Septic arthritis

195 Which organism can colonize the stomach of humans?

- ❑ (A) *Bacteroides*
- ❑ (B) *Escherichia*
- ❑ (C) *Lactobacillus*
- ❑ (D) *Malassezia*
- ❑ (E) Viridans streptococci

196 A 35-year-old man is admitted to the hospital with a temperature of 40°C and difficulty breathing. Physical examination reveals decreased breath sounds on the right side and oral thrush. Infiltrates in both lung fields are observed by chest radiography, and cavitation is seen on the right side. Bronchoalveolar lavage (BAL) fluid is collected and submitted for culture and Gram stain; blood is drawn for three sets of blood cultures. Preliminary tests are positive for HIV, and the patient's CD4 lymphocyte count is 100/mm^3. Gram stain of the BAL fluid shows pleomorphic gram-positive rods. After 48 h of incubation, the BAL fluid is positive for abundant colonies of gram-positive coccobacilli. During the next 2 days, the colonies take on a salmon-pink color. Because the organism stains irregularly, a modified acid-fast stain is performed and is positive. The organism is catalase- and urease-positive but fails to ferment any carbohydrates. Which organism is most likely responsible for this man's infection?

- ❑ (A) *Gordonia*
- ❑ (B) *Legionella*
- ❑ (C) *Mycobacterium*
- ❑ (D) *Nocardia*
- ❑ (E) *Rhodococcus*

197 A 28-year-old woman develops pain when urinating and increased frequency of urination. Over the next few days, she notices that the pain has intensified and now radiates to her lower back. She also notices that she feels hot and has had low-grade fevers ranging from 38° to 39°C. Her physician suspects she has an infection and collects urine cultures. The next day, the laboratory calls the physician and reports the urine culture as positive with a bacterial count of 10^5/ml of urine. The organism grows on both blood agar and MacConkey agar, with spreading colonies on the blood agar and colorless colonies on the MacConkey agar. The organism is also strongly urease-positive. Which organism is responsible for this woman's infection?

- ❑ (A) *Escherichia coli*
- ❑ (B) *Klebsiella pneumoniae*
- ❑ (C) *Proteus mirabilis*
- ❑ (D) *Pseudomonas aeruginosa*
- ❑ (E) *Salmonella typhi*

198 Which organism would be considered an opportunistic pathogen?

- ❑ (A) *Escherichia coli*
- ❑ (B) *Francisella tularensis*
- ❑ (C) *Mycobacterium tuberculosis*
- ❑ (D) *Neisseria gonorrhoeae*
- ❑ (E) *Salmonella typhi*

199 A 63-year-old man sees a physican at the Veterans Administration Hospital with complaints of dizziness. During the preceding 6 months, he has had night sweats, low-grade fevers, and a 20-lb weight loss. A physical examination reveals that he is afebrile with normal vital signs. The physician notes that the patient's teeth are in poor condition, and she hears a grade III/VI holosystolic cardiac murmur. Blood cultures are drawn because the physician suspects subacute infectious endocarditis. After 3 days of incubation, all blood cultures are reported to be positive for an anaerobic gram-positive rod. Preliminary biochemical tests are consistent with *Lactobacillus*. Which antibiotic should be used to treat this infection?

- ❑ (A) Ampicillin
- ❑ (B) Ceftazidime
- ❑ (C) Oxacillin plus metronidazole
- ❑ (D) Penicillin plus gentamicin
- ❑ (E) Vancomycin

200 An isolate of *Staphylococcus aureus* is found to be resistant to oxacillin. Which mechanism is most likely causing this resistance?

- ❑ (A) Production of an extended spectrum beta-lactamase (ESBL)
- ❑ (B) Production of an AmpC beta-lactamase
- ❑ (C) Production of penicillinase
- ❑ (D) Production of the *mec*A gene product
- ❑ (E) Production of a modified outer membrane porin protein

201 Quantitation of the number of bacteria is useful for differentiating between colonization and significant infection for which specimen?

- ❑ (A) Blood
- ❑ (B) Cerebrospinal fluid
- ❑ (C) Sputum
- ❑ (D) Stool
- ❑ (E) Urine

202 Which statement about Lyme disease is correct?

- ❑ (A) The disease is transmitted by fleas.
- ❑ (B) The reservoirs for infection are the white-footed mouse and ground squirrel.
- ❑ (C) Disease is most common in the very young and very old.
- ❑ (D) Late manifestations of disseminated disease include arthritis, cardiac abnormalities, and neurologic disease.
- ❑ (E) The diagnostic tests of choice are microscopy and culture.

203 Members of the viridans group of *Streptococcus* have been most commonly associated with which disease?

- ❑ (A) Gastroenteritis
- ❑ (B) Meningitis
- ❑ (C) Osteomyelitis
- ❑ (D) Septic arthritis
- ❑ (E) Subacute endocarditis

204 Which disinfectant is active against mycobacteria and spores?

- ☐ (A) Alcohol
- ☐ (B) Formaldehyde
- ☐ (C) Iodophors
- ☐ (D) Phenolics
- ☐ (E) Quaternary ammonium compounds

205 Historically, *Haemophilus influenzae* type B was a major pediatric pathogen, causing meningitis, epiglottitis, and cellulitis. In the late twentieth and early twenty-first centuries, these infections have been eliminated through the introduction of a conjugated vaccine. This vaccine is directed against which bacterial component?

- ☐ (A) Endotoxin
- ☐ (B) Phospholipase C
- ☐ (C) Pilin proteins
- ☐ (D) Polyribitol phosphate
- ☐ (E) Somatic O antigen

206 The majority of infections caused by *Campylobacter jejuni* have been associated with which foods?

- ☐ (A) Chicken
- ☐ (B) Ham
- ☐ (C) Potato salad
- ☐ (D) Rice
- ☐ (E) Seafood

207 A resident of Wisconsin sees her physician because of a skin lesion that she notices on her arm. It began as a small papule and then enlarged during the next 10 days (see figure). When she presents this lesion to her physician, the involved area is 30 cm in diameter, has a flat red border, and has an area of central clearing. She also has a headache, low-grade fever, and myalgias. Her activities during the weeks before the rash and symptoms developed included hunting with her dog, gardening, and swimming in the local lake. Which organism is most likely responsible for this infection?

- ☐ (A) *Borrelia burgdorferi*
- ☐ (B) Brown recluse spider bite
- ☐ (C) *Leptospira interrogans*
- ☐ (D) *Sporothrix schenckii*
- ☐ (E) *Trichophyton mentagrophytes*

208 *Neisseria gonorrhoeae* can escape phagocytic clearance by which mechanism?

- ☐ (A) Capsule-mediated inhibition of phagocytosis
- ☐ (B) Inhibition of phagosome/lysosome fusion
- ☐ (C) Inhibition of opsonization mediated by protein A
- ☐ (D) Lysis of phagosome and replication in cytoplasm
- ☐ (E) Replication in fused phagosome/lysosome

209 A 35-year-old man with advanced HIV presents to his physician with cutaneous lesions that were first noticed 1 month previously. The lesions started as small, reddened nodules that first appeared in a cluster. During the course of the month, the lesions expanded in size, and additional lesions appeared. At the time the patient sees his physician, the lesion has a purple surface, and serous sanguinous exudate is present. The exudate is collected for Gram stain and bacterial culture. Small gram-negative rods are observed on Gram stain and grow after prolonged incubation. Which organism is most likely responsible for this infection?

- ☐ (A) *Bartonella henselae*
- ☐ (B) *Burkholderia cepacia*
- ☐ (C) *Capnocytophaga ochracea*
- ☐ (D) *Mycobacterium avium*
- ☐ (E) *Pseudomonas aeruginosa*

210 Which antibiotic inhibits protein synthesis by binding to the 50S ribosome?

- ☐ (A) Ciprofloxacin
- ☐ (B) Erythromycin
- ☐ (C) Imipenem
- ☐ (D) Rifampin
- ☐ (E) Tetracycline

211 A 43-year-old woman goes to her physician with a 4-day history of low-grade fevers, fatigue, and a painful sore throat. A gray-colored membrane is observed over both tonsils and extends over the uvula and soft palate. Adenopathy and cervical swelling are also present. When the physician attempts to remove the membrane, he notices that the underlying mucosa is edematous and bleeding. Which organism is most likely responsible for this infection?

- ☐ (A) *Bordetella pertussis*
- ☐ (B) *Corynebacterium diphtheriae*
- ☐ (C) *Neisseria gonorrhoeae*
- ☐ (D) *Staphylococcus aureus*
- ☐ (E) *Streptococcus pyogenes*

212 Which structure is unique to gram-negative bacteria?

- ❏ (A) Cytoplasmic membrane
- ❏ (B) Endoplasmic reticulum
- ❏ (C) Golgi apparatus
- ❏ (D) Nuclear membrane
- ❏ (E) Outer membrane

213 Vaccination is used to stimulate immunity to *Bordetella pertussis*. Which antibiotic is used to protect an individual exposed to a patient with active pertussis?

- ❏ (A) Ampicillin
- ❏ (B) Ciprofloxacin
- ❏ (C) Doxycycline
- ❏ (D) Erythromycin
- ❏ (E) Vancomycin

214 A 36-year-old woman with a history of rheumatic heart disease undergoes dental extractions for severely decayed teeth. Prophylactic antibiotics are not administered before the procedure. Approximately 6 weeks after the procedure, the woman develops fevers, chills, and night sweats. After 1 week of symptoms, the patient sees her physician, who notes that she has experienced a 10-lb weight loss since her last visit. Which organism is most likely responsible for this patient's clinical presentation?

- ❏ (A) *Candida albicans*
- ❏ (B) *Staphylococcus aureus*
- ❏ (C) *Staphylococcus epidermidis*
- ❏ (D) *Streptococcus pneumoniae*
- ❏ (E) *Streptococcus mutans*

215 *Mycobacterium tuberculosis* can escape phagocytic clearance by which mechanisms?

- ❏ (A) Capsule-mediated inhibition of phagocytosis
- ❏ (B) Inhibition of phagosome/lysosome fusion
- ❏ (C) Inhibition of opsonization mediated by protein A
- ❏ (D) Lysis of phagosome and replication in cytoplasm
- ❏ (E) Replication in fused phagosome/lysosome

216 Approximately 4 hours after eating a breakfast of scrambled eggs, ham, custard-filled Danish roll, and orange juice, a husband and wife develop nausea and start vomiting. They rapidly develop severe abdominal pain and diarrhea. The couple goes to the local hospital. They are dehydrated but have no evidence of fever, rash, or other signs. Which antibiotic should be used to treat this couple for food poisoning?

- ❏ (A) Amoxicillin
- ❏ (B) Dicloxacillin
- ❏ (C) Erythromycin
- ❏ (D) Vancomycin
- ❏ (E) No antibiotic

217 Approximately 2 weeks after birth, an infant develops watery discharge from both eyes. During the next few days, this discharge becomes purulent, and the conjunctiva becomes erythematous (see figure). The mother returns to the hospital, and her pediatrician orders cultures and Gram stain of the exudates. No organisms are observed on Gram stain; cultures on blood agar, chocolate agar, MacConkey agar, and Sabouraud agar are negative. The organism responsible for this infection would be susceptible to which drug?

From Morse S et al: *Atlas of sexually transmitted diseases and AIDS*, ed 3, St Louis, 2003, Mosby.

- ❏ (A) Ciprofloxacin
- ❏ (B) Erythromycin
- ❏ (C) Imipenem
- ❏ (D) Penicillin
- ❏ (E) Tetracycline

218 *Legionella pneumophila* can escape phagocytic clearance by which mechanism?

- ❏ (A) Capsule-mediated inhibition of phagocytosis
- ❏ (B) Inhibition of phagosome/lysosome fusion
- ❏ (C) Inhibition of opsonization mediated by protein A
- ❏ (D) Lysis of phagosome and replication in cytoplasm
- ❏ (E) Replication in fused phagosome/lysosome

219 A young boy develops symptoms that are characteristic of pertussis. Which specimen would be best for confirming this diagnosis?

- ❏ (A) Blood culture
- ❏ (B) Cough plate
- ❏ (C) Expectorated sputum
- ❏ (D) Induced sputum
- ❏ (E) Nasopharyngeal aspirate

220 One day after a premature delivery, a baby boy has become unresponsive, tachypnic, and cyanotic. Blood and cerebrospinal fluid are collected for culture, and the baby is started on antibiotic therapy. No bacteria are seen in the initial Gram stain of CSF; however, after 1 day of incubation, both the blood and CSF cultures are positive with gram-negative rods. The organism is beta-hemolytic on blood agar and forms purple colonies on MacConkey agar. Which organism is most likely responsible for this infection?

- ❑ (A) *Enterobacter aerogenes*
- ❑ (B) *Escherichia coli*
- ❑ (C) *Klebsiella pneumoniae*
- ❑ (D) *Pseudomonas aeruginosa*
- ❑ (E) *Salmonella typhi*

221 Which statement about *Clostridium* is correct?

- ❑ (A) Spore formation is an important feature of these organisms.
- ❑ (B) Botulinum toxin blocks the release of neurotransmitters for inhibitory synapses.
- ❑ (C) Infection with *Clostridium botulinum* confers lifelong immunity.
- ❑ (D) *Clostridium perfringens* can produce a disease that is identical to tetanus.
- ❑ (E) Clindamycin is the drug of choice for treating *Clostridium difficile* infections.

222 In late 2001 and early 2002, four infants residing in Staten Island, New York, became ill with the same bacterial pathogen. The infants were between the ages of 3 weeks and 18 weeks. All had been in good health following uneventful pregnancies. Two infants were breast-fed, and two were formula-fed. Upon presentation to the hospital, all infants were irritable, lethargic, and constipated. Two infants had sluggishly reactive pupils, and two were described as having loss of facial expression. Three of the infants required mechanical ventilation. Specimens of blood, stool, urine, and cerebrospinal fluid were collected for microbiologic testing. Which organism was most likely responsible for these infections?

- ❑ (A) *Bordetella pertussis*
- ❑ (B) *Campylobacter jejuni*
- ❑ (C) *Clostridium botulinum*
- ❑ (D) *Salmonella choleraesuis*
- ❑ (E) *Streptococcus pneumoniae*

223 A mother brings her 6-week-old infant to his pediatrician with concerns about a developing respiratory infection. The mother explains that the baby developed a nasal discharge and cough that worsened during the preceding week. The baby has become progressively more irritable, and the cough (a staccato pattern) was beginning to interfere with the baby's eating and sleeping. No temperature has been noted. Auscultation reveals good breath sounds and no wheezing, but rales are noted. A chest radiograph demonstrates bilateral interstitial infiltrates (see figure). Which test would be expected to determine this infant's disease?

- ❑ (A) Gram stain of the nasal discharge
- ❑ (B) Culture on blood, chocolate, and Thayer-Martin agars
- ❑ (C) Culture in tissue culture cells
- ❑ (D) Serology for specific IgM and IgG antibodies
- ❑ (E) Urine antigen test

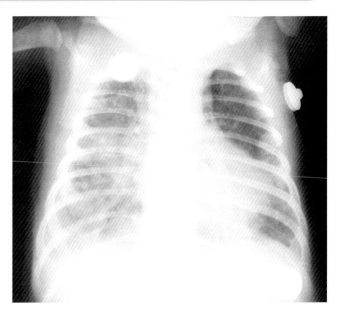

From Morse S et al: *Atlas of sexually transmitted diseases and AIDS*, ed 3, St Louis, 2003, Mosby.

224 *Enterococcus* is inherently resistant to sulfonamides by which mechanism?

- ❑ (A) Use of exogenous thymidine
- ❑ (B) Active efflux out of cell
- ❑ (C) Decreased affinity of dihydrofolate reductase
- ❑ (D) Enzymatic degradation of antibiotics
- ❑ (E) Presence of permeability barrier

225 During a military conflict in Somalia, soldiers develop a febrile illness characterized by the abrupt onset of fever with rigors, severe headache, myalgias, arthralgias, lethargy, photophobia, and coughing. Observed are conjunctival suffusion and a petechial rash that develop 4 days into the illness and then fade after 1 to 2 days at the time the symptoms wane. Splenomegaly and hepatomegaly are also characteristically present. After 1 week to 10 days, the symptoms recur. The tentative diagnosis of this disease is relapsing fever. Which vector is most likely the cause of this disease?

- ❑ (A) Flea
- ❑ (B) Hard tick
- ❑ (C) Louse
- ❑ (D) Mite
- ❑ (E) Mosquito

226 Which antibiotic can be used to treat infections caused by *Listeria*?

- ❑ (A) Ampicillin
- ❑ (B) Ceftazidime
- ❑ (C) Gentamicin
- ❑ (D) Tetracycline
- ❑ (E) Trimethoprim

227 A 73-year-old diabetic man is brought to the hospital by his daughter because he is complaining of intense pain in his left ear. The ear is edematous with erythema and a purulent discharge present. A CT scan of the ear reveals soft tissue swelling and destruction of the underlying temporal bone. Which organism is most likely responsible for this infection?

- ☐ (A) *Moraxella catarrhalis*
- ☐ (B) *Pseudomonas aeruginosa*
- ☐ (C) *Staphylococcus aureus*
- ☐ (D) *Streptococcus pneumoniae*
- ☐ (E) *Streptococcus pyogenes*

228 Which statement is correct?

- ☐ (A) *Bacteroides fragilis* colonizes the pharynx.
- ☐ (B) Acceptable specimens for anaerobic culture include lung aspirates, biopsied tissue, and clean voided, midstream urine.
- ☐ (C) Clinical clues of anaerobic infections include a wound with foul odor, gas in the tissue, and presence of a sinus tract with sulfur granules.
- ☐ (D) *Peptostreptococcus* is typically resistant to penicillin.
- ☐ (E) *Actinomyces* is a gram-negative, non–spore-forming rod.

229 A 30-year-old woman goes to her physician complaining of a persistent nonproductive cough and low-grade fevers. A chest radiograph shows bilateral infiltrates with no signs of consolidation. Blood cultures and induced sputum are collected for culture. The blood cultures are negative, no organisms are observed on Gram stain of the sputum specimen, and routine bacterial and fungal cultures are negative after 48 h. Growth of a bacterium, however, is observed after 7 days on a special medium supplemented with serum, yeast extract, and glucose. Which bacterial organism is most likely responsible for this woman's infection?

- ☐ (A) *Chlamydophila (Chlamydia) pneumoniae*
- ☐ (B) *Klebsiella pneumoniae*
- ☐ (C) *Legionella pneumophila*
- ☐ (D) *Mycoplasma pneumoniae*
- ☐ (E) *Streptococcus pneumoniae*

230 A sexually active 20-year-old woman sees her primary care physician with complaints of a vaginal discharge that has a "fishy" odor. The discharge is collected; when potassium hydroxide (KOH) is added to the sample, the distinct odor is confirmed ("whiff test"). The pH of the discharge is elevated, and a Gram stain reveals bacterial organisms (see figure). Which organism is most likely the one observed in the Gram stain and is also associated with bacterial vaginosis (also called vaginitis)?

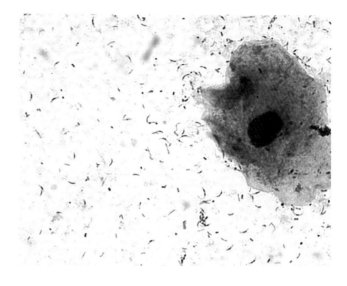

- ☐ (A) *Actinomyces*
- ☐ (B) *Bacteroides*
- ☐ (C) *Lactobacillus*
- ☐ (D) *Mobiluncus*
- ☐ (E) *Prevotella*

231 A 55-year-old woman who has suffered extensive burns in a house fire is hospitalized in a university hospital burn unit. Approximately 1 week after hospitalization, she develops fevers to 39.5°C, erythema and tenderness at the site of her femoral catheter, and pain in her leg. The catheter is removed and sent with blood for culture. The laboratory reports 2 days later that a gram-negative pleomorphic rod is growing in the blood culture (see figure). Upon subculture of the blood culture bottle, the organism grows only anaerobically. The catheter is cultured on aerobic blood and chocolate agars, and these cultures remain negative. Which organism is most likely responsible for this infection?

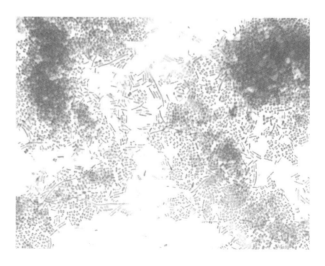

❏ (A) *Bacteroides fragilis*
❏ (B) *Campylobacter fetus*
❏ (C) *Enterobacter cloacae*
❏ (D) *Fusobacterium nucleatum*
❏ (E) *Pseudomonas aeruginosa*

232 Which organism commonly colonizes the surface of the eyes?

❏ (A) *Escherichia coli*
❏ (B) *Pseudomonas aeruginosa*
❏ (C) *Staphylococcus aureus*
❏ (D) *Staphylococcus epidermidis*
❏ (E) *Streptococcus pneumoniae*

233 A 68-year-old woman is brought to the hospital because she is complaining of feeling ill and has a low-grade temperature. When the woman arrives in the emergency department, she is disoriented and agitated. Her temperature is 39.5°C, blood pressure is 140/90 mm Hg, and heart rate is 36 bpm. Her chest radiograph is clear, but a new heart murmur is heard. Blood cultures are collected and, after 48 h of incubation, are reported to be positive with a thin, curved, gram-negative rod. Preliminary testing indicates the organism grows slowly at 37°C but not at 42°C. Which organism is most likely responsible for this woman's infection?

❏ (A) *Campylobacter coli*
❏ (B) *Campylobacter fetus*
❏ (C) *Campylobacter jejuni*
❏ (D) *Campylobacter lari*
❏ (E) *Campylobacter upsaliensis*

234 A 28-year-old man with AIDS develops a 1-cm tender erythematous skin nodule on his right leg. An aspirate of the nodule is collected by his physician and sent for stains and culture. Abundant PMNs but no organisms are seen on Gram stain; however, abundant short acid-fast rods are observed on the acid-fast stain. After 4 weeks of incubation, the routine bacterial cultures and acid-fast cultures are negative. During this period, additional nodules appear on the skin surface of both legs. Acid-fast organisms are present in these nodules as well. Which organism is most likely responsible for this infection?

❏ (A) *Mycobacterium avium*
❏ (B) *Mycobacterium chelonae*
❏ (C) *Mycobacterium haemophilum*
❏ (D) *Nocardia asteroides*
❏ (E) *Rhodococcus equi*

235 A young girl is bitten on her hand by her pet cat. The wound is cleaned with soapy water, and a topical disinfectant is applied for 1 day. Approximately 3 days later, erythema is noticed at the bite wound; within 1 more day, the area becomes indurated and painful. Axillary lymphadenopathy is also noticed. The girl is taken to the local hospital. The wound is opened, and 3 cc of purulent material is drained. The exudate is

sent to the microbiology laboratory for Gram stain and culture. Small, gram-negative coccobacilli are seen on Gram stain (see figure), and the organism grows the next day on blood agar and chocolate agar, but organisms do not grow on MacConkey agar. The organism has a musty odor, is catalase-positive, and ferments glucose. Antimicrobial susceptibility tests demonstrate the organism is susceptible to penicillin, tetracycline, and ciprofloxacin. Which organism is most likely responsible for this girl's infection?

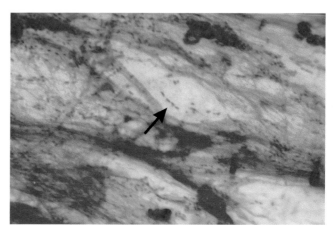

❏ (A) *Brucella melitensis*
❏ (B) *Escherichia coli*
❏ (C) *Francisella tularensis*
❏ (D) *Haemophilus influenzae*
❏ (E) *Pasteurella multocida*

236 Which factor is responsible for endotoxin activity?

❏ (A) Core polysaccharide
❏ (B) Lipid A
❏ (C) Lipoteichoic acid
❏ (D) O antigen
❏ (E) Peptidoglycan

237 A 33-year-old woman visits her physician because she has been feeling tired and has muscle aches, a low-grade fever, and a loss of appetite during the last month. Prior to this condition, she had been in good health since she was a teenager, although she did have rheumatic fever when she was young. Approximately 3 weeks before her current condition developed, she had a dental extraction. She tells the physician that her dentist did not give her any prophylactic antibiotics at the time of the procedure. The concern about subacute endocarditis is confirmed by the presence of a heart murmur. Three sets of blood cultures are collected and are reported to be positive after 3 days of incubation. Small gram-negative rods are observed on Gram stain of the blood culture broths, and these organisms grow when the blood is subcultured to chocolate, blood, and anaerobic blood agars but not to MacConkey agar. The organism on the aerobic and anaerobic blood agars is noted to pit the agar and has a bleach-like odor. Which organism is most likely responsible for this woman's infection?

- ❑ (A) *Actinobacillus*
- ❑ (B) *Cardiobacterium*
- ❑ (C) *Eikenella*
- ❑ (D) *Haemophilus*
- ❑ (E) *Kingella*

238 Antimicrobial susceptibility tests are performed for *Klebsiella pneumoniae* isolated from a blood culture. The organism is determined to be an extended spectrum beta-lactamase (ESBL) producing strain. Which susceptibility pattern would most likely be observed for this organism?

- ❑ (A) Resistant to aztreonam, ceftazidime, and piperacillin; susceptible to cephalothin, ceftazidime, cefoxitin, imipenem, and piperacillin-tazobactam
- ❑ (B) Resistant to aztreonam, cephalothin, ceftazidime, and piperacillin; susceptible to cefoxitin, imipenem, and piperacillin-tazobactam
- ❑ (C) Resistant to aztreonam, cephalothin, ceftazidime, cefoxitin, and piperacillin; susceptible to imipenem and piperacillin-tazobactam
- ❑ (D) Resistant to aztreonam, cephalothin, ceftazidime, cefoxitin, and piperacillin, and piperacillin-tazobactam; susceptible to imipenem
- ❑ (E) Resistant to all antibiotics

239 Isolation of *Campylobacter* was originally accomplished by which method?

- ❑ (A) Culture on BCYE medium
- ❑ (B) Culture in McCoy cells
- ❑ (C) Culture in Thioglycolate broth
- ❑ (D) Filtration through a 0.45-μm filter
- ❑ (E) Use of differential centrifugation

240 Approximately 2 weeks after orthopedic surgery for repair of a compound fracture of the femur, a 27-year-old man develops purulent drainage and redness at the surgical site. During the next week, the drainage increases, the surgical incision becomes warm and tender to the touch, and he develops a low-grade fever. When this patient sees his physician, the clinical diagnosis of a surgical wound infection is made, and cultures are obtained. The laboratory calls the physician 24 h later and reports the growth of gram-positive cocci in pairs and short chains. The preliminary test for catalase production is negative. Which causal organism is the most likely cause of this man's condition?

- ❑ (A) *Enterococcus faecalis*
- ❑ (B) *Staphylococcus aureus*
- ❑ (C) *Staphylococcus epidermidis*
- ❑ (D) *Streptococcus pneumoniae*
- ❑ (E) *Streptococcus pyogenes*

241 A 37-year-old man living in New Mexico is well until he suddenly develops a fever, chills, and a headache. Within a few hours of the onset of these symptoms, he has exquisite tenderness in his groin and notices swelling in the area. This becomes so painful that it hurts to move his legs. The skin overlying the swelling is erythematous and edematous. He is taken to the hospital, and he is extremely agitated upon arrival. His temperature is 40°C, heart rate is 115 bpm, and his blood pressure is 100/60 mm Hg. Approximately 5 days before the patient became ill, he had removed a number of dead rodents from a shed on his farm. At the time, he remembers being bitten by fleas from the rodents. Blood cultures and an aspirate from the swelling in the groin are collected for culture. Gram-negative coccobacilli are observed on Gram stain of the aspirate, and the same organism grows from both the blood and aspirate cultures. Which antibiotic would be most effective for treating this infection?

- ❑ (A) Ampicillin
- ❑ (B) Ceftriaxone
- ❑ (C) Erythromycin
- ❑ (D) Streptomycin
- ❑ (E) Vancomycin

242 Which virulence factor is considered important for *Enterococcus faecium?*

- ❑ (A) Antibiotic resistance
- ❑ (B) Capsule formation
- ❑ (C) Endotoxin production
- ❑ (D) Enterotoxin production
- ❑ (E) Pyrogenic factor

243 Which statement is correct?

- ❑ (A) *Staphylococcus aureus* food poisoning is mediated by a heat-labile enterotoxin.
- ❑ (B) Staphylococcal exfoliative toxins are responsible for gas gangrene.
- ❑ (C) Staphylococcal scalded skin syndrome is a toxin-mediated infection seen primarily in immunocompromised patients.
- ❑ (D) Infections with coagulase-negative staphylococci are characterized by an acute onset and a rapidly fatal course.
- ❑ (E) Staphylococci that are resistant to oxacillin are resistant to all penicillins, cephalosporins, and carbapenems.

244 The wife of a 65-year-old man with COPD brings him to the hospital because he is complaining of difficulties in breathing and an increase in his coughing. Sputum and blood cultures are collected for culture. The blood cultures are negative, but tiny gram-negative rods are seen on Gram stain (see figure) and from the culture. The organism grows on chocolate agar but not on blood agar or MacConkey agar. The organism also grows on trypticase soy agar supplemented with hematin and nicotinamide adenine dinucleotide (NAD) but not if either factor is missing. Which organism is responsible for this man's pulmonary infection?

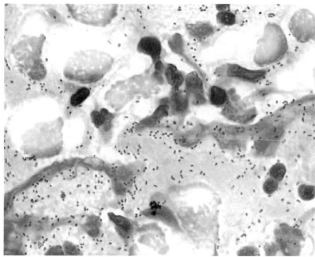

- [ ] (A) *Haemophilus aphrophilus*
- [ ] (B) *Haemophilus ducreyi*
- [ ] (C) *Haemophilus influenzae*
- [ ] (D) *Haemophilus parainfluenzae*
- [ ] (E) *Moraxella catarrhalis*

245 Which specimen is appropriate for anaerobic culture?

- [ ] (A) Catheterized urine
- [ ] (B) Expectorated sputum
- [ ] (C) Lung aspirate
- [ ] (D) Rectal swab
- [ ] (E) Urethral swab

246 Which virulence factor is responsible for the persistent cough caused by *Mycoplasma pneumoniae* infections?

- [ ] (A) Endotoxin
- [ ] (B) Exotoxin A
- [ ] (C) P1 adhesin protein
- [ ] (D) Phospholipase C
- [ ] (E) Tracheal cytotoxin

247 Which antibiotic inhibits protein synthesis by binding to the 30S ribosome?

- [ ] (A) Ciprofloxacin
- [ ] (B) Erythromycin
- [ ] (C) Imipenem
- [ ] (D) Rifampin
- [ ] (E) Tetracycline

248 Which organism is commonly found on the skin's surface?

- [ ] (A) *Actinomyces*
- [ ] (B) *Bacteroides*
- [ ] (C) *Bifidobacterium*
- [ ] (D) *Fusobacterium*
- [ ] (E) *Peptostreptococcus*

249 Which diagnostic test would be most useful for the identifying the associated staphylococcal disease?

- [ ] (A) Endocarditis: blood culture
- [ ] (B) Food poisoning: stool culture
- [ ] (C) Impetigo: blood culture
- [ ] (D) Scalded skin syndrome: blood culture
- [ ] (E) Toxic shock syndrome: blood culture

250 A hard tick, *Ixodes scapularis*, transmits which infectious agent?

- [ ] (A) *Borrelia burgdorferi*
- [ ] (B) *Leptospira interrogans*
- [ ] (C) *Yersinia pestis*
- [ ] (D) *Rickettsia prowazekii*
- [ ] (E) *Plasmodium falciparum*

251 A 64-year-old man with a recent history of fatigue, weakness, shortness of breath, and easy bruising is admitted to the local hospital. Acute myelogenous leukemia is diagnosed, and chemotherapy is initiated. The patient develops a fever of 40°C 2 weeks later, and three sets of blood cultures are collected. Two of the three cultures are reported to be positive with gram-positive rods. Subcultures of the blood culture broths grow only on anaerobic blood agar plates. The organism is catalase-negative and resistant to vancomycin. Which organism is most likely responsible for this patient's infection?

- [ ] (A) *Actinomyces*
- [ ] (B) *Bifidobacterium*
- [ ] (C) *Eubacterium*
- [ ] (D) *Lactobacillus*
- [ ] (E) *Propionibacterium*

252 A laboratory rat bites a technician on his left thumb. He cleans his thumb with a disinfectant and continues his research work. The technician develops a high-grade fever accompanied with a headache and severe arthralgias and myalgias 3 days later. He thinks he has the flu and remains in bed for the next day; however, the headache becomes more severe, and he decides to go to his physician. By the time he arrives in his physician's office, he has developed a rash over his arms and legs, including the palms of his hands and soles of his feet. Blood and joint fluid are collected for culture. The joint fluid culture is negative after 5 days, but the blood culture is positive with pleomorphic gram-negative rods (see figure). Which organism is most likely responsible for this man's infection?

- ☐ (A) *Capnocytophaga*
- ☐ (B) *Eikenella*
- ☐ (C) *Leptospira*
- ☐ (D) *Spirillum*
- ☐ (E) *Streptobacillus*

253 A 56-year-old man has been hospitalized for 3 weeks for treatment of leukemia when he develops a persistent low-grade fever. It is noted that the skin overlying an intravenous catheter is warm and red. Two blood cultures are collected, and the catheter is removed and cultured. After 2 days of incubation, cultures of the blood and catheter are positive for coagulase-negative staphylococci. Which virulence factor is important for coagulase-negative staphylococci?

- ☐ (A) Cytotoxin
- ☐ (B) Enterotoxin
- ☐ (C) Protein A
- ☐ (D) Slime layer
- ☐ (E) TSST-1

254 Which antibiotic would be expected to be active against both *Neisseria gonorrhoeae* and *Chlamydia trachomatis?*

- ☐ (A) Azithromycin
- ☐ (B) Ceftriaxone
- ☐ (C) Ciprofloxacin
- ☐ (D) Erythromycin
- ☐ (E) Penicillin

255 Which property is considered a major virulence factor in *Bacteroides fragilis?*

- ☐ (A) Cytotoxin
- ☐ (B) Enterotoxin
- ☐ (C) Endotoxin
- ☐ (D) Metronidazole resistance
- ☐ (E) Polysaccharide capsule

256 A 34-year-old man develops an inflammatory skin lesion on his hand. He suffered an injury to the hand 4 days previously. The edge of the lesion is raised and erythematous, with discol-oration in the central area. When he sees his physician, he describes the lesion as painful with a burning sensation and intensely pruritic. There is no evidence of suppuration. His physician biopsies the wound and submits the specimen for Gram stain, as well as for aerobic and anaerobic bacterial cultures. Slender, gram-variable rods are observed in the Gram stain, and the cultures are positive after 2 days of incubation. Which organism is most likely responsible for this patient's infection?

- ☐ (A) *Bacteroides fragilis*
- ☐ (B) *Enterococcus faecalis*
- ☐ (C) *Erysipelothrix rhusiopathiae*
- ☐ (D) *Pseudomonas aeruginosa*
- ☐ (E) *Streptococcus pyogenes*

257 The exotoxin produced by *Corynebacterium diphtheriae* works by which mechanism?

- ☐ (A) Blocks release of acetylcholine
- ☐ (B) Blocks release of gamma-aminobutyric acid
- ☐ (C) Inactivates EF-2 and prevents protein synthesis
- ☐ (D) Stimulates increased adenylate cyclase activity
- ☐ (E) Stimulates release of proinflammatory cytokines

258 Which factor is important for *Streptococcus pneumoniae* virulence?

- ☐ (A) Endotoxin
- ☐ (B) Exotoxin A
- ☐ (C) M protein adhesin
- ☐ (D) Polysaccharide capsule
- ☐ (E) Pyrogenic exotoxin

259 Which factor is associated with pyelonephritis and renal calculi ("kidney stone") formation?

- ☐ (A) Endotoxin production
- ☐ (B) Presence of specific pili that bind to host cell surfaces
- ☐ (C) Resistance to antibiotic killing
- ☐ (D) Resistance to serum killing
- ☐ (E) Urease production

260 Three patients present to an inner city hospital with infections subsequently demonstrated to be caused by the same organism. The first patient, a 23-year-old prostitute, presents with a temperature of 38.5°C, hypotension, icterus, pulmonary rales, and muscle tenderness. The second patient, a 38-year-old male, has a temperature of 38.5°C, icterus, mild upper quadrant tenderness, and muscle tenderness. The third patient, a 28-year-old male, has flu-like symptoms, a low-grade fever, and muscle tenderness. The first and third patients cut their feet on glass in a city alley, whereas the second patient cut his hand on glass in an alley. The patients have not been in contact with each other and no one has a significant travel history. All three patients have elevated serum bilirubin levels. Two of the patients develop acute renal failure in the second week of hospitalization; one patient develops meningitis. A fourth patient is subsequently reported to the public health department with the same illness. This patient's illness develops after swimming in a city reservoir. Which organism is most likely responsible for these illnesses?

- ❑ (A) *Aeromonas hydrophila*
- ❑ (B) *Leptospira interrogans*
- ❑ (C) *Mycobacterium marinum*
- ❑ (D) *Streptococcus pyogenes*
- ❑ (E) *Vibrio vulnificus*

261 Approximately 4 h after eating at a family picnic, three people develop nausea and abdominal cramps, followed by severe diarrhea and vomiting shortly after the onset of the initial symptoms. None of them has a fever. Within 24 h, the ill family members have recovered from their illness. Which toxin is most likely responsible for this illness?

- ❑ (A) Alpha-toxin
- ❑ (B) Enterotoxin A
- ❑ (C) Exfoliative toxins
- ❑ (D) Leukocidin
- ❑ (E) TSST-1

262 Which structure is characteristic of a prokaryotic cell?

- ❑ (A) Golgi apparatus
- ❑ (B) Linear strands of DNA
- ❑ (C) Mitochondria
- ❑ (D) Peptidoglycan
- ❑ (E) 80S ribosome

263 *Coxiella burnetii* infect a variety of animals, including birds, farm animals (e.g., sheep, cattle, goats), domestic pets (e.g., dogs, cats), rabbits, and humans. Which route of infection is the most common for humans?

- ❑ (A) Ingestion
- ❑ (B) Inhalation
- ❑ (C) Mosquito bite
- ❑ (D) Tick bite
- ❑ (E) Penetration through unbroken skin

264 A sexually active man living in Brazil notices a small painless papule along the shaft of his penis. During the next few weeks, the papule enlarges and then ulcerates. The ulcer appears erythematous with raised edges (see figure). Additional papules appear on the penis during the next week and coalesce with the primary lesion, forming a large granulomatous ulcer. Despite the appearance, the ulcer remains painless with no purulence, although it bleeds easily upon contact. Which diagnostic test should be ordered to confirm the diagnosis of this infection?

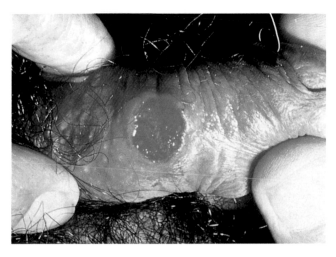

From Morse SA et al: *Atlas of sexually transmitted diseases and AIDS*, ed 3, 2003, Mosby.

- ❑ (A) Culture of the ulcer exudate on Thayer-Martin medium
- ❑ (B) Culture of the ulcer exudate on McCoy cells
- ❑ (C) Culture of the ulcer exudate on MacConkey agar
- ❑ (D) Darkfield examination of the ulcer
- ❑ (E) Giemsa stain of the ulcer exudate

265 Which test should be ordered to confirm the clinical diagnosis of leptospirosis?

- ❑ (A) Gram stain
- ❑ (B) Darkfield examination
- ❑ (C) Culture of blood
- ❑ (D) Culture of urine
- ❑ (E) Serology

266 Lysozyme is able to degrade which bacterial component and kill the organism?

- ❑ (A) Capsule
- ❑ (B) Cytoplasmic membrane
- ❑ (C) DNA
- ❑ (D) Outer membrane
- ❑ (E) Peptidoglycan

267 A sexually active 16-year-old girl notices a vaginal discharge and pain when urinating. Despite her use of a vaginal douche, the discharge increases. Approximately 3 days after the start of the discharge, she notices increased lower abdominal pain that radiates to both sides of the abdomen. A physical exam at the health clinic demonstrates enlargement of the liver with hepatic tenderness and right upper quadrant pain. The clinical diagnosis of gonorrhea is made and confirmed by culture of the vaginal discharge. This patient most likely has which condition?

- ❑ (A) Endotoxemia
- ❑ (B) Fitz-Hugh-Curtis syndrome
- ❑ (C) Hepatic abscess
- ❑ (D) Reiter's syndrome
- ❑ (E) Toxic shock syndrome

268 A 34-year-old woman develops blurred vision, a dry mouth, constipation, and abdominal pain 5 days after consuming canned tomatoes. The woman's physician suspects she has botulism. The toxin produced by *Clostridium botulinum* acts by which one mechanism?

- ☐ (A) Catalyzes hydrolysis of membrane phospholipids
- ☐ (B) Integrates into cell membranes, leading to pore formation with cell lysis
- ☐ (C) Stimulates macrophages to release proinflammatory cytokines
- ☐ (D) Blocks release of the neurotransmitter acetylcholine
- ☐ (E) Blocks release of neurotransmitters for inhibitory synapses

269 An elderly homeless man notices a firm, swollen mass along his jaw line. The jaw is not painful, so he initially ignores the mass. Over the next 4 weeks, the swelling increases and then a pimple appears. The pimple enlarges in size and then breaks down. A small amount of drainage collects at the lesion (see figure). Additional ulcers subsequently form adjacent to the original ulcer. Because of the progression of these lesions, the man goes to the local health clinic where the drainage is collected for Gram stain and culture. Which test would be useful to establish the diagnosis of this man's infection?

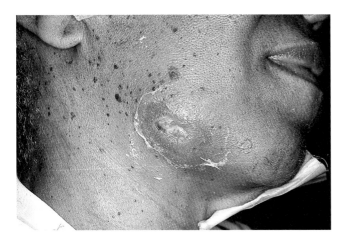

- ☐ (A) Culture on aerobic blood agar
- ☐ (B) Culture on anaerobic blood agar
- ☐ (C) Culture on BCYE agar
- ☐ (D) Cryptococcal latex agglutination test
- ☐ (E) Histoplasma antigen test

270 Which pathogen is susceptible to metronidazole?

- ☐ (A) *Actinomyces*
- ☐ (B) *Bacteroides*
- ☐ (C) *Clostridium*
- ☐ (D) *Mobiluncus*
- ☐ (E) *Peptostreptococcus*

271 A 60-year-old woman living in Connecticut presents to her physician with a 5-day history of high fevers (up to 40°C),

headaches, myalgia, and malaise. She remembers that 12 days before the start of her illness, she removed two engorged ticks from her legs. Leukopenia and thrombocytopenia were documented at the time she is admitted into the hospital. During the course of her illness, no evidence of a rash develops. The fever, however, is persistent despite intravenous treatment with ceftazidime and vancomycin, and she becomes increasingly confused and somnolent. Bacterial cultures of blood, cerebrospinal fluid, and stool are negative. Giemsa stains of peripheral blood demonstrate intracellular organisms in granulocytic cells. Which organism is most likely responsible for this infection?

- ☐ (A) *Anaplasma phagocytophilum*
- ☐ (B) *Babesia microti*
- ☐ (C) *Coxiella burnetii*
- ☐ (D) *Plasmodium vivax*
- ☐ (E) *Rickettsia rickettsii*

272 Acute glomerulonephritis is a complication of infection with *Streptococcus pyogenes*. It is characterized by inflammation of the renal glomeruli with edema, hypertension, hematuria, and proteinuria. Which test would be most useful for the diagnosis of acute glomerulonephritis if the primary infection is pyoderma?

- ☐ (A) Blood culture
- ☐ (B) Measurement of ASO antibodies
- ☐ (C) Measurement of anti-DNase B antibodies
- ☐ (D) Measurement of streptokinase antibodies
- ☐ (E) Urine culture

273 Which bacterium has mycolic acids in its cell wall?

- ☐ (A) *Actinomyces*
- ☐ (B) *Rhodococcus*
- ☐ (C) *Rothia*
- ☐ (D) *Streptomyces*
- ☐ (E) *Tropheryma*

274 A skin test measuring cellular immunity is a useful screening test to determine exposure to *Mycobacterium tuberculosis*. Which mycobacterial antigen is used to elicit this response?

- ☐ (A) N-acetylglucosamine
- ☐ (B) Arabinogalactan
- ☐ (C) Cell wall proteins
- ☐ (D) M-diaminopimelic acid
- ☐ (E) Mycolic acid

275 An acutely ill 69-year-old man presents to the hospital complaining of pain in the left arm. The patient states that he noticed on the previous day a small area of redness on the left elbow that was associated with tenderness. This area became progressively more painful. He denies an insect bite or trauma to the area. The physician notices crepitance and skin mottling extending over the upper left arm and involving the adjacent chest wall. Fluid is aspirated from the swollen elbow and arm, and spore-forming gram-positive rods are observed (see figure) in the absence of neutrophils. The patient is rushed to surgery, where his arm is amputated and extensive débridement of the chest wall is necessary. Despite the surgical intervention and administration of antibiotics, the patient expires the next day. Postmortem examination reveals the patient had colon cancer. Which organism is most likely responsible for this infection?

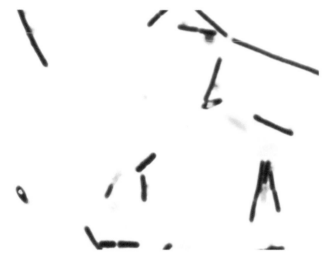

- ❏ (A) *Bacillus anthracis*
- ❏ (B) *Bacillus cereus*
- ❏ (C) *Clostridium perfringens*
- ❏ (D) *Clostridium septicum*
- ❏ (E) *Erysipelothrix rhusiopathiae*

276 An 85-year-old man with non-Hodgkin's lymphoma is admitted to the hospital with a 1-week history of low-grade fevers, productive cough, malaise, and weakness. Upon examination, he has a temperature of 39.5°C, WBC of 12,600 per mm³ with 85% PMNs, and an elevated sedimentation rate. A chest radiograph reveals infiltrates in the left upper lung field. Neurological examination shows lower extremity weakness, more pronounced on the right, with diminished reflexes in both lower limbs. A CT scan of his brain shows multiple lesions. Expectorated sputum is sent to the clinical microbiology laboratory. Filamentous, branching organisms that stain weakly with the Gram stain are observed the specimen is examined. The organisms also stain with the modified acid-fast stain. After 4 days, abundant, intensely white colonies are observed on blood agar, Sabouraud agar, and Middlebrook medium. After additional incubation, the colonies develop an orange color and aerial hyphae. Which organism is most likely responsible for this man's infection?

- ❏ (A) *Actinomyces*
- ❏ (B) *Mycobacterium*
- ❏ (C) *Nocardia*
- ❏ (D) *Rhodococcus*
- ❏ (E) *Streptomyces*

277 Most clinically important species of *Brucella* share two surface antigens, A and M antigens, that stimulate an immune response in infected patients. Which *Brucella* species does not have these antigens and is not detected by the serologic assays that are used to detect the other species?

- ❏ (A) *Brucella abortus*
- ❏ (B) *Brucella canis*
- ❏ (C) *Brucella melitensis*
- ❏ (D) *Brucella suis*
- ❏ (E) All *Brucella* species are detected

278 Sexually active individuals may have multiple infections with *Neisseria gonorrhoeae*. Which surface protein contributes to the antigenic variation that is responsible for reinfection with this organism?

- ❏ (A) Opa protein (protein II)
- ❏ (B) Pilin protein
- ❏ (C) Por protein (protein I)
- ❏ (D) Rmp protein (protein III)
- ❏ (E) Transferrin-binding protein

279 A 32-year-old man with HIV presents to his physician with a 3-week history of low-grade fevers, chest pain, and a progressively worsening productive cough. His CD4 lymphocyte cell count is 50/mm³. Chest radiograph shows bilateral infiltrates in his lung fields. Sputum is collected for bacterial, fungal, and mycobacterial stains and cultures. The Gram stain and fungal stains are negative, but large, acid-fast rods are seen in the specimen. After 3 weeks of incubation, acid-fast rods are recovered in the Lowenstein-Jensen medium and Middlebrook broth. After exposure to light, the colonies on the Lowenstein-Jensen medium develop a yellow pigment (see figure). Which organism is most likely responsible for this man's infection?

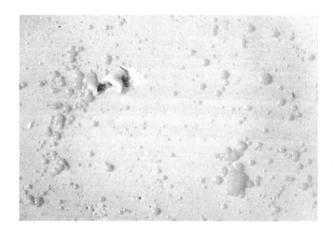

From Baron EJ, Peterson LR, Finegold SM: *Bailey and Scott's diagnostic microbiology*, ed 9, St Louis, 1994, Mosby.

- ❏ (A) *Mycobacterium avium*
- ❏ (B) *Mycobacterium fortuitum*
- ❏ (C) *Mycobacterium haemophilum*
- ❏ (D) *Mycobacterium kansasii*
- ❏ (E) *Mycobacterium tuberculosis*

280 Approximately 4 days after intraabdominal surgery, the patient develops spiking fevers and increased abdominal tenderness. The patient returns to surgery, and the physician drains 50 cc of foul-smelling, purulent material. The pus is submitted for culture; after 2 days, growth is present on the anaerobic media. Gram stain of the colonies shows pleomorphic gramnegative rods. Preliminary identification test results show resistance to kanamycin, vancomycin, and colistin, as well growth stimulated by 20% bile. Which virulence factor produced by this organism is responsible for abscess formation?

- ☐ (A) Capsule
- ☐ (B) Endotoxin
- ☐ (C) Fimbria
- ☐ (D) Phospholipase C
- ☐ (E) Superoxide dismutase

281 The exotoxin produced by *Clostridium tetani* works by which mechanism?

- ☐ (A) Blocks release of acetylcholine
- ☐ (B) Blocks release of GABA
- ☐ (C) Inactivates EF-2 and prevents protein synthesis
- ☐ (D) Stimulates increased adenylate cyclase activity
- ☐ (E) Stimulates release of proinflammatory cytokines

282 A mother notices that her 18-month-old boy is unusually irritable and is pulling at his left ear. Approximately 5 days earlier, he had an upper respiratory tract infection with nasal congestion and a dry, nonproductive cough. The respiratory symptoms have resolved, but the ear pain persists. When the boy's pediatrician examines the child's ear, the membrane is swollen and red. The diagnosis of otitis media is made. Which organism is most likely responsible for this infection?

- ☐ (A) *Pseudomonas aeruginosa*
- ☐ (B) *Staphylococcus aureus*
- ☐ (C) *Streptococcus pneumoniae*
- ☐ (D) *Streptococcus pyogenes*
- ☐ (E) *Streptococcus salivarius*

283 Bacteria become resistant to imipenem by which mechanism?

- ☐ (A) Acetylation of the antibiotic
- ☐ (B) Active efflux of the antibiotic out of the cell
- ☐ (C) Modification of pentapeptide side chain in the cell wall peptidoglycan
- ☐ (D) Modification of a ribosomal binding site
- ☐ (E) Production of metallo beta-lactamase

284 A sexually active 23-year-old man presents to his physician with the complaint that he has a small ulcer that has formed on the shaft of his penis (see figure). A small papule was initially present that enlarged and then broke down, forming an ulcer with raised margins. The ulcer is painless. Painless swellings of the regional lymph nodes are noted on physical examination. The physician considers syphilis as the most likely cause of the infection. Which test would be the most sensitive one to confirm the diagnosis of syphilis at this stage of the infection?

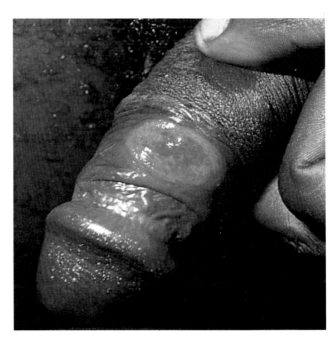

From Morse S et al: *Atlas of sexually transmitted diseases and AIDS*, ed 3, St Louis, 2003, Mosby.

- ☐ (A) Culture
- ☐ (B) Darkfield examination
- ☐ (C) Gram stain
- ☐ (D) FTA-ABS test
- ☐ (E) VDRL test

285 A 33-year-old woman suffers a cut on the back of her hand while cleaning her fish tank. Approximately 3 weeks after the injury, she notices the area that she injured is red, swollen, and painful to her touch. During the next month, a subcutaneous nodule develops that enlarges and eventually ruptures with serous drainage. Additional nodules also develop along the lymphatics. When she goes to her physician, the initial nodule has evolved into a verrucous, crusted plaque. She has no systemic symptoms. Biopsies of the lesion and one nodule are performed and sent for histopathology and culture. Which diagnostic test would most likely reveal the organism responsible for her symptoms?

- ☐ (A) Culture in Middlebrook broth at 30°C
- ☐ (B) Culture on Lowenstein-Jensen medium at 37°C
- ☐ (C) Culture on BCYE agar at 37°C
- ☐ (D) Culture on Sabouraud agar at room temperature
- ☐ (E) Gram stain

286 Which medium is optimum for the recovery of *Corynebacterium diphtheriae*?

- ❑ (A) Bordet-Gengou agar
- ❑ (B) Cysteine-tellurite agar
- ❑ (C) MacConkey agar
- ❑ (D) Sheep blood agar
- ❑ (E) Thayer-Martin agar

287 Which statement about *Peptostreptococcus* is correct?

- ❑ (A) Most infections are monomicrobic.
- ❑ (B) *Peptostreptococcus* is an important cause of gas gangrene.
- ❑ (C) *Peptostreptococcus* is responsible for abscesses connected with sinus tracks.
- ❑ (D) *Peptostreptococcus* is responsible for urinary tract infections (UTIs).
- ❑ (E) Penicillin is the drug of choice for treating infections caused by *Peptostreptococcus*.

288 Which statement about *Staphylococcus aureus* is accurate?

- ❑ (A) Gram-positive cocci are arranged in pairs and short chains.
- ❑ (B) The organism is characterized by a positive catalase reaction and negative coagulase reaction.
- ❑ (C) The organism is capable of producing heat-stable enterotoxins.
- ❑ (D) Cytotoxins mediate tissue damage in rheumatic heart disease.
- ❑ (E) PV leukocidin is responsible for scalded skin syndrome.

289 Which genus was originally classified as a "nutritionally deficient *Streptococcus*"?

- ❑ (A) *Abiotrophia*
- ❑ (B) *Aerococcus*
- ❑ (C) *Lactococcus*
- ❑ (D) *Leuconostoc*
- ❑ (E) *Pediococcus*

290 A 20-year-old male student is brought by his girlfriend to the emergency department of a local hospital. Upon physical examination, the patient is found obtunded, has a temperature of 39°C, a blood pressure of 104/52 mm Hg, and a heart rate of 148 bpm. He has a stiff neck and generalized petechial rash with two areas of purpura. CSF is collected. The opening pressure is 180 mm H_2O, WBCs are 4300/mm^3 with 91% neutrophils, glucose is 10 mg/dl, and protein is 755 mg/dl. A Gram stain and culture of CSF is performed, with the Gram stain positive for the organism shown in the figure. Which organism is most likely responsible for this patient's infection?

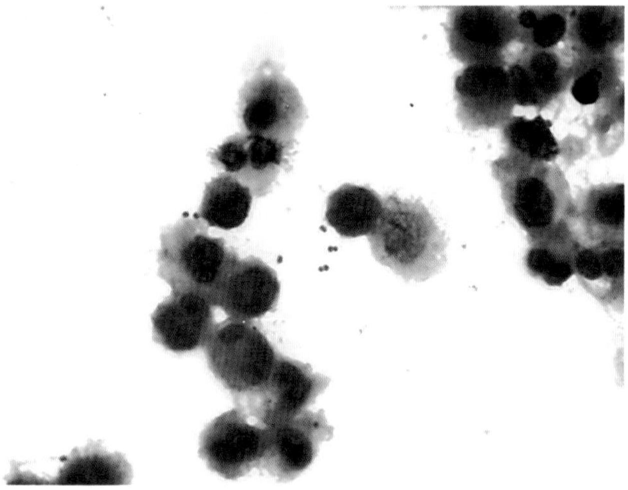

- ❑ (A) *Cryptococcus neoformans*
- ❑ (B) *Haemophilus influenzae*
- ❑ (C) *Listeria monocytogenes*
- ❑ (D) *Neisseria meningitidis*
- ❑ (E) *Streptococcus pneumoniae*

291 Bacteria become resistant to ciprofloxacin by which mechanism?

- ❑ (A) Acetylation of the antibiotic
- ❑ (B) Active efflux of the antibiotic out of the cell
- ❑ (C) Modification of a DNA gyrase
- ❑ (D) Modification of a pentapeptide side chain in cell wall peptidoglycan
- ❑ (E) Modification of a ribosomal binding site

1 (E) *Pasteurella.* *Pasteurella multocida* is commonly associated with animal bite wounds, particularly cat bites. Cats can inflict a deep puncture wound that is difficult to clean adequately. *P. multocida* is a facultative anaerobe that grows on blood and chocolate agars but generally grows poorly or not at all on MacConkey agar. *Capnocytophaga* organisms, particularly *C. canimorsus* and *C. cynodegmi*, are associated with animal bites; however, these bacteria are long, thin gram-negative rods that grow best in a microaerophilic atmosphere. *Eikenella* is gram-negative coccobacillus associated with human bite wounds but not animal bites. The Gram stain morphology and poor growth on MacConkey agar are inconsistent with *Escherichia*. *Fusobacterium* is a strict anaerobe.
MM5 374-375

2 (B) Culture of the baby's stool. Infant botulism is the most common form of botulism reported in the United States. Most infants acquire the infection by ingesting foods contaminated with spores of the clostridium. The most common contaminated food product is honey. Although spores and toxin may be recovered in honey or other contaminated foods, detecting these in the foods is an insensitive way to confirm the clinical diagnosis. The most sensitive method for confirming the clinical diagnosis is culturing stool specimens for the bacterium. Blood cultures should not be processed. Serum and stool specimens should also be collected and assayed for toxin, with stool specimens being considered as more reliable than serum specimens. Antibodies against the toxin would not be detected.
MM5 410-411

3 (B) *Campylobacter fetus.* Although patients with *C. fetus* infections may initially experience gastroenteritis, the most common presentation is septicemia with dissemination of the bacteria to multiple organs. *C. fetus* has an affinity for the vascular endothelium and is associated with septic thrombophlebitis, endocarditis, and pericarditis. *C. coli*, *C. jejuni*, and *C. upsaliensis* primarily cause gastroenteritis, with dissemination to the blood very uncommon. *H. pylori* is a cause of gastritis, gastric ulcers, gastric adenocarcinoma, and gastric mucosa–associated lymphoid-type lymphomas. This organism is also rarely recovered in blood.
MM5 350

4 (C) Phagocytized bacteria inhibit phagosome/lysosome fusion. Infection with *M. tuberculosis* is initiated by introduction of the bacterium into the lower respiratory tract followed by phagocytosis by inactivated alveolar macrophages. The phagocytized bacteria inhibit phagosome/lysosome fusion and initiate replication in the macrophage. The macrophage is eventually destroyed, and new cycles of phagocytosis, replication, and cell death are initiated. Infected macrophages can spread to the regional lymph nodes and to distal tissues (e.g., bone marrow, spleen, kidneys, central nervous system). Circulating macrophages and lymphocytes are attracted to the infected cells and

cellular debris, leading to the formation of granulomas (a characteristic of these infections).
MM5 298-300

5 (C) Assay of stool filtrates for toxin. Detection of *C. difficile* toxins is most reliable by using one of a number of commercial immunoassays for the toxins. The specimen that must be tested is a stool filtrate; toxin is not present in the blood. A Gram stain may provide an early clue that the disease is caused by *C. difficile*, but the stain is insensitive and nonspecific. Culture and NAA tests (e.g., polymerase chain reaction [PCR]) do not differentiate between colonization with *C. difficile* and disease caused by this organism.
MM5 411-413

6 (A) *Actinomyces.* Characteristic of infections caused by *Actinomyces* is the production of macroscopic colonies or granules. The granules can appear white or have pigment (hence the name *sulfur granules*). The granules are found in the exudates from wounds or sinus tracts that form during the course of the disease. None of the other genera listed in this question forms macroscopic colonies or sulfur granules.
MM5 417-419

7 (C) *Escherichia coli.* The patient's clinical symptoms are consistent with a urinary tract infection. The presence of fever and lower back pain would localize the infection to the kidneys (i.e., pyelonephritis). *E. coli* is the most common cause of urinary tract infections, although each of the other organisms in the answers to this question can produce the same symptoms. Most strains of *E. coli* produce beta-hemolytic colonies on blood agar and ferment lactose, producing pink-colored colonies on MacConkey agar (acid produced during fermentation causes a color shift in the neutral red indicator incorporated in the agar). MacConkey agar is a selective, differential agar for gram-negative bacteria. *P. mirabilis* is the only other gram-negative rod that is listed; however, it fails to ferment lactose and produces translucent or colorless colonies on MacConkey agar. *S. aureus* and *E. faecalis* are gram-positive bacteria that fail to grow on MacConkey agar. *S. aureus* is typically beta-hemolytic, whereas *E. faecalis* is only rarely beta-hemolytic. *C. albicans* is the most common fungus associated with urinary tract infections; however, disease caused by *C. albicans* is most commonly present in hospitalized patients, patients receiving antibacterial antibiotics, or patients with indwelling urinary catheters.
MM5 327, 337

8 (D) Inhibits initiation of RNA synthesis. Rifampin binds to DNA-dependent RNA polymerase and inhibits the initiation of RNA synthesis. Resistance to rifampin can develop rapidly if the drug is used alone. Rifampin resistance in gram-positive bacteria results from a mutation in the chromosomal gene that codes for the beta subunit of RNA polymerase. Gram-negative bacteria are resistant intrinsically to rifampin as the result of decreased uptake of the hydrophobic antibiotic.
MM5 211

9 **(A) Capsule-mediated inhibition of phagocytosis.** *Streptococcus pneumoniae* is covered with a complex polysaccharide capsule. This is the major virulence factor for these bacteria because the presence of the capsule prevents phagocytosis. Encapsulated strains are associated with disease in humans and experimental animals, whereas nonencapsulated strains are avirulent. Free capsular polysaccharides can be released from the bacteria and bind opsonic antibodies, further protecting the bacteria from phagocytosis.
MM5 198-201, 253-254

10 **(B) *Listeria monocytogenes*.** Although *L. monocytogenes* is most likely the bacterium that caused the meningitis, it is important to note first that all five of the bacteria listed in this question can also cause the disease. *E. coli* and group B *S. agalactiae* are primarily restricted to babies less than 1 month of age, whereas *L. monocytogenes*, *N. meningitidis*, and *S. pneumoniae* can cause meningitis in all age groups (*N. meningitidis* is most common in young adults, whereas the other two bacteria cause disease most commonly in the young and the very old). The baby's meningitis is most likely caused by *L. monocytogenes* because the organism is a slow-growing, weakly beta-hemolytic, gram-positive coccobacillus. In contrast with other organisms, *L. monocytogenes* grows slowly in CSF and typically is not observed in a Gram stain of CSF because relatively few organisms are present. When observed by Gram stain, *L. monocytogenes* may be mistaken for *S. pneumoniae*. Organisms isolated in culture are readily differentiated by colonial morphology (*S. pneumoniae* is alpha-hemolytic) and simple phenotypic tests. *E. coli* and *N. meningitidis* are gram-negative and should not be mistaken for *L. monocytogenes*. *S. agalactiae* is a gram-positive cocci but grows well on blood agar and appears as long chains rather than single cells or pairs.
MM5 274-276

11 **(E) Urethral discharge.** The urethral discharge is collected on a swab and transferred to appropriate media or transport systems. Blood should not be collected on a swab because relatively few organisms are typically present in the blood of a septic patient (i.e., an organism count of less than 1/ml of blood). A large volume of blood (i.e., 10 to 20 ml) should be cultured. Although a large amount of bacteria is typically present in the cerebrospinal fluid of a patient with meningitis, the organisms most commonly responsible for meningitis (e.g., *Streptococcus pneumoniae, Neisseria meningitidis*) are very labile and will die rapidly on a swab. Multiple media must be inoculated with fecal material, so the quantity collected on a swab is generally inadequate. Sputum must be carefully examined macroscopically to select a portion of specimen that is not contaminated with upper respiratory tract secretions. This cannot be done if the specimen is collected on a swab.
MM5 213-218

12 **(A) Ciprofloxacin.** Ciprofloxacin inhibits the DNA gyrases or topoisomerases that are required for DNA replication, recombination, and repair. Tetracycline and erythromycin inhibit protein synthesis by binding to the 30S and 50S ribosomal subunits; imipenem disrupts the synthesis of the peptidoglycan layer of the cell wall; and rifampin binds to DNA-dependent RNA polymerase to inhibit the initiation of RNA synthesis.
MM5 210-211

13 **(D) *Pseudomonas aeruginosa*.** The Gram stain morphology, colonial morphology, and preliminary biochemical test results are consistent with *P. aeruginosa*. *A. haemolyticus* and *S. maltophilia* are oxidase-negative. *M. catarrhalis* are gram-negative cocci arranged in pairs that resemble *Neisseria*. *B. cepacia* is typically susceptible to trimethoprim/sulfamethoxazole.
MM5 357, 362-363

14 **(C) *Mycoplasma pneumoniae*.** The boy presents with community-acquired pneumoniae. The presentation of this disease is protean; however, patients commonly develop symptoms after a 2- to 3-week incubation period. The patient typically presents with a low-grade fever, malaise, headache, and a dry, nonproductive cough. Pharyngitis may be present. Chest radiographs are typically more impressive than the clinical presentation. *C. (Chlamydia) pneumoniae* and *L. pneumophila* are also responsible for community-acquired "atypical pneumonia." *S. pneumoniae* is a common cause of community-acquired pneumonia, but the presentation will be more acute and patients will typically have a productive cough. *T. pallidum*, the etiologic agent of syphilis, would not present in this fashion. The negative Gram stain and culture would rule against *S. pneumoniae* but would be expected for *M. pneumoniae*, *C. pneumoniae*, and *L. pneumophila*. The important clue here is the positive cold agglutinin test. Positive tests are observed in 50% of the infections with *M. pneumoniae*, but this positive test is not seen with *C. pneumoniae* or *L. pneumophila*. The false-positive VDRL is also observed with *M. pneumoniae*. Despite the positive cold agglutinin test, this is an insensitive and relatively nonspecific indicator of *M. pneumoniae*. Culture in specialized media is available, but the test is slow (requiring incubation for 2 weeks or longer) and insensitive. Specific serology, such as through complement fixation and enzyme-linked immunoassays (ELISA), is available but is also slow (peak titers may require 4 weeks or longer). The most sensitive and specific test involves the use of molecular probes, either with or without nucleic acid amplification.
MM5 445-446

15 **(D) *Staphylococcus aureus*.** The boy has septic arthritis. In a child this age with no evidence of an open wound from the fall, the most common cause of septic arthritis is *S. aureus*. The Gram stain results are consistent with this diagnosis. *E. faecalis* and *S. pyogenes* (group A *Streptococcus*) are also gram-positive cocci; however, they are not as commonly associated with septic arthritis. In addition, the Gram stain morphology of *E. faecalis* is cocci arranged in pairs and short chains, and *S. pyogenes* appears as cocci arranged in long chains. *B. cereus* is a

gram-positive rod and would not be suspected unless the patient has an open lesion with evidence of soil contamination of the wound. *N. gonorrhoeae*, a gram-negative cocci arranged in pairs, is a common cause of septic arthritis in sexually active patients.
MM5 232-233

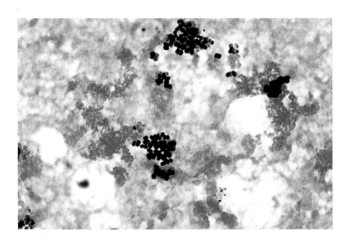

16 **(E) Penicillin.** Treatment of diphtheria requires the use of penicillin (or erythromycin) to eliminate the toxin-producing bacteria, as well as the early administration of diphtheria antitoxin, to neutralize the exotoxin before it is bound by the host cells.
MM5 279-283

17 **(D) Resistance to penicillin is mediated by beta-lactamases.** More than 80% to 90% of staphylococcal isolates produce beta-lactamases that are able to hydrolyze penicillin. Dicloxacillin, oxacillin, and ampicillin/sulbactam resistance is mediated by alterations in the penicillin-binding proteins and not by beta-lactamase production. Vancomycin resistance is related to changes in the outer cell wall of the bacteria or acquisition of resistance genes that modify the peptidoglycan structure.
MM5 204-208

18 **(D) Nucleic acid-based tests.** *Tropheryma whipplei* is the etiologic agent of Whipple disease, a disorder characterized by arthralgia, diarrhea, abdominal pain, weight loss, lymphadenopathy, fever, and increased skin pigmentation. Historically, the disease was diagnosed on the basis of the clinical presentation and the detection of periodic acid-Schiff stain (PAS) positive inclusion in foamy macrophages that infiltrated the lamina propria of the small intestine. Although these inclusions were plentiful in tissues, the organism has not been reliably grown in culture. The bacterial etiology of this infection was confirmed by molecular diagnostic tests, specifically amplification and sequencing of ribosomal DNA of this bacterium that was present in the infected macrophages. Although PAS staining can still be used for confirming the diagnosis, nucleic acid–based tests are used to document definitively that *Tropheryma* is involved in the disease process.
MM5 294

19 **(B) Lice.** Trench fever is a disease that has occurred during military conflicts. No animal reservoir has been identified; rather, the disease is spread person-to-person by the human body louse.
MM5 397-399

20 **(D) *Streptococcus pneumoniae.*** Patients that are asplenic are at increased risk of developing overwhelming infections with encapsulated organisms. The spleen is responsible for producing opsonizing antibodies, required for the removal of encapsulated organisms such as *S. pneumoniae* and *H. influenzae*. In the absence of a functional spleen, infection with these organisms can reach a magnitude that allows the organisms to be observed directly in blood specimens (an organism count of more than 10^5/ml of blood compared with an organism count of less than 1/ml of blood in septic patients with functional spleens). The vast majority of these infections are caused by *S. pneumoniae*. Observation of gram-positive cocci in the blood confirms the diagnosis. The other organisms listed in the answers for this question are not associated with an increased risk of infection in these patients and would not reach a magnitude that would permit direct observation in peripheral blood smears.
MM5 252-257

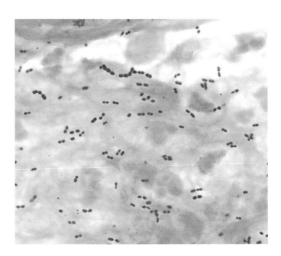

21 **(B) *Peptostreptococcus* and *Fusobacterium.*** This man has multiple brain abscesses, which are most commonly caused by invasion of normal oral bacteria into the brain by either direct extension or bacteremia. The immunocompromised status of the man made him more susceptible to this infection. All of the organisms listed in this question can be found in the oropharynx and can cause a brain abscess. *Staphylococcus*, *Streptococcus*, and *Haemophilus*, however, can be excluded from causing this man's infection because the organisms did not grow on the aerobic media. *Peptostreptococcus* is the most commonly isolated anaerobic gram-positive cocci. *Bacteroides*, *Fusobacterium*, and *Prevotella* can be differentiated by the size of these anaerobic gram-negative rods: *Fusobacterium* are typically long and thin, *Bacteroides* are pleomorphic, and *Prevotella* are short rods.
MM5 415-416, 424

22 **(B)** *Propionibacterium* **is found on the skin's surface.** With the exception of *Propionibacterium* and *Peptostreptococcus*, relatively few anaerobes are found on the surface of the skin. *B. fragilis* is a gram-negative bacillus. *Lactobacillus* colonizes the genitourinary tract but is rarely associated with infections at this site. Most anaerobic infections are polymicrobic and caused by the patient's endogenous organisms, with the exception of a *Clostridial* infection.
MM5 416, 419

23 **(A)** **Beef stew.** *Clostridium perfringens* food poisoning is a common but underappreciated bacterial disease and is characterized by a short incubation and duration with symptoms of abdominal cramps and watery diarrhea. The disease is mediated by a heat-labile enterotoxin, so disease can be avoided by heating the contaminated food immediately before serving. The food products most commonly associated with *C. perfringens* infections are meats and gravies.
MM5 405

24 **(B)** **Chicken.** The most common source of *Campylobacter* is contaminated chicken and other poultry products. *Campylobacter* infections have also been associated with contaminated milk and water.
MM5 350

25 **(A)** **Intraabdominal abscesses.** *B. fragilis*, the most virulent anaerobe in the colon, causes intraabdominal infections after intestinal perforations. Gas gangrene or myonecrosis can be caused by *B. fragilis*, but *Clostridium* species (particularly *C. perfringens* and *C. septicum*) are a more common cause. Anaerobes responsible for brain abscesses are typically present as a polymicrobic infection caused by aerobic and anaerobic bacteria that colonize the upper respiratory tract, such as streptococci, peptostreptococci, *Porphyromonas*, *Prevotella*, and *Fusobacterium*. Pelvic inflammatory disease is most commonly caused by *Neisseria gonorrhoeae* or *Chlamydia trachomatis*. *Clostridium difficile* causes pseudomembranous colitis.
MM5 423-425

26 **(E)** **Blocks release of the neurotransmitters for inhibitory synapses.** The neurotoxin of *Clostridium tetani* is called tetanospasmin. It acts by blocking the release of the neurotransmitters gamma-aminobutyric acid (GABA) and glycine that are important regulators of inhibitory synapses. This action causes excitatory synaptic activity that is unregulated (spastic paralysis), producing symptoms such as contraction of facial muscles, drooling, sweating, irritability, and cardiac arrhythmias.
MM5 406-407

27 **(B)** *Clostridium difficile* **can survive in an environment (e.g., hospital floors, medical instruments) for a prolonged period.** *C. difficile* is a spore-forming organism that frequently colonizes the environment surrounding an infected patient.

Lactobacillus is an opportunistic pathogen but is not associated with intravascular catheters. After tetanus toxin binds to the nerve endings, the toxin is internalized. Therefore an antibody response is not associated with tetanus. The primary virulence factor found in *B. fragilis* is its polysaccharide capsule; this bacterium does not produce endotoxin or exfoliative toxin. *B. fragilis* is typically resistant to penicillin.
MM5 411-413

28 **(E)** *Nocardia asteroides.* All of the organisms listed in the answers to this question are bacteria. Despite that fact, these organisms either do not stain with the Gram stain or stain poorly. Only *N. asteroides* can be reliably stained with the Gram stain even though the pattern is beaded; that is, the organism will partially retain the stain. This staining characteristic, coupled with the ability to stain with weak acid-fast stains, is very useful for a preliminary identification of this organism. *C. pneumoniae* has an inner and outer membrane structure similar to gram-negative bacteria, but this bacterium lacks a rigid peptidoglycan layer and does not retain the Gram stain. *L. pneumophila* has a gram-negative cell wall but is too thin to be detected by Gram stain when present in clinical specimens. This property contributed to the problems encountered when the first major outbreak occurred with this organism (at the Legionnaire's convention in Philadelphia in 1976). After *L. pneumophila* bacteria are grown in culture, they thicken and can be seen as thin, gram-negative rods. *M. tuberculosis* has a cell wall similar in structure to the cell wall of gram-positive bacteria; however, a major component of the cell wall is lipids that render the bacteria hydrophobic. The hydrophobic nature of the cell wall prevents uptake of the Gram stain, so these bacteria typically appear as "ghosts" or nonstaining halos. *M. pneumoniae* does not retain the Gram stain because the bacterium lacks a cell wall.
MM5 287-290

29 **(A)** *Bacillus cereus.* The clinical presentation of this disease is consistent with food poisoning caused by *B. cereus*. Disease is mediated by a heat-stable enterotoxin. *B. cereus* can grow in contaminated foods, releasing the enterotoxin. Subsequent reheating of the food does not inactivate the enterotoxin. Because the enterotoxin is present in the food, the incubation period between ingestion and disease is short, and the duration of disease is also short. Each of the other organisms in the answers to this question produces gastroenteritis 1 to 2 days after ingestion of the contaminated foods. The delay occurs because the organisms must grow in the intestines before they invade the intestinal mucosa or produce enteric toxins. Diseases caused by these other bacteria are self-limiting, but symptoms may persist for up to 1 week after onset.
MM5 269-270

30 **(B)** **Bile solubility.** *S. pneumoniae* is unique among the streptococci in its sensitivity to bile. The ability of bile to dissolve colonies of *S. pneumoniae* is a rapid, specific identification test. Susceptibility to optochin is also used to identify *S. pneumoniae*.

This test, however, requires culturing the isolated organism on a blood agar plate, placing a disk with optochin on the plate, and then examining the plate after overnight incubation for inhibition of the bacteria. All streptococci are catalase-negative, so this test is not helpful. Production of coagulase is used to identify *S. aureus*. Oxidase is primarily used for the identification of gram-negative bacteria.

MM5 256

31   (B) Clarithromycin. The organism responsible for this man's infection is *Mycobacterium avium* complex, which is the most common nontuberculous mycobacterium responsible for disseminated disease in AIDS patients. *Mycobacterium tuberculosis* can be excluded here because it generally has a more acute presentation and is niacin-positive and nitrate reductase-positive. A point that underscores the low level of virulence of *M. avium* complex is the observation that extremely high concentrations of the bacteria are present in tissues and the blood before patients develop significant symptoms. In addition, disease with *M. avium* complex is only seen when the CD4 cell count falls below $100/mm^3$. *M. avium* complex is generally resistant to all antibiotics except the macrolides: clarithromycin and azithromycin.

MM5 303-305, 308-309

32   (C) Imipenem. The beta-lactam antibiotics (e.g., imipenem) bind to the enzymes responsible for the assembly of the peptidoglycan layer in the bacterial cell wall. Ciprofloxacin disrupts DNA replication by binding to the alpha subunit of DNA gyrase. Erythromycin binds to the 50S ribosomal subunit and blocks polypeptide elongation. Rifampin binds to the DNA-dependent RNA polymerase and inhibits the initiation of RNA synthesis. Tetracycline inhibits protein synthesis by binding to the 30S ribosomal subunits, thus blocking the binding of aminoacyl-transfer RNA (tRNA) to the 30S ribosome/mRNA complex.

MM5 204-207

33   (A) *Actinomyces*. This woman has pelvic actinomycosis, which is most commonly associated with IUDs that have been in place for more than 1 year. *Actinomyces* is part of the normal flora of the mouth, gastrointestinal tract, and vagina. In the presence of the IUD, the organism is able to localize on the foreign body and incite an inflammatory response. As the disease progresses, sinus tract formation and spread to adjacent tissues can occur. *Lactobacillus*, *Mobiluncus*, and *Propionibacterium* are also found in the vagina but have not been associated with disease similar to this woman's presentation. *Nocardia* is an aerobic environmental organism that typically forms filamentous gram-positive rods. *Nocardia* is weakly acid-fast, which is a useful test to differentiate *Nocardia* from *Actinomyces*.

MM5 417-419

34   (D) *Streptococcus pneumoniae*. Sinusitis typically develops in patients who have respiratory allergies or a history of a preceding viral respiratory infection (e.g., respiratory syncytial virus infection). In each situation, inflammation and swelling of the passages cause the sinuses to become occluded, trapping nasopharyngeal flora in the sinuses, which permits the growth of bacteria. The most common causes of chronic sinusitis are *S. pneumoniae*, nontypable strains of *Haemophilus influenzae*, *Moraxella catarrhalis*, and a mixture of aerobic and anaerobic bacteria. *Haemophilus influenzae* type b is rarely found in the nasopharynx. *N. neningitidis* is present in the nasopharynx of healthy individuals but has not been associated with sinusitis. *S. aureus* can cause sinusitis, but the patient would have a more acute presentation. *S. pyogenes* is a common cause of pharyngitis but rarely causes sinusitis.

MM5 255-256

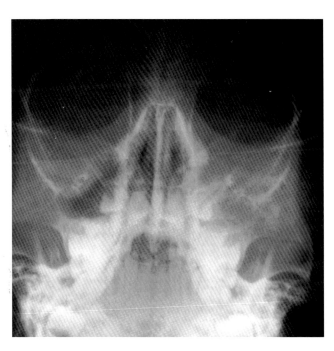

From Cohen J, Powderly WG: *Infectious diseases*, ed 2, St Louis, 2004, Mosby.

35   (C) Erythromycin. Mycoplasmas lack a cell wall; therefore antibiotics that interfere with cell wall biosynthesis would be inactive. This would include the beta-lactamases (e.g., ampicillin-sulbactam, ceftazidime, imipenem) and vancomycin. Erythromycin interferes with protein synthesis and is effective in treating infections caused by *M. pneumoniae*. The tetracyclines can also be used to treat infections caused by this organism.

MM5 443, 446-447

36   (E) Tick. Ticks are the primary vector of tularemia in the United States. Other sources of infection with *Francisella tularensis* are contact with an infected animal or domestic pet that is host to the tick carrying this disease or inhalation of infectious aerosols (e.g., aerosolized blood from an infected rabbit during dressing). Deer flies are also a vector of tularemia but are believed to be infrequently associated with human disease.

MM5 386-389

37 **(E) Urease.** The most likely organism responsible for this disease is *Helicobacter pylori*. Virtually all cases of type B gastritis and most gastric and duodenal ulcers are produced by this organism. *H. pylori* produces a number of virulence factors, but the most important one is urease. The product of this enzyme neutralizes stomach acids, allowing the organism to pass through the gastric mucosa and adhere to the gastric surface. The activity of this enzyme is also measured in a variety of diagnostic tests.

MM5 351-354

38 **(A) Bartonella henselae.** This girl has "cat-scratch disease" (CSD) caused by *B. henselae*. Although a variety of other organisms can cause a similar clinical picture, the negative cultures provide strong evidence that the girl has CSD. Generally, relatively few organisms are present at the scratch site or in the lymph node, with most of the symptoms related to the vigorous inflammatory reaction to the organism. *B. henselae* is a fastidious, slow-growing organism requiring incubation for up to 6 weeks before growth is detected. The diagnostic test of choice for this disease is serology. *K. granulomatis* (formally *Calymmatobacterium granulomatis*) is the etiologic agent of granuloma inguinale, a granulomatous disease affecting the genitalia and inguinal nodes. This organism has not been reliably grown in cell-free culture. *C. ochracea* is a slow-growing facultative anaerobe associated with periodontitis, bacteremia, and rarely endocarditis. *E. corrodens* is a normal resident of the human oropharynx and has been associated with bite wounds, pulmonary infections, bacteremia, and endocarditis. *P. multocida* is a normal resident in the oropharynx of cats and dogs and has been associated with bite wounds, pulmonary infections, and bacteremia in immunocompromised patients.

MM5 397-398

39 **(B) Tick.** Lyme disease is the leading vector-borne disease in the United States. The major reservoir hosts in the United States are the white-footed mouse and white-tailed deer. The white-footed mouse is the primary host of larval and nymph stages of hard ticks (primarily the *Ixodes* species), and the adult tick stage infest the white-tailed deer. More than 90% of human infections are caused by bites of the nymph stages, so the mouse is the more important reservoir host for human infections. The tick larvae become infected when they feed on the mouse reservoir. When the larva molts to a nymph stage, it takes a second blood meal, and humans can be the accidental host. Although adult stages can cause disease, this form is generally large and will be noticed and removed before the tick can transmit the *Borrelia* organism (i.e., requires a period of feeding for 48 h or more).

MM5 433-438

40 **(B) Clostridium difficile.** All five organisms in the answers to this question can cause gastrointestinal disease; however, the important clue is that the symptoms developed after the patient started antibiotics. Beta-lactam antibiotics (e.g., ceftazidime) and clindamycin have been most commonly associated with disease caused by *C. difficile*. The antibiotics suppress the bacteria normally present in the gastrointestinal tract and allow proliferation of *C. difficile*, which may have been present in the intestine or acquired during hospitalization. The presence of white plaques over the colonic mucosa is consistent with the more severe form of disease, pseudomembranous colitis. This early stage of *C. difficile* disease is referred to as "antibiotic-associated diarrhea."

MM5 411-413

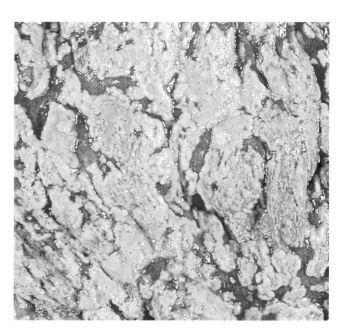

41 **(C) Kinyoun stain.** The Kinyoun stain is an acid-fast stain. Acid-fast organisms include *Mycobacterium, Nocardia, Rhodococcus, Tsukamurella, Gordonia, Cryptosporidium, Cyclospora,* and *Isospora,* as well as those from the phylum Microsporidia. The calcofluor white stain is a nonspecific fluorochrome that binds to chitin in the cell wall of fungi. Mycobacteria can stain weakly with the Gram stain (gram-positive), but most isolates will not retain the stain. The trichrome stain is used to detect intestinal and urogenital protozoa. The Giemsa stain is used to detect blood-borne pathogens (e.g., *Borrelia, Ehrlichia, Anaplasma, Rickettsia, Plasmodium, Babesia, Microfilaria*).

MM5 173-174

42 **(A) Actinobacillus actinomycetemcomitans.** This woman has a previously damaged heart valve and should have received antimicrobial prophylaxis before her dental procedure. During the dental procedure, organisms from her oropharynx were introduced into her blood and attached to her damaged heart valve. The organisms were able to proliferate and cause further damage. Slow-growing organisms, such as the ones listed in the

incorrect answers to this question, produce a subacute form of endocarditis, with symptoms developing over weeks to months. *S. epidermidis* and *S. mutans* can be excluded as a cause because these are gram-positive cocci. *A. actinomycetemcomitans* is the correct answer because these organisms characteristically form adherent colonies on the surface of glass and plastic, such as the material of a heart valve.
MM5 374

43 (B) Lipooligosaccharide (LOS). LOS is a major antigen in the cell wall of *N. gonorrhoeae.* This antigen is composed of lipid A and a core oligosaccharide, similar to gram-negative lipopolysaccharide (LPS), and possesses endotoxin activity. However, LOS does not have the antigenically diverse O polysaccharide antigens found in LPS. LOS stimulates the inflammatory response and release of tumor necrosis factor-α that causes most of the symptoms associated with gonococcal disease. *N. gonorrhoeae* does not have a true carbohydrate capsule such as that found in *N. meningitidis.* The Opa protein mediates attachment to epithelial cells, RMP protects the bacteria from bactericidal antibodies, and teichoic acid is not found in *N. gonorrhoeae.*
MM5 311-315

44 (E) *Staphylococcus saprophyticus.* The patient's clinical illness is consistent with a urinary tract infection. It could be restricted to the bladder (cystitis) or, more likely, involve the kidneys (acute pyelonephritis). The latter is indicated by the flank pain (over the kidney) and fever. *S. saprophyticus* causes urinary tract infections primarily in young, sexually active women. This organism can also produce upper tract infection with urinary tract stone formation (due to production of urease, leading to alkalization of the urine and mineral precipitation). The Gram stain result is also consistent with *S. saprophyticus. C. albicans* is a cause of vaginitis and can cause urinary tract infections but most commonly in catheterized patients and patients receiving broad-spectrum antibacterial agents. In a setting such as this young woman's, the presence of *C. albicans* in urine would most likely be insignificant. Although *C. albicans* can stain gram-positive, the cells are much larger than bacteria and would not be mistaken for bacteria. *E. faecalis* is a gram-positive coccus that colonizes the gastrointestinal tract and can cause urinary tract infections. This organism, however, typically produces infections in patients who have been treated with broad-spectrum antibiotics and are either catheterized or have a history of urinary tract manipulations. Neither situation exists in this woman. *E. coli* is the most common cause of urinary tract infections, including those in young adult women. However, *E. coli* is a gram-negative rod. *N. gonorrhoeae* is one of the most prevalent causes of sexually transmitted diseases. An infection of the urethra would produce pain on urination and pyuria; however, symptoms of an upper tract infection would not be common, and the Gram stain is inconsistent with *N. gonorrhoeae.*
MM5 233

45 (D) Resistant to all beta-lactam antibiotics; susceptible to vancomycin. If a *Staphylococcus* is oxacillin-resistant, it is resistant to all beta-lactam antibiotics. Vancomycin is the drug of choice for treating these organisms. At present, vancomycin-resistant *S. aureus* is very uncommon.
MM5 234-235

46 (A) *Mycobacterium fortuitum.* This opportunistic infection is caused by *M. fortuitum.* Infections with this organism were historically restricted to traumatic accidents where contaminated soil was introduced into subcutaneous tissues. This organism, however, is now more commonly associated with iatrogenic infections, such as this line-related infection. Diagnosis is sometimes complicated because these organisms are generally not seen on Gram stain, and the growth can require extended incubation of cultures. The uniform staining and lack of branching are inconsistent with *N. asteroides or N. brasiliensis. R. equi* would appear as a coccus or coccobacillus. *M. haemophilum* would grow on both sheep blood agar and chocolate agar but not in 2 days (growth requires 2 or more weeks).
MM5 305

47 (A) Penicillin. The organism isolated in this man's culture is *Eikenella corrodens.* This is an organism that is a normal resident in the human oropharynx and has been associated with human bite infections and fistfight injuries and less commonly with endocarditis, sinusitis, meningitis, brain abscesses, pneumonia, and lung abscesses. Most bite or fistfight infections are polymicrobic and involve aerobic, facultative anaerobic, and strict anaerobic bacteria. *E. corrodens* is a slow-growing facultative anaerobe. It grows slowly on nonselective aerobic media but generally grows poorly or not at all on selective media such as MacConkey agar. Characteristics that help to identify this organism are the bleach-like odor it produces and the ability to pit ("corrode") agar. In contrast with most gram-negative bacteria, penicillin is active against this organism and is considered the drug of choice for treating infections. Other active antibiotics include ampicillin, extended-spectrum cephalosporins, tetracyclines, and fluoroquinolones. Antibiotics that are generally inactive include oxacillin, first-generation cephalosporins (e.g., cephalothin), clindamycin, erythromycin, and aminoglycosides.
MM5 320-321

48 (C) *Escherichia coli* O157. Antibiotic treatment of patients infected with *E. coli* O157 has been associated with an increased risk of developing hemolytic uremic syndrome. Infection with *C. jejuni* is generally self-limiting, but antibiotic therapy is recommended for treatment of severe gastroenteritis or disseminated disease. *C. difficile* disease is managed by discontinuing the antibiotics that induced the disease and treatment with either metronidazole or vancomycin to eliminate the bacteria. *H. pylori* infections are managed by using a combination of a proton pump inhibitor (e.g., omeprazole) and one or more antibiotics (e.g., tetracycline, clarithromycin, amoxicillin, metronidazole).

S. sonnei infections are treated with antibiotics to limit the spread of organisms to contacts.

MM5 329-330, 337-338

49 **(D)** *Nocardia asteroides.* An infection with *N. asteroides* typically presents as a bronchopulmonary infection, with dissemination to the central nervous system or subcutaneous tissues as a common complication. These bacteria are gram-positive but characteristically stain poorly. *N. asteroides* organisms have mycolic acids in their cell wall and are weakly acid-fast. This property is useful to distinguish *N. asteroides* from *A. israelii* and *C. jeikeium* (non–acid-fast) as well as *M. tuberculosis* (strongly acid-fast). *R. equi* is weakly acid-fast and is associated with cavitary lung disease, but it typically appears as coccobacilli or cocci.

MM5 287-292

50 **(E)** **Replication in fused phagosome/lysosome.** The virulence of *Salmonella* is related to the ability of the organism to replicate in phagocytic cells. The bacteria accomplish this by their ability to replicate in fused phagosome/lysosome. Other bacteria that are resistant to lysosomal enzymes include *Coxiella*, *Ehrlichia*, and *Mycobacterium leprae*.

MM5 198-201, 330

51 **(D)** *Legionella micdadei.* Only a few bacteria exist that are acid-fast or partially acid-fast (i.e., retain the acid-fast stain after decolorization with a weak but not a strong acid solution). Mycobacteria are strongly acid-fast, and the following bacteria are the only other genera that are weakly acid-fast: *Nocardia*, *Rhodococcus*, *Tsukamurella*, *Gordonia*, and *Legionella micdadei*. *L. micdadei* is unique in that it is the only *Legionella* species that is weakly acid-fast and that it loses this property when the organism is grown in culture.

MM5 325

52 **(E)** **Replication in fused phagosome/lysosome.** *Coxiella burnetii* is an obligate intracellular pathogen. Intracellular multiplication is initiated after the bacteria are phagocytized,

and the phagosome fuses to form a phagolysosome. The acidic environment activates the bacterial metabolic machinery.

MM5 198-201, 460-462

53 **(A)** **This organism is typically susceptible to penicillin.** The drug of choice for treating an infection with *E. rhusiopathiae* is penicillin. Although cephalosporins, erythromycin, and clindamycin are active, aminoglycosides and vancomycin are not. *E. rhusiopathiae* isolates are catalase-positive, gram-positive rods and should not be mistaken for *Streptococcus*. Infections caused by this organism are zoonotic, associated with exposure to infected animals or their by-products. *E. rhusiopathiae* grows aerobically and anaerobically (facultative anaerobe) and does not contain endotoxin (this is found only in gram-negative bacteria).

MM5 276-277

54 **(B)** *Cardiobacterium hominis.* The chronic course, clinical signs, and persistent bacteremia are consistent with the diagnosis of subacute bacterial endocarditis. The chronic, subacute course of this infection is also consistent with the fact that the etiologic agent, *C. hominis*, grows slowly in culture. This organism is part of the normal oral flora in children and adults. As the name would suggest, this organism is almost exclusively associated with endocarditis. Disease is typically initiated in patients with either poor oral hygiene or those who have just undergone a dental procedure and most commonly is found in patients with a previously damaged heart valve. The course of disease is slow, with nonspecific symptoms developing over the period of months. Although the organism can be recovered on common, nonselective laboratory media, prolonged incubation is required. Because many microbiology laboratories do not incubate blood cultures beyond 4 or 5 days, a specific request for prolonged incubation (7 to 10 days) should be made for each patient with suspected subacute bacterial endocarditis. Keys for identifying this organism include the slow growth on nonselective media; inability to grow on MacConkey agar; and catalase-negative, oxidase-positive, and a weakly positive indole reaction results. *A. baumanni* can be excluded because this organism will grow on MacConkey agar, is oxidase-negative, and is a coccobacillus. *C. ochracea* is oxidase-negative and is rarely associated with endocarditis. *E. corrodens* can cause subacute bacterial endocarditis but can be excluded because it is catalase-positive. *H. parainfluenzae* requires V factor (NAD) for growth, so it will grow on chocolate agar but not blood agar.

MM5 399

55 **(C)** *Legionella pneumophila.* This patient has atypical pneumonia. The clinical symptoms can be caused by a group of bacteria that include *L. pneumophila*, *M. pneumoniae*, and *C. pneumoniae* (formerly classified in the genus *Chlamydia*). Microscopy is not useful for the diagnosis of this disease because *L. pneumophila* is too thin to be easily seen, *M. pneumoniae* lacks a cell wall so it does not retain the stain, and *C. pneumoniae* lacks a rigid peptidoglycan cell wall layer. *L. pneumophila* requires L-cysteine and has enhanced growth in the presence of iron, both factors present in BCYE agar. *C. pneumoniae* and *M. pneumoniae* will not grow on BCYE agar. *K. pneumoniae* and *S. pneumoniae* are both common causes of pneumonia; however, the chest radiograph is inconsistent with disease caused by these organisms. Abscess formation and production of blood-tinged sputum are typically seen in *K. pneumoniae* infections. Consolidated lung masses (lobar pneumonia) are characteristically observed in *S. pneumoniae* infections.

MM5 391-395

56 (D) Metronidazole. Virtually all strains of the *Bacteroides fragilis* group, and many members of the genera *Porphyromonas*, *Prevotella*, and *Fusobacterium*, produce beta-lactamases that inactivate penicillin and carbenicillin. Approximately 20% to 30% of *Bacteroides* are resistant to clindamycin, and 5% to 10% of *Bacteroides* produce a specific beta-lactamase that inactivates imipenem. At the present time, metronidazole is the only antibiotic that is consistently active against the anaerobic gram-negative rods.

MM5 426

57 (B) Inhibition of phagosome/lysosome fusion. *Francisella tularensis* is an intracellular pathogen that can survive in macrophages of the reticuloendothelial system because the organism inhibits phagosome/lysosome fusion. Other bacteria that can survive because of their ability to inhibit fusion include *Legionella*, *Mycobacterium tuberculosis*, and *Chlamydophila*.

MM5 198-201, 386

58 (B) *Corynebacterium urealyticum*. *C. urealyticum* is one of the few corynebacteria that can cause urinary tract infections. Characteristically, this organism produces urease and is able to lyse urea (hence its name), producing an alkaline urine. This can then lead to the formation of urinary tract calculi. *E. faecium* is a gram-positive coccus, and *E. coli* is a gram-negative rod, so these answers can be eliminated. *C. perfringens* is an anaerobic gram-positive rod, but is an uncommon cause of urinary tract infections (as are all anaerobes). Lactobacilli, such as *L. acidophilus*, are gram-positive rods that are present in the urethra and vagina in large numbers, but when they are isolated in urine, they commonly represent contaminants.

MM5 283-284

59 (E) Spore formation. Formation of spores is only reported for gram-positive bacteria. The two most clinically important genera of bacteria that form spores are *Bacillus*, including *B. anthracis*; the pathogen responsible for anthrax; and *Clostridium*, a large genus composed of many species responsible for a wide range of infections including botulism, tetanus, gas gangrene, and pseudomembraneous colitis. The cytoplasmic membrane and peptidoglycan layer are found in both gram-positive and gram-negative bacteria. Endotoxin and an outer membrane are unique to gram-negative bacteria and are not found in gram-positive organisms.

MM5 22-23

60 (E) Toxic shock syndrome toxin-1. Toxic shock syndrome toxin-1 (TSST-1) was originally described as an enterotoxin (enterotoxin F) and is still associated with diarrhea. The first report of toxic shock syndrome was in children after injection of a vaccine contaminated with *S. aureus*. In the 1980s, the syndrome was observed in menstruating women who had localized infections with *S. aureus* in hyperabsorbent tampons. With the removal of the tampons from the market, most reports of toxic shock syndrome are associated with wound infection. Characteristic of toxic shock syndrome is multiorgan dysfunction, skin desquamation, shock, and death. *Staphylococcus aureus* produces a variety of toxins that mediate disease. Alpha-toxin is an example of a cytotoxic toxin produced by this organism. This toxin is an important mediator of tissue damage and is toxic for many cells (e.g., erythrocytes, leukocytes, platelets), but it does not produce the clinical pictures described here. Leukocidin is also a cytotoxic toxin. Enterotoxin A is one of eight serologically distinct, heat-stable enterotoxins described for *S. aureus*. Enterotoxin A is the toxin most commonly associated with staphylococcal food poisoning. Because this condition is mediated by ingestion of preformed toxin, the incubation period after ingestion of the contaminated food is only a few hours, and the duration of condition is less than 24 h. Two exfoliative toxins (A and B) have also been described, each of which can mediate scalded skin syndrome in babies. These are serine proteases that split the intercellular bridges in the stratum granulosum epidermis. Cytolysis and inflammation are not present in the involved skin, so Gram stains and culture are not useful.

MM5 224-226

61 (E) Host immune response to bacteria. The tissue destruction and lesions observed in syphilis are primarily caused by the patient's immune response to infection. Other virulence factors, such as those listed in the answers to this question, are important for permitting the survival of the bacteria in their human host, but the factors do not directly contribute to the pathology observed in syphilis. Virulent strains of *Treponema pallidum* produce hyaluronidase, which may facilitate perivascular infiltration. Likewise, outer membrane proteins are associated with adherence of the bacteria to the surface of host cells, and the bacteria can be coated with host fibronectin that can protect the spirochetes from phagocytosis.

MM5 427-428

62 (E) Immunoassay for toxins. Although *C. difficile* will grow on blood agar (incubated anaerobically), the preferred diagnostic test is detection of the bacterial enterotoxin and cytotoxin by an immunoassay. Presence of the toxins differentiates colonization of an individual with the organism (as demonstrated by culture) and disease. MacConkey agar is incubated aerobically and is used for the recovery of organisms such as *Salmonella* and *Shigella*. Sorbitol/MacConkey agar is a special formulation of MacConkey agar (sorbitol replaces lactose) that is used for the detection of enterohemorrhagic *Escherichia coli* (EHEC) O157 (which does not ferment sorbitol in contrast with

microaerophilic = Campylobacter

other *E. coli* strains). *Campylobacter* species are detected by culturing the specimens on selective agar incubated in a micro-aerophilic atmosphere.
MM5 337, 350, 411-413

63 (A) *Bartonella.* *B. henselae* and *B. quintana* have been associated with febrile bacteremia. In contrast with immunocompetent patients who can have an acute febrile illness, these organisms can produce a nonspecific febrile illness in HIV-infected patients. Localizing signs are generally not present, and the only way to definitively make the diagnosis is to grow the organism in culture. The difficulty with this process is the organism grows slowly and requires an atmosphere of carbon dioxide enrichment and high humidity (40% or greater). The fact that this gram-negative, curved rod grows slowly both in the blood culture broth and on solid media and that it is associated with negative catalase and oxidase tests is adequate to make the presumptive diagnosis of *Bartonella* bacteremia. All of the other organisms listed in the answers to this question will grow rapidly, although *Prevotella* is an anaerobe and requires the appropriate anaerobic atmosphere.
MM5 397-398

64 (C) *Nocardia brasiliensis.* This patient has most likely contracted mycetoma, which is a chronic, localized infection of the subcutaneous tissues that spreads into adjacent structures. The infection is often painless, although secondary infections with suppurative bacteria are common. Specimens must be collected for microscopy and culture because a variety of bacteria and fungi can cause this disease. *N. brasiliensis* is the most common cause of this disease in the Americas. *N. brasiliensis* is a relatively slow-growing bacterium and generally requires 3 to 5 days of incubation before good growth is obtained. One characteristic of *N. brasiliensis* colonies is they produce aerial hyphae, the filamentous projections seen in the figure shown here. *A. israelii* can produce subcutaneous infections but requires anaerobic incubation for growth. *S. schenckii* produces subcutaneous lesions, but these typically follow the lymphatics and are not localized to the foot. *M. avium* and *V. vulnificus* do not produce a condition such as this patient's.
MM5 291-292

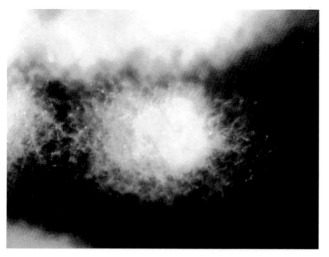

65 (C) Inhibition of opsonization mediated by protein A. Protein A is a surface protein present in most strains of *S. aureus*. The protein has an affinity for binding to the Fc receptor of immunoglobulins IgG_1, IgG_2, and IgG_4. This effectively prevents antibody-mediated immune clearance of the bacteria. Extracellular protein A can also bind antibodies, thereby forming immune complexes with the subsequent consumption of complement.
MM5 198-201, 223

66 (E) Soft cheese. *L. monocytogenes* can be isolated from soil, water, vegetation, and the intestinal contents of a variety of animals. Fecal carriage in healthy individuals is low, probably less than 5%. Most infections with *L. monocytogenes* have been associated with consumption of contaminated milk, soft cheese, undercooked meats, raw vegetables, and cabbage. Because *L. monocytogenes* can grow at 4°C, listeriae can multiply to large numbers in contaminated foods stored in the refrigerator for a prolonged period.
MM5 273-276

67 (E) Stimulates release of proinflammatory cytokines. The lethal toxin produced by *B. anthracis* consists of two protein subunits: protective antigen (PA) and lethal factor (LF). PA is responsible for binding to receptors on the surface of host cells. After binding to the surface receptors, PA is cleaved and the 63-kDa fragment remains on the cell surface. The surface fragments self-associate, forming a ring complex of seven fragments that both bind LF and act as a pore for entry of LF into the cell. LF is a zinc metalloprotease that cleaves MAP kinase kinases, leading to release of proinflammatory cytokines.
MM5 198-201, 265-266

68 (A) *Chlamydophila (Chlamydia) pneumoniae.* *C. pneumoniae* is an obligate intracellular bacterium that grows in cell cultures such as Hep-2 cells. Infections caused by this organism can also be detected by serologic tests. None of the other bacteria listed in this question can grow in monolayered cells. *K. pneumoniae* and *S. pneumoniae* grow on media used for routine sputum and blood cultures; *L. pneumophila* requires specialized media supplemented with iron and L-cysteine (e.g., BCYE agar).
MM5 470

69 (B) *Clostridium.* *Clostridium* produces spores that allow it to survive in its environment. The other anaerobes in the answers to the question are unable to survive exposure to oxygen and are associated with endogenous infections.
MM5 401

70 (C) Doxycycline. This man has an infection with *Brucella*, probably *B. melitensis* that is associated with goats (hence the name). *Brucella* is an organism that has a predilection for infecting organs rich in erythritol, a sugar metabolized by many *Brucella*. Animal tissues that are rich in erythritol include breast, uterus, placenta, and epididymis. Human disease primarily

results from consumption of contaminated unpasteurized milk and other dairy products. The drug of choice for treating this infection is doxycycline. If a pregnant woman is infected, then trimethoprim/sulfamethoxazole is an acceptable alternative.
MM5 383-386

71 (B) Corynebacterium jeikeium. C. jeikeium is an opportunistic pathogen, causing infections in immunocompromised patients, patients receiving broad spectrum antibiotics, or patients with intravenous catheters. The organism colonizes the skin surface and then gains access to the blood through the compromised skin surface (e.g., at the insertion site of the catheter). Treatment of infections caused by C. jeikeium is complicated because the organism is generally resistant to most antibiotics except vancomycin. A. haemolyticum is a "coryneform-shaped" organism that is catalase-negative and susceptible to most antibiotics. L. casei is generally resistant to vancomycin; L. monocytogenes is generally susceptible to most antibiotics; and P. acnes is an anaerobe that is generally susceptible to most antibiotics.
MM5 283-284

72 (C) A syphilic patient's immune response may lead to tissue damage. T. pallidum does not produce any significant virulence factors; rather, it produces pathology by stimulating the patient's immune system. The other answers to this question are incorrect because bacteria are extremely thin (0.1 to 0.2 μm); bacteria fail to grow in culture; early but not late syphilis is characterized by ulcers and rash; and penicillin is uniformly active.
MM5 427-430

73 (C) Sinus aspirate. Because the organisms responsible for sinusitis originate from a complex mixture of bacteria in the nasopharynx, cultures of specimens from the nasopharynx, throat, and lungs would not be helpful. The only reliable specimen would be a direct aspirate from the involved sinus. Because this is uncommonly done, except at the time of surgical drainage of the sinuses, most infections are treated empirically. Blood cultures would rarely be positive.
MM5 214

74 (E) 20 ml. The success of a blood culture is directly related to the volume of blood that is cultured. Because the majority of patients with clinical sepsis have an organism count of less than 1/ml of blood, the incidence of positive blood cultures increases as the volume of blood that is cultured is increased. It is recommended that approximately 20 ml of blood should be collected from an adult for each blood culture. Proportionally smaller volumes should be collected from children and neonates.
MM5 213-216

75 (C) Rickettsia prowazekii. R. prowazekii is the etiologic agent of epidemic typhus or louse-borne typhus. In contrast with other rickettsial infections, typhus primarily affects

humans. Infections are spread in crowded, unclean conditions. Recrudescent disease (Brill-Zinsser disease) with this organism can occur years after the initial exposure. C. burnetii infections (Q fever) are primarily spread by the airborne route, although ticks can be an uncommon vector. E. chaffeensis (ehrlichiosis) and R. rickettsii (Rocky Mountain spotted fever) are spread by ticks, whereas R. typhi (murine typhus) is spread by fleas.
MM5 453-454

76 (D) Only one serotype has been identified. A single serotype has been identified for C. pneumoniae. This bacterium is a human pathogen, with no recognized animal reservoir. Infections are spread by the respiratory route, with mild infections believed to occur commonly. Most infections are either asymptomatic or present as a mild respiratory disease. More severe infections present as atypical pneumonia, and C. pneumoniae has been associated with atherosclerosis. In contrast with Chlamydia trachomatis, C. pneumoniae does not have plasmid DNA and is resistant to sulfonamides. Macrolides, tetracyclines, and fluoroquinolones are active against C. pneumoniae. Moreover, C. pneumoniae inclusions in infected tissue culture cells do not contain glycogen, so iodine staining cannot be used as a rapid diagnostic tool.
MM5 470

77 (C) Interferes with protein synthesis. The disease produced by C. diphtheriae is mediated by a two-component (A-B) exotoxin that inhibits protein synthesis. The gene for this toxin, tox gene, is introduced into strains of C. diphtheriae by a lysogenic bacteriophage (beta-phage). The receptor for the toxin is the heparin-binding epidermal growth factor, which is present on the surface of many eukaryotic cells, particularly heart and nerve cells. Its presence on these cells explains the cardiac and neurologic symptoms observed in patients with severe diphtheria. After the toxin is transported into the cell, it terminates protein synthesis by inactivating elongation factor-2 (EF-2).
MM5 279-283

78 (B) Enterococcus faecalis. Organisms responsible for peritonitis have demonstrated an ability to produce disease in the intestinal tract (i.e., they have specific, relevant virulence factors). Even though hundreds of different species of bacteria are present in the intestines, relatively few produce peritonitis. Enterococcus organisms, both E. faecalis and E. faecium, can cause peritonitis. The Gram stain result for the patient is consistent with this organism. Two additional organisms that commonly cause peritonitis are Escherichia coli (which is treated effectively by ceftazidime) and Bacteroides fragilis (which is treated by metronidazole). Yeasts such as C. albicans could also be responsible for infection in this setting; however, the organism would not grow anaerobically. P. anaerobius is associated with polymicrobic abdominal infections, but this organism would not grow aerobically. Streptococci and staphylococci are uncommon causes of peritonitis in this setting.
MM5 259-262

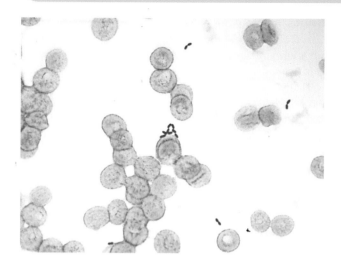

79 **(C) *Clostridium*.** Clostridia, particularly *C. perfringens* and *C. septicum*, are associated with soft tissue infections including cellulitis, fasciitis, and myonecrosis (gas gangrene). Gas gangrene is not associated with the other organisms listed in the answers to this question.
MM5 404-406, 413

80 **(D) *Mycobacterium kansasii*.** As with many bacteria, fungi, and parasites, the initial key for the specific identification of an organism is based on the appearance of the organism. Specifically, many bacteria have characteristic microscopic and macroscopic morphologies. These key characteristics can be quite useful for an accurate, preliminary identification of the organism and can provide information that can guide the management of a patient. Pigment-producing organisms can be separated into those that produce pigments only after exposure to light (photochromogens) and those that produce pigments in light or dark (scotochromogens). In the case of mycobacteria, *M. kansasii* and *M. marinum* are clinically important photochromogens, and most scotochromogens are clinically insignificant. *M. tuberculosis* is nonpigmented (e.g., referred to as "buff-colored"). Thus, if a pigmented organism is isolated, it cannot be *M. tuberculosis*. *M. avium* is also nonpigmented or will have a faint yellow color. *M. fortuitum* and *M. haemophilum* are also nonpigmented. These organisms can be separated by other growth characteristics: *M. avium* grows slowly, whereas *M. fortuitum* grows rapidly; *M. haemophilum* grows only at cool temperatures and on media supplemented with iron products.
MM5 297-298

81 **(E) *Streptococcus*.** At the present time, all isolates of *Streptococcus* are susceptible to vancomycin. Reports of vancomycin-resistant streptococci were the result of incorrectly identified bacteria in the genera *Enterococcus*, *Leuconostoc*, and *Pediococcus*. All gram-negative bacteria (e.g., *Escherichia*) are resistant to vancomycin.
MM5 247, 250, 252, 256-257, 262

82 **(D) Strict anaerobic gram-negative rod: *Bacteroides*.** Of the bacteria listed in this question, *Bacteroides*, *Peptostreptococcus*, and *Clostridium* are strict anaerobes; *Bacteroides* is a gram-negative rod; *Peptostreptococcus* is a gram-positive coccus; and *Clostridium* is a spore-forming, gram-positive rod. *Enterococcus* is a facultative anaerobe (grows aerobically and anaerobically), and *Chlamydia* is a strict aerobic organism.
MM5 421

83 **(B) Coagulase.** The most likely organism responsible for wound infections that develop immediately after surgery is *Staphylococcus aureus*. If the infection has a delayed onset (developing weeks to months after the surgery), then the less virulent staphylococcal species that colonizes the skin would be considered important. Coagulase is an important virulent factor for *S. aureus*, responsible for converting fibrinogen to fibrin that can interfere with the removal of the organism by phagocytic cells. The presence of coagulase is the primary enzymatic marker that separates *S. aureus* from other staphylococci (coagulase-negative staphylococci). All staphylococci produce catalase, so this enzyme is not a useful diagnostic marker for *S. aureus*. Endotoxin is produced only by gram-negative rods, which are relatively uncommon causes of postsurgical wound infections. Exotoxin A is produced by the gram-negative rod, *Pseudomonas aeruginosa*. Lecithinase is produced by a variety of bacteria, including *Clostridium perfringens*. This organism can cause serious postsurgical wound infection and is beta-hemolytic on blood agar; however, *C. perfringens* is an anaerobe and fails to grow in an aerobic atmosphere.
MM5 221-234

84 **(E) Urease.** The most common cause of gastritis in patients who are not using nonsteroidal anti-inflammatory drugs is *Helicobacter pylori*. An important virulence factor for this organism is urease. *H. pylori* produces high concentrations of urease and is able to convert the urea to alkaline by-products, thus neutralizing the stomach acids. This fact has been exploited in diagnostic tests that measure either urease or the by-products. The other toxins listed in the question (cytotoxin produced by *Clostridium difficile*, emetic enterotoxin produced by *Bacillus cereus*, and endotoxin produced by gram-negative rods) and coagulase produced by *Staphylococcus aureus* do not have a role in gastritis.
MM5 351-354

85 **(D) Lysis of phagosome and replication in cytoplasm.** *S. sonnei* is capable of invading and replicating in cells lining the colonic mucosa and macrophages. The bacteria secrete a class of proteins (IpaA, IpaB, IpaC, and IpaD) that induce membrane ruffling on the host cell, leading to phagocytosis of the bacteria. *S. sonnei* then lyses the phagocytic vacuole and initiates replication in the host cell cytoplasm.
MM5 198-201, 332-333

86 **(A)** ***Campylobacter.*** *Campylobacter* organisms are curved gram-negative rods, appearing as a single cell or (more commonly) as pairs of bacteria arranged in an S shape. The most common *Campylobacter* species that cause gastroenteritis in humans grow at 42°C in an atmosphere of 5% O_2, 10% CO_2, and 85% N_2. *Escherichia, Salmonella, Shigella,* and *Yersinia* are members of the family Enterobacteriaceae and have all been associated with gastroenteritis. The Enterobacteriaceae typically appear as gram-negative rods with bipolar staining (i.e., they stain most intensely at their ends). All of the Enterobacteriaceae grow on MacConkey agar and have no special growth requirements.

MM5 337, 347-351

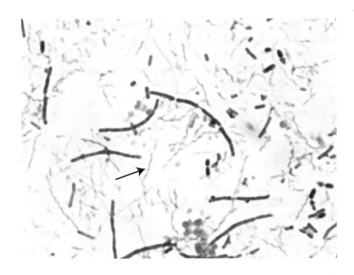

87 **(C)** ***Legionella pneumophila.*** The BCYE agar was developed for the isolation of *Legionella*. Although other organisms can grow on this medium (e.g., *Nocardia*), only *L. pneumophila* would selectively grow on this medium. All of the organisms listed in the answers can cause pneumonia, particularly in a patient with compromised pulmonary function. *K. pneumoniae* and *S. pneumoniae*, however, would readily grow in the bacterial cultures and be seen on the Gram stain. *C. pneumoniae* requires growth in special cell cultures, and *M. pneumoniae* would not grow on routine bacterial media, including BCYE agar.

MM5 391-395

88 **(B) Azithromycin.** *Mycoplasma* species are unique among bacteria because they do not have a cell wall and because their cell membrane contains sterols. The absence of the cell wall renders *Mycoplasma* organisms resistant to antibiotics that interfere with synthesis of the cell wall, such as penicillins (e.g., ampicillin-sulbactam, penicillin), cephalosporins, carbapenems (e.g., imipenem), and vancomycin. Azithromycin is a macrolide antibiotic that inhibits bacterial growth by disrupting protein synthesis.

MM5 210, 446-447

89 **(B) Serogroup B.** Vaccines for *N. meningitidis* are directed against the capsular polysaccharides. Most, with the exception of serogroup B, have proved to be effective antigens.

MM5 319-320

90 **(A)** ***Arcanobacterium haemolyticum.*** *A. haemolyticum* is a gram-positive rod that was formerly classified as a *Corynebacterium* species. This organism has been implicated in wound infections, abscess formation, septicemia, and endocarditis. The most common presentation, however, is pharyngitis with a scarlet fever-like rash. The organism grows slowly and is weakly hemolytic on sheep blood agar. Better hemolysis is seen on media with human or rabbit blood, but these media are not commonly used in clinical laboratories. Thus, most infections are likely to be misdiagnosed as culture-negative scarlet fever. *A. haemolyticum* is susceptible to penicillin and erythromycin, drugs commonly used to treat *S. pyogenes* infections. *C. diphtheriae* can produce a sore throat with fever and headaches but does not cause an erythematous rash. *L. monocytogenes* is a beta-hemolytic, gram-positive rod but is not associated with pharyngitis and a rash. *S. aureus* and *S. dysgalactiae* are gram-positive cocci. *S. aureus* can cause a retropharyngeal abscess but is not associated with pharyngitis. *S. dysgalactiae* can cause pharyngitis, but a rash is not typical with this infection.

MM5 284

91 **(C) Infection is associated with consumption of soft cheeses and undercooked meats.** The organism responsible for this infection is *Listeria monocytogenes*. Pregnant women in their last trimester are particularly susceptible to infections with this organism. Although the bacteremia can be self-limiting, prompt treatment is indicated to spare the fetus. *L. monocytogenes* is an intracellular pathogen that grows primarily in macrophages. Once the bacteria enter the cell, the phagolysosome is lysed, and the organism grows in the cell cytosol. Release of the bacteria from the cell is typically by cell-to-cell contact, so free bacteria are not common in the extracellular spaces. Thus, cellular immunity rather than humoral immunity is important for control of infection. Food products that are the source of infections include meats (e.g., turkey franks, cold cuts), soft cheeses, and raw vegetables. The organism is able to grow at refrigerator temperatures and in a wide range of pH, so contaminated foods stored in the refrigerator for a prolonged period are a common source of infection.

MM5 274-275

92 **(A) Blocks release of acetylcholine.** *C. botulinum* toxins are A-B toxins. The B subunit binds to specific sialic acid receptors and glycoproteins on the surface of motor neurons and stimulates endocytosis of the toxin molecule. Botulinum toxin remains at the neuromuscular junction. With acidification of the endosome, the A subunit is transported into the cytosol. The A subunit has endopeptidase activity that inactivates the proteins that regulate release of acetylcholine. This release in turn blocks neurotransmission at peripheral cholinergic synapses.

MM5 409

93 (B) *Clostridium perfringens.* Massive hemolysis is a rare but well-recognized complication of a *C. perfringens* infection, which this patient acquired. It is surprising that this complication is not seen more commonly, in light of the variety of hemolytic toxins that are produced by this organism. The most important toxin is alpha toxin, a lecithinase that lyses erythrocytes, platelets, leukocytes, and endothelial cells. This toxin can produce enhanced vascular permeability and result in massive hemolysis and bleeding. Although the other organisms listed in the answers to this question produce hemolytic toxins, none have been associated with the massive hemolysis seen in this patient.

MM5 402-406

94 (D) Giemsa stain of blood. Demonstrating the organisms in peripheral blood using the Giemsa stain enables the diagnosis of relapsing fever. The organism responsible for epidemic relapsing fever, *Borrelia recurrentis*, is present during the febrile period but not the days between fevers. Relatively few organisms may be present; therefore care must be used to examine the blood smears (both thick and thin smears should be prepared), and multiple blood specimens may need to be examined. *B. recurrentis* has been grown in specialized blood cultures but this is an insensitive, slow technique and is not performed in clinical laboratories. Enzyme immunoassays have not been developed for the diagnosis of relapsing fever. Proteus OXK agglutinin titers are elevated in a patient with a relapsing fever, but this assay is insensitive and nonspecific.

MM5 437-438

95 (B) *Clostridium difficile* cytotoxin. White plaques of fibrin, mucus, and inflammatory cells overlying the normal interstinal mucosa are characteristic of the more advanced form of *C. difficile* disease: pseudomembraneous colitis. The enteric toxins of *B. cereus* and *S. aureus* produce a disease characterized by rapid onset, explosive diarrhea, and vomiting. These two diseases are intoxications caused by ingestion of the toxin. Thus, the onset is within 4 to 6 h after ingestion of the toxin, and the duration is generally 24 h or less. *E. coli* verotoxin and *Shigella dysenteriae* toxin are responsible for the hemorrhagic colitis produced by these organisms. Neither disease, however, would present with plaques over the colonic mucosa.

MM5 411-413

96 (D) *Shigella dysenteriae.* *S. dysenteriae* produces an exotoxin, Shiga toxin. This toxin disrupts protein synthesis in the intestinal epithelium and can mediate damage to the glomerular endothelial cells, resulting in renal failure. This complication has also been reported with enterohemorrhagic *Escherichia coli*. In contrast, the complication is not observed with the other enteric pathogens listed in this question (*B. cereus*, *C. difficile*, *S. enterica*, and *Y. enterocolitica*).

MM5 328-330, 332-333

97 (D) Serologic detection of specific antibodies. Most clinical infections are confirmed using serology (i.e., indirect hemag-glutination test, enzyme-linked immunosorbent assay, microscopic agglutination test). Serologic tests are both sensitive and specific, with detectable antibodies developing in the second week of illness (although some patients may not mount a serologic response for weeks into the illness). Use of microscopic stains (e.g., Gram, Giemsa) is not useful because the bacteria are too thin to be seen with the Brightfield microscope. Cultures of blood and cerebrospinal fluid can be positive during the first week of clinical illness; however, special selective media (e.g., Fletcher, Tween 80-albumin broths) must be inoculated and held for up to 4 weeks. Culture of urine can be positive after the first week, and the bacteria can persist for weeks in this specimen. This culture is also insensitive and time-consuming. PCR amplification is potentially a useful test although rarely used.

MM5 440-441

98 (B) *Corynebacterium jeikeium.* *C. jeikeium* is a well-recognized opportunistic pathogen in immunocompromised patients, particularly those with hematologic disorders. Predisposing conditions for infection with this organism include prolonged hospitalization, granulocytopenia, prior or concurrent antimicrobial therapy, and the presence of intravenous catheters (all conditions present in this patient). *C. diphtheriae* is the cause of diphtheria; *C. macginleyi* is an uncommon cause of eye infections; *C. pseudotuberculosis* is associated with lymphadenitis, ulcerative lymphangitis, and abscess formation; and *C. ulcerans* can also cause respiratory diphtheria.

MM5 283-284

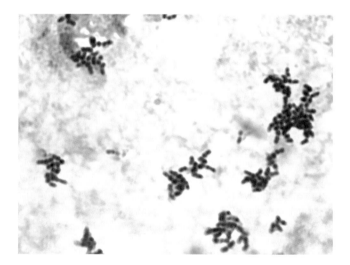

99 (D) *Mycobacterium tuberculosis.* A live vaccine with attenuated *M. bovis* (bacille Calmette-Guérin [BCG]) is commonly used in countries where tuberculosis is endemic and is responsible for significant morbidity and mortality. The *Bordetella pertussis* vaccine is an acellular vaccine containing the inactivated pertussin toxin and one or more other bacterial components (e.g., filamentous hemagglutinin, pertactin, fimbriae). Inactivated whole cell vaccines and partially purified antigen vaccines have been used for *Coxiella* infections (Q fever).

The antigen in the *H. influenzae* vaccine is the purified capsular polyribitol phosphate (PRP) of *H. influenzae* serotype B. The vaccine for *S. pneumoniae* uses a mixture of purified capsular antigens conjugated to proteins.
MM5 162-163, 309

100   (E) *Yersinia enterocolitica.* *Y. enterocolitica* is a relatively uncommon enteric pathogen in the United States, but it is seen more commonly in colder areas of the United States and other countries. It grows preferentially at cooler temperatures where it is more active metabolically. This feature has been exploited in the laboratory where stool specimens can be mixed in a nutrient broth and stored in the refrigerator. Most other bacteria will die at this temperature, whereas *Y. enterocolitica* is able to replicate. This selective culture method is called **cold enrichment**. Another bacterium with this property is *Listeria monocytogenes.* The other enteric pathogens listed in the answers to this question do not grow at cold temperatures. For example, *C. jejuni* preferentially grows at 42°C—another form of selective isolation of a bacterium by temperature.
MM5 334-335

101   (C) Culture on sorbitol/MacConkey agar. *E. coli* O157 will grow on MacConkey agar but cannot be differentiated from the many other strains of *E. coli* that are present in the intestines. Most strains of *E. coli* O157 do not ferment sorbitol (in contrast with other strains of *E. coli*), so a sorbitol/MacConkey agar is a common medium used for the detection of this organism. Most enteric bacteria grow on blood agar, so *E. coli* O157 would be overgrown with the normal intestinal bacterial flora. The important virulence factors produced by this organism are Shiga toxin and Shiga-like toxin (formerly known as verotoxins because they cause a cytopathic effect in the Vero cell line). These toxins can be detected by immunoassays; however, performing an immunoassay for A and B toxins is not the correct test because these toxins are found in *Clostridium difficile*, not *E. coli* O157. *Campylobacter*, not *E. coli*, is cultured on selective agar incubated in a microaerophilic atmosphere.
MM5 337-338, 350, 411-413

102   (D) Lysis of phagosome and replication in cytoplasm. *L. monocytogenes* is a facultative intracellular pathogen that can grow in macrophages and epithelial cells. Following penetration into the cells, the acid pH of the phagolysosome activates a bacterial exotoxin (listeriolysin O) and two phospholipase C enzymes. The activities of this toxin and two enzymes lead to lysis of the phagolysosome and release of the bacteria into the cell cytosol.
MM5 198-201, 273-274

103   (B) Detection of specific antibodies. Although *C. burnetii* can be grown in vitro, this is rarely performed. The bacteria do not grow on blood agar. Likewise, the bacteria stain poorly with the Gram stain, so this would be an unreliable test. The most commonly used test for documenting *C. burnetii* infections,

particularly in chronic disease such as endocarditis, is the serological detection of specific antibodies directed against the bacterial LPS antigen. *C. burnetii* undergoes a phase variation in expressing the cell wall LPS antigen. Two phases of this antigen are typically expressed (phase I and phase II antigens). Phase I antigens are weakly immunogenic; therefore the antibody response in acute disease is typically directed against the phase II antigen. In chronic disease, antibodies against both antigens are detected, the phase I antibodies typically at a higher level. These antibodies may also contribute to the pathology of *C. burnetii* disease (Q fever) because high antibody levels lead to the formation of immune complexes that have been implicated in some of the observed pathology. Although cellular immunity is important in clinical recovery, a skin test documenting human disease is not available. Likewise, antigen detection tests have not been developed.
MM5 460-462

104   (D) L-pyrrolidonyl-arylamidase (PYR) test. The PYR test is a rapid identification test for enterococci. The other important gram-positive coccus that is PYR-positive is *Streptococcus pyogenes* (group A *Streptococcus*). The PYR test, in combination with the Gram stain and a few other simple, rapid tests, can also be used to identify the enterococci. Bile solubility is used to identify *Streptococcus pneumoniae;* coagulase to identify *Staphylococcus aureus;* germ tube formation to identify *Candida albicans;* and bacitracin susceptibility to identify *Streptococcus pyogenes.*
MM5 246-247

105   (D) Lyme disease. Lyme disease is the most common vector-borne disease in the United States, with 15,000 to 20,000 cases of disease reported each year and many more infections undiagnosed or reported. Ticks are the vector responsible for this disease. Infections from *Babesia microti*, the etiologic agent of babesiosis, and *Ehrlichia*, the agent of ehrlichiosis, are transmitted by ticks. *Yersinia pestis*, the agent responsible for plague, is transmitted by fleas. None of these diseases is as common as Lyme disease. Legionnaire's disease, caused by *Legionella*, is not vector-borne.
MM5 435-437

106   (D) Group B *Streptococcus agalactiae.* The bacteria associated with meningitis in newborns are *S. agalactiae* and *Escherichia coli*. *H. influenzae* was at one time a common cause of meningitis in children ages 3 months to 5 years; however, immunization of infants has essentially eliminated this disease in developed countries. *N. meningitidis* and *S. pneumoniae* are common causes of bacterial meningitis but in older children and adults. *S. enteritidis* is an uncommon cause of meningitis and does cause disseminated disease in children.
MM5 474, 484

107   (A) Endothelial cells. After transmission of *Rickettsia rickettsii* from an infected tick to a human host, the *Rickettsia* organisms multiply in the endothelial cells at the site of the bite.

Subsequent cycles of replication lead to further endothelial cell damage, as well as damage to the vascular smooth muscle cells. The primary clinical manifestations of Rocky Mountain spotted fever are caused by vascular leakage with resulting hypovolemia and hypoproteinemia caused by reduced perfusion of various organs and the loss of plasma into tissues. The characteristic rash is caused by dilation of small blood vessels at the site of rickettsial replication. Pulmonary symptoms result from damage to the pulmonary vascular system with resulting leakage of fluid into the interstitial tissue, pneumonitis, and pulmonary edema. Encephalitis can result from damage to the vascular system of the brain.
MM5 449-451

108   (C) *Salmonella typhi.* MacConkey agar is a selective, differential agar. Only gram-negative rods grow on this agar, and if the organism ferments lactose, pink-purple colonies will be seen. Nonlactose-fermenting organisms will form colorless colonies on this agar. *E. coli* O157 and *Y. enterocolitica* will be pink on this agar (*Y. enterocolitica* is a slow fermenter of lactose). *S. choleraesuis*, *S. typhi*, and *S. sonnei* will form colorless colonies on MacConkey agar and red colonies on XLD agar; *E. coli* will be yellow on XLD, and *Y. enterocolitica* will not grow on this medium. Both *Salmonella* species will have an alkaline over acid reaction with hydrogen sulfide production on TSI; *S. sonnei* does not produce hydrogen sulfide. In contrast with *S. choleraesuis*, *S. typhi* produces minute quantities of hydrogen sulfide. *S. choleraesuis* produces gas on TSI, whereas *S. typhi* does not. The appearance of the TSI agar slant is very characteristic of *S. typhi*. If this is observed, agglutination tests with the organism should be performed to demonstrate the presence of the somatic group D antigen and the heat-labile capsular Vi antigen (definitive tests for *S. typhi*).
MM5 337

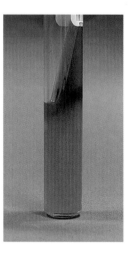

109   (E) Initiates premature release of peptide chains from ribosome. Quinupristin-dalfopristin is a member of the streptogramin class of antibiotics. Dalfopristin binds to the 50S ribosomal subunit and induces a conformational change that facilitates binding of quinupristin. Dalfopristin prevents peptide chain elongation, and quinupristin initiates premature release of peptide chains from the ribosome.
MM5 210

110   (C) The organism does not have a capsule. Bacteria that are part of the normal nasopharyngeal flora cause most sinus infections; these bacteria include *Haemophilus influenzae*, *Streptococcus pneumoniae*, *Moraxella catarrhalis*, and *Staphylococcus aureus*. The most common *H. influenzae* strains in the nasopharynx and associated with sinusitis are nontypeable strains. That is, the bacteria do not have a capsule or, if a capsule is present, do not have PRP in the capsule. This fact is important because the agglutination tests used to detect *H. influenzae* will only detect *H. influenzae* type B, which is the only strain that has PRP in the capsule.
MM5 369-372

111   (A) Binds to globotriaosylceramide (Gb₃) receptors. The patient is infected with *Escherichia coli* O157 and has the complication of HUS. *E. coli* O157 produces Shiga and Shiga-like toxins. These toxins bind to Gb₃ surface receptors and are transported into the specific cells. The receptors are on a number of cells but most commonly in the intestinal epithelium and the renal endothelium. Internalization of the toxin leads to termination of protein synthesis and cell death. *Clostridium difficile* produces two toxins: (i) an enterotoxin that is chemotactic for neutrophils (as described in answer B) and responsible for the hemorrhagic necrosis characteristic of *C. difficile* pseudomembranous colitis and (ii) a cytotoxin that produces actin depolymerization (as described in answer D). *Shigella* and other bacteria are able to introduce bacterial proteins into host cells via a type III secretion system (as described in answer C). In the example of *Shigella*, four proteins are transferred into epithelial cells and macrophages, which induce membrane rearrangements and phagocytosis of the bacteria. In their intracellular location, the bacteria are able to proliferate. Toxigenic *E. coli* and other enteric pathogens produce toxins that stimulate an increase in cAMP levels with resulting hypersecretion of fluid (as described in answer E).
MM5 329-330, 332-333

112   (C) Measurement of antistreptolysin O (ASO) antibodies. Rheumatic fever is an immunologically based reaction to *Streptococcus pyogenes* infection of the pharynx. Antibodies develop 3 to 4 weeks after the initial infection. An elevated ASO titer is observed in patients with a pharyngeal infection. Two forms of streptokinase are produced by *S. pyogenes*, but these do not appear to be sensitive or specific markers for rheumatic fever. Because this disease is an immunologic reaction to strains producing pharyngitis, culture of blood and synovial fluid and the microscopic examination of skin nodules are not helpful.
MM5 247

113 (D) Neisseria meningitidis. Although *N. gonorrhoeae* is the most common species responsible for urethritis, which is this man's condition, the growth properties and biochemical test results are inconsistent with this organism. *N. gonorrhoeae* does not produce acid in maltose and does not grow on blood agar or nutrient agar. In contrast, *N. meningitidis* can grow on nutrient agar (not all strains) and produces acid in both glucose and maltose. *N. lactamica* can grow on Thayer-Martin medium as well as nutrient agar and produces acid in glucose and maltose but also in lactose. *N. sicca* does not grow on Thayer-Martin medium and produces acid in glucose and maltose as well as in sucrose. *M. catarrhalis* does not grow on Thayer-Martin agar and does not produce acid in any of the listed sugars.
MM5 316-317

114 (E) Stenotrophomonas maltophilia. *S. maltophilia* is a ubiquitous environmental organism that is isolated with increasing frequency as a source of hospital-acquired pulmonary infections. The organism is resistant to many antibiotics, which pose treatment problems. The typical setting for infections with this organism is as described in this case—a patient with a prolonged hospitalization who has received a variety of broad-spectrum antibiotics. The morphology of the organism and the biochemical properties separate *S. maltophilia* from the other organisms listed in the answers to this question. *A. baumannii* is typically susceptible to imipenem (although resistance has been described); *B. pseudomallei* is oxidase positive; *L. pneumophila* has specialized growth requirements and would not grow on blood agar or MacConkey agar; and *P. aeruginosa* is resistant to trimethoprim/sulfamethoxazole and has a fluorescent green color and sweet fruity odor.
MM5 364

115 (B) Endocarditis of a prosthetic heart valve. The coagulase-negative staphylococci are associated with infections localized on foreign bodies, such as catheters, shunts, and prosthetic valves and joints. The bacteria are able to adhere to the surface of the synthetic materials by production of a slime layer. This layer in turn protects the bacteria from phagocytosis and the effects of antibiotics. A brain abscess is typically caused by a polymicrobic infection of aerobic and anaerobic bacteria. Intraabdominal infections or abscesses are most commonly caused by *Bacteroides fragilis*, whereas osteomyelitis and wound infections are most commonly the result of *Staphylococcus aureus*.
MM5 233

116 (E) Vancomycin. This woman's infection is caused by *Staphylococcus*, with *S. aureus* being the most likely organism because the infection develops shortly after the surgery. Oxacillin resistance in staphylococci develops as a result of acquisition of the *mec*A gene that codes for a novel penicillin-binding protein, PBP2′. Oxacillin interferes with bacterial cell wall synthesis by binding to enzymes (i.e., penicillin-binding proteins, PBPs) that catalyze construction of the cell wall peptidoglycan layer. PBP2′

retains its enzymatic activity but is not bound and inactivated by oxacillin or other beta-lactam antibiotics. Thus production of PBP2′ renders the organism resistant to all beta-lactam antibiotics. Only vancomycin would be active against this organism.
MM5 234-235

117 (A) Acetylation of an antibiotic. Chloramphenicol is a bacteriostatic antibiotic that binds reversibly to the peptidyl-transferase component of the 50S ribosomal subunit, thus blocking peptide elongation. Resistance to chloramphenicol is observed in bacteria producing plasmid-encoded chloramphenicol acetyltransferase, which catalyzes the acetylation of the 3-hydroxy group of chloramphenicol. The resulting antibiotic molecule is unable to bind to the 50S subunit.
MM5 210

118 (C) Campylobacter jejuni. The Guillain-Barré syndrome is an autoimmune disorder of the peripheral nervous system characterized by the development of symmetrical weakness over a period of several days and recovery requiring weeks to months. It is believed that antibodies directed against *Campylobacter* oligosaccharides cross-react with glycosphingolipids present on the surface of neural tissues.
MM5 347-349

119 (D) Rice. The most commonly implicated source of infection with *B. cereus* is contaminated rice. *Bacillus* spores contaminate rice. When the rice is cooked, the spores are stimulated to germinate. If the rice is left in a warmer, the spores can release an enterotoxin. Reheating the rice will not destroy the preformed toxin even though the bacteria may be killed. Hence, diagnosis of *B. cereus* food poisoning is based on clinical and epidemiologic evidence rather than on laboratory tests such as stool cultures.
MM5 369-370

120 (B) Elastase. This patient has an infection with *Pseudomonas aeruginosa*. The lesions described are characteristic of ecthyma gangrenosum. Although *P. aeruginosa* produces a variety of toxins and other virulence factors, two elastases are thought to be responsible for the skin lesions: LasA, a serine protease, and LasB, a zinc metalloprotease. They act synergistically to degrade elastin, resulting in damage to elastin-containing tissues. The enzymes also degrade complement components and inhibit neutrophil chemotaxis and function, leading to further spread and tissue damage. Alkaline protease produces localized tissue damage; endotoxin mediates the various biologic effects of the sepsis syndrome; exotoxin A inhibits host cell protein synthesis; and pyocyanin mediates tissue damage through production of toxic oxygen radicals.
MM5 357-360

121 (D) Nocardia asteroides. *Nocardia* organisms are slow-growing, filamentous gram-positive rods. Although *Nocardia* can resemble *Actinomyces* on Gram stain, *N. asteroides* is differentiated from *A. israelii* by the ability of *N. asteroides* to grow aerobically and stain with the acid-fast stain. *Nocardia* is not fastidious and can grow on a variety of media, including BCYE (developed for *Legionella*), Sabouraud dextrose agar (used for fungi), and Lowenstein-Jensen agar (used for mycobacteria). *L. micdadei* is acid-fast when the clinical specimen is stained but loses this property when grown in culture. *L. micdadei* species can grow on BCYE agar but not on the other media listed in this question. *M. chelonae* is acid-fast and will grow on most media, but it is not filamentous and has not been associated with the clinical picture described here. *R. equi* will stain weakly with acid-fast stains and can grow on all the media listed, but it is also not filamentous. When *R. equi* is observed in young cultures, it will appear rod-like; however, in older cultures the organism will appear coccoid.

MM5 287-292

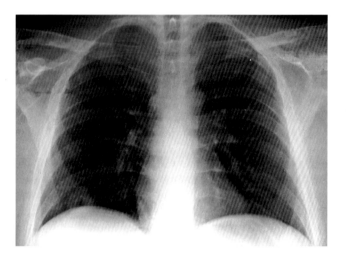

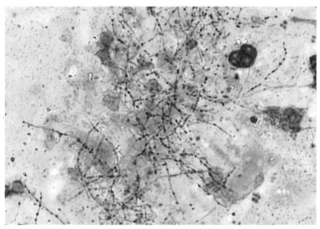

122 **(E) Transpeptidases.** The beta-lactam antibiotics function by binding to the enzymes responsible for construction of the peptidoglycan layer in the bacterial cell wall. If the enzymes are inactivated, then construction of the peptidoglycan layer is disrupted. These enzymes include transpeptidases, carboxypeptidases, and endopeptidases. These enzymes are collectively referred to as penicillin-binding proteins or PBPs. Gram-positive bacteria use an amino acid bridge (e.g., pentaglycine bridge) to cross-link the peptidoglycan chains. Although the assembly of the peptidoglycan is affected by the beta-lactamas, the antibiotics do not bind to the major components of the peptidoglycan (e.g., glycan chains, peptide cross-links). The antibiotics only bind to the proteins (enzymes) responsible for the assembly of the peptidoglycan layer. The antibiotics also do not bind to LPS or teichoic acid (other important structural components of the bacterial cell wall).

MM5 18-19

123 **(D) DNA/DNA hybridization.** Bacterial classification was performed historically by defining a number of phenotypic properties (e.g., Gram stain morphology, macroscopic morphology, biochemical reactivity) that could be used to separate organisms into discrete groups. The medical microbiology field has realized that this system has practical applications in the clinical laboratory but that it also has significant limitations as a taxonomic tool. Bacteria can lose a specific property (e.g., most strains of *Escherichia coli* can ferment lactose, but this property is lost by some strains). Sequencing of the 16S rRNA gene is used commonly in clinical laboratories for classification of organisms at the species or genus level, but this method cannot be used for all organisms. The best example of this is the observation that *Bacillus anthracis* and *Bacillus cereus* have the same 16S rRNA gene sequence. Use of the G + C ratio is helpful for placing organisms in large categories (e.g., families or orders), but the ratio is not useful for separating species or genera. Analysis of DNA fragments by PFGE is a valuable technique for separating organisms at a subspecies level for epidemiologic purposes, but this technique cannot be used for classification of species or genera. DNA-DNA hybridization is a method that assesses the total homology of the genomes of organisms. As total genome sequencing becomes more widespread, this method will replace DNA-DNA hybridization as the definitive method for taxonomic classification of bacteria.

MM5 8

124 **(E) *Mycobacterium tuberculosis.*** Two key tests for the biochemical identification of *M. tuberculosis* are the niacin and nitrate reductase tests. *M. tuberculosis* is the only commonly isolated mycobacterium that is positive with both tests. Some strains of *M. chelonae* will be niacin-positive, but all the other bacteria listed in the answers to this question will be negative. In addition to *M. tuberculosis*, *M. kansasii* and *M. fortuitum* are positive for nitrate reductase. Although biochemical identification of some common mycobacteria have now been replaced with molecular-based identification tests, many small laboratories still rely on the biochemical tests for a definitive identification.

MM5 305-308

125 **(B) Enterohemorrhagic *E. coli.*** All five groups of *E. coli* in the answers to this question have been implicated as causes of gastroenteritis. Infections with ETEC, EPEC, and EAEC are generally restricted to the small intestine, whereas infections with

EHEC and EIEC primarily involve the colon. The patients in this report had colitis, with or without blood. The other 10% of the patients developed hemolytic uremic syndrome (HUS), which is characterized by acute renal failure, microangiopathic hemolytic anemia, thrombocytopenia, hypertension, and central nervous system manifestations. EHEC but not EIEC is frequently associated with HUS in children.

MM5 326-330

126 (D) Panton-Valentine (PV) leukocidin. PV leukocidin has been associated with strains of methicillin-resistant *S. aureus* that cause severe necrotizing pneumonia and skin lesions. Alpha-toxin is a cytotoxin that is important in staphylococcal infections, but it has not been specifically associated with necrotizing pneumonia. Enterotoxins produced by *S. aureus* are responsible for staphylococcal food poisoning. Exfoliative toxin is responsible for scalded skin syndrome, and TSST-1 is responsible for toxin shock syndrome.

MM5 223-226, 232

127 (E) Use of respiratory therapy equipment. *P. aeruginosa* is a ubiquitous organism that is present in and on moist surfaces throughout hospitals. These areas would include sinks, drains, and moist reservoirs, such as respiratory therapy equipment. Care must be used to maintain the equipment so nosocomial infections such as this one do not occur. Because *P. aeruginosa*, like other gram-negative bacteria, has an outer lipid membrane, the organism must remain moist for it to survive. For this reason, acquisition of infections in aerosols is unlikely for gram-negative bacteria. Infection can occur by contact with medical personnel or by ingestion of contaminated hospital food, but these are less likely sources. Intravenous line infections with *P. aeruginosa* can occur but would not present initially as bronchopneumonia.

MM5 360

128 (C) Bacteria are phagocytosed but then prevent phagosome/lysosome fusion. Members of the family Chlamydiaceae are intracellular parasites. They are able to escape intracellular killing by preventing fusion of phagosomes and lysosomes. If the outer membrane of the bacteria is damaged or the bacteria are inactivated by heat, phagolysosome fusion can occur with subsequent bacterial death. During the replication cycle, the infectious elementary body of the bacteria is reorganized into the noninfectious, replicating reticulate body. Toward the end of the replication cycle, the bacteria are reorganized into the elementary bodies that are released when the infected cell ruptures and then infect other cells.

MM5 463-464

129 (E) *Streptococcus pyogenes*. This is a classic presentation of scarlet fever, caused by *S. pyogenes* (group A *Streptococcus*). Infection initially develops as pharyngitis, although a wound infection may occur. The distribution of the rash and the more intense inflammation along the skin folds (Pastia sign) is characteristic of the scarlatiniform rash. *B. pertussis* produces a primary infection of the throat and emits a toxin that mediates the systemic signs of disease (whooping cough); however, the clinical presentation of the rash is not consistent with *B. pertussis* infection. *H. influenzae*, *S. aureus*, and *S. pneumoniae* colonize the oropharynx but do not typically cause pharyngitis or an associated rash.

MM5 243

130 (E) *Vibrio vulnificus*. *V. vulnificus*, a particularly virulent species of *Vibrio*, is associated with serious wound infections and septicemia. Exposure to contaminated seawater and consumption of contaminated raw shellfish are the most common sources of infection. Infections are most severe in patients with hepatic disease, hematopoietic disease, or chronic renal failure and in those patients receiving immunosuppressive drugs. *Vibrio* species are oxidase-positive and are able to ferment glucose, a relatively uncommon trait. *A. baumannii* and *S. maltophilia* oxidize glucose but are oxidase-negative. *B. cepacia* oxidizes glucose and is oxidase-positive. *E. coli* ferments glucose and is oxidase-negative.

MM5 343

131 (B) Soft tick. Endemic relapsing fever can be caused by more than 15 species of *Borrelia*. Many rodents, small animals (e.g., rabbits, squirrels), and soft ticks are the reservoir for these *Borrelia* organisms. Transmission of *Borrelia* organisms from animal-to-animal or to humans is by the bite of an infected tick. The bacteria multiply in the tick and are present in the saliva and feces of the tick. The other arthropods listed in the answers to this question (i.e., flea, louse, mite, mosquito) do not transmit this disease.

MM5 435-436

132 (D) Urine refrigerated at 4° to 8°C after collection. Refrigeration of urine prevents overgrowth with small numbers of bacteria that can contaminate the specimen during collection. The bacteria that commonly cause urinary tract infections are not adversely affected by refrigeration. Preservatives (e.g., boric acid) can also be used to suppress the contaminants. A midstream urine specimen should not be submitted for anaerobic culture. All anaerobic specimens must be collected in a way to avoid any contamination with the patient's normal bacterial flora. In the case of a urine culture, this means that the specimen should be collected by suprapubic aspiration. The collection of sputum during a period of 24 h for a mycobacterial culture should not be processed because large numbers of contaminating bacteria are usually present. Although respiratory specimens processed for mycobacteria are typically treated with agents to eliminate contaminating organisms, the treatment of specimens with large numbers of contaminants will frequently need to be prolonged, resulting in the loss of mycobacteria, as well as the contaminating bacteria. Patients with bacteremia typically have very few organisms in the blood. Therefore a large volume of blood (e.g., approximately 10 ml for a 10-year-old boy) must be cultured. *Streptococcus pneumoniae* and *Neisseria meningitidis* are important causes of meningitis. Both of these organisms are sensitive to cold temperatures and will not survive in refrigerated specimens, such as cerebrospinal fluid.

MM5 213-219

133 **(A)** *Acinetobacter baumannii.* All organisms listed in the answers are gram-negative rods that can grow on the media listed in the question. *Acinetobacter* is an important cause of nosocomial pneumonia and is oxidase-negative, a nonfermenter, as well as a strict aerobic bacterium. *B. cepacia* is oxidase-positive; *E. cloacae* is a fermenter that grows aerobically and anaerobically (i.e., facultative anaerobe); *P. aeruginosa* is oxidase-positive; and *S. maltophilia* is one of the few organisms that is always resistant to imipenem.

MM5 364-365

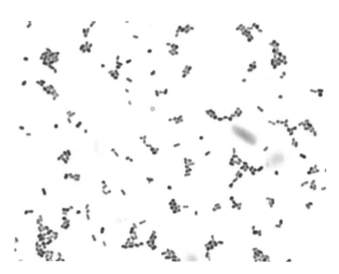

134 **(D)** **Modification of the pentapeptide side chain in cell wall peptidoglycan.** Vancomycin disrupts cell wall peptidoglycan synthesis in growing gram-positive bacteria. The antibiotic interacts with the D-alanine-D-alanine termini of the pentapeptide side chains and interferes sterically with the formation of the bridges between the peptidoglycan chains. Vancomycin is inactive against gram-negative bacteria because the molecule is too large to pass through the outer membrane and reach the peptidoglycan target site. Gram-positive bacteria that are resistant to vancomycin have an alteration in the pentapeptide chain. For example, the pentapeptide chain in *Leuconostoc, Lactobacillus, Pediococcus,* and *Erysipelothrix* terminates in D-alanine-D-lactate, which does not bind vancomycin. The pentapeptide chain in *Enterococcus gallinarum* and *Enterococcus casseliflavus* terminate in D-alanine-D-serine.

MM5 207-208

135 **(A)** *Enterococcus avium.* Vancomycin disrupts cell wall synthesis of gram-positive bacteria by interacting with the D-alanine-D-alanine termini of the pentapeptide bridges that cross-link the peptidoglycan chains. *E. casseliflavus* and *E.*

gallinarum have chromosomally mediated intrinsic resistance to vancomycin (they have intrinsic genes that code for D-alanine-D-serine termini). *E. faecalis* and *E. faecium* have acquired resistance that is most commonly represented with the acquisition of a plasmid with either the *van*A or *van*B gene (that encodes the D-alanine-D-lactate termini). All other species of *Enterococcus* are currently considered susceptible to vancomycin.

MM5 207-208, 259, 262

136 **(B)** *Burkholderia cepacia.* *B. cepacia* is a ubiquitous environmental organism. Although all individuals are exposed to this organism and transient colonization can occur, patients with cystic fibrosis are particularly susceptible to colonization, which causes them to develop pneumonia. *B. cepacia* and to a lesser extent *P. aeruginosa* are responsible for the overwhelming majority of pulmonary infections in cystic fibrosis patients. The dirt-like odor and slow growth of the organism on MacConkey agar are useful differential characteristics that separate *B. cepacia* and *P. aeruginosa*. Like *P. aeruginosa*, *B. cepacia* is oxidase-positive and uses carbohydrates oxidatively but not fermentatively. *A. baumannii* is an oxidative gram-negative rod that is oxidase-negative; *K. pneumoniae* is an oxidase-negative, fermentative gram-negative rod; *S. maltophilia* is an oxidase-negative, oxidative gram-negative rod that is characteristically resistant to imipenem and other carbapenems.

MM5 363-364

137 **(B)** **Epiglottitis: blood culture.** The general rule is that specimens submitted for culture should be collected from the site of the infection. The exception to this rule is epiglottitis. The opening of the epiglottis is narrow, particularly in children. An attempt to collect a specimen from this site can result in spasms and complete airway obstruction. A reliable and safer specimen would be blood because most patients with epiglottitis are bacteremic. Pus collected from an abscess frequently contains few viable organisms. A preferred specimen would be to collect material at the edge of the lesion, where the bacteria should be actively growing. Otitis media is an infection of the middle ear. A swab of the outer ear does not represent the organism(s) responsible for the infection. The middle ear should be aspirated by tympanocentesis. Likewise, specimens from the nasopharynx do not represent the organisms responsible for sinusitis. A bacteriologic diagnosis can only be made by aspirating the sinus. To determine urethritis, the laboratory will analyze the first voided portion of urine that contains the organisms responsible for the infection of the urethra. Because most organisms are eliminated with the initial voided specimen, a midstream urine specimen cannot be used to diagnose urethritis. In contrast, a midstream specimen is preferred for diagnosing cystitis and pyelonephritis.

MM5 214

138 **(D)** **Streptomycin.** Streptomycin is the drug of choice for treating infections with *F. tularensis*. Ceftriaxone and penicillin are ineffective because they are inactivated by beta-lactamases

produced by *F. tularensis*. Chloramphenicol and tetracycline have been associated with a high rate of relapse.
MM5 386-389

139 (E) Rabbits. *F. tularensis* is able to infect a wide variety of animals including many wild mammals, domestic dogs and cats, birds, fish, and blood-sucking arthropods. The most common reservoirs of *F. tularensis* in the United States are rabbits, muskrats, and ticks. Most human infections are acquired by the bite of a tick or contact with an infected rabbit or with a pet that has caught an infected rabbit. Birds, cattle, deer, and fleas do not serve as a natural reservoir or vector for tularemia.
MM5 386-389

140 (C) Inhibits DNA topoisomerase. Levofloxacin is a fluoroquinolone antibiotic with excellent activity against gram-positive and gram-negative bacteria. This antibiotic inhibits the activity of DNA topoisomerases, which are required for DNA replication, recombination, and repair.
MM5 210-211

141 (B) *Francisella tularensis*. This man's condition is an example of pulmonary tularemia. Clues to this answer are exposure to a sick rabbit (rabbits and ticks are important hosts for *F. tularensis* in endemic areas in the United States, including Missouri); slow growth on chocolate and BCYE agars (both contain cysteine that is required by *F. tularensis* for growth); and the Gram stain morphology. *B. parapertussis* causes a mild pertussis-like illness; *L. pneumophila* will grow on BCYE agar (originally developed for the isolation of *Legionella*) but not on chocolate agar; *N. meningitidis* is a gram-negative diplococci; and *P. aeruginosa* is a gram-negative rod that is significantly larger than *F. tularensis*.
MM5 386-389

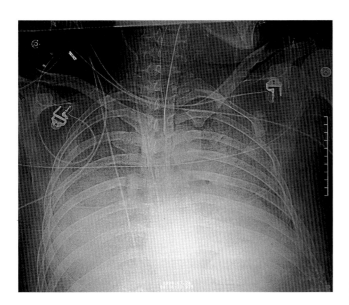

142 (E) Modification of the ribosomal binding site. Clindamycin blocks protein elongation by binding to the 50S ribosome. It inhibits peptidyltransferase by interfering with the binding of the aminoacyl-tRNA complex. Methylation of the 23S ribosomal RNA prevents binding of clindamycin to the 50S ribosome and is the source of bacterial resistance.
MM5 210

143 (B) Inhibition of phagosome/lysosome fusion. Bacteria have developed a number of mechanisms by which they either avoid phagocytosis or avoid intracellular death once they have been phagocytosed. Two examples of bacteria that can survive phagocytosis and replicate in a protected intracellular environment are *Brucella* and *Francisella*. Both organisms are able to prevent phagosome/lysosome fusion. *Francisella* and many other organisms, such as *Streptococcus pneumoniae*, have capsules that protect them from phagocytosis. *Bordetella* produces an adenylate cyclase toxin that inhibits leukocyte chemotaxis. *Listeria* is able to grow intracellularly because it is able to lyse the phagosome before it is fused with the lysosome. Many bacteria (e.g., *Clostridia*, *Pseudomonas*) produce phospholipase C that is capable of lysing cell membranes (e.g., red blood cell and white blood cell membranes).
MM5 383, 387

144 (D) *Streptococcus pneumoniae*. Most species of streptococci are susceptible to penicillin; however, resistance is being reported for some species of streptococci in the viridans group. This group of organisms consists of at least 24 heterogeneous species that are organized taxonomically into five subgroups. Some of the most important species belong to the mitis group and include *S. pneumoniae*. Penicillin resistance has primarily been restricted to this group of streptococci. Group B *S. agalactiae* and group A *S. pyogenes* are not classified with the viridans streptococci and are uniformly susceptible to penicillin. *S. anginosus* is a viridans streptococcus that causes pyogenic infections (e.g., intraabdominal abscesses). All strains are susceptible to penicillin. Likewise, *S. bovis*, an intestinal streptococcus associated with colonic carcinoma, is susceptible to penicillin.
MM5 256-257

145 (B) *Haemophilus influenzae*. The major serotype of *H. influenzae* associated with disease is type B. *H. influenzae* type B was a major cause of pediatric morbidity and mortality before the conjugated, polysaccharide vaccine was introduced. The major virulence factor in *H. influenzae* type B is the antiphagocytic polysaccharide capsule, which contains ribose, ribitol, and phosphate (referred to as polyribitol phosphate or PRP). Antibodies directed against the capsule stimulate bacterial phagocytosis and complement-mediated bactericidal activity. The immunogenicity of polysaccharides can be enhanced by chemical linkage to a protein carrier (conjugated vaccine). Conjugated vaccines are used to stimulate immunity against diphtheria toxin, *N. meningitidis*, *Corynebacterium diphtheriae*, as well as *H. influenzae*.
MM5 160-162, 369-370

146 **(B)** *Haemophilus ducreyi.* *H. ducreyi* is responsible for chancroid or soft chancre. This sexually transitted disease presents as a painful ulcer with associated lymphadenopathy. Recovery of this organism in culture can be difficult. The best medium appears to be guanine and cytosine (GC) agar supplemented with hemoglobin, fetal bovine serum, CVA enrichment, and vancomycin incubated at 33°C in a carbon dioxide–enriched atmosphere for up to 1 week. The clinical diagnosis for this patient is confirmed by the Gram stain results. *C. trachomatis,* herpes simplex virus, and *T. pallidum* would not be seen by Gram stain. *N. gonorrhoeae* would appear as gram-negative diplococci and is not associated with genital ulcers.

MM5 368-372

147 **(E)** **Toxin-mediated disruption of protein synthesis with destruction of intestinal microvilli.** *E. coli* O157 is considered an enterohemorrhagic *E. coli,* referring to the colitis with bloody stools that is characteristic of this infection. The pathology is mediated by the Shiga (Stx-1) or Shiga-like (Stx-2) toxins. The toxins bind to specific glycolipid receptors on the surface of many cells, most notably in the intestinal villi and renal endothelial cells. Transfer of a toxin subunit into the cell leads to disruption of protein synthesis and cell death. Various other strains of *E. coli* can produce gastrointestinal disease by a variety of mechanisms. These include enteroaggregative *E. coli* (such as in answer A), enterotoxigenic *E. coli* that produce a heat-labile (answer B) and a heat-stable (answer C) enterotoxin, and enteroinvasive *E. coli* (answer D) that can invade the colonic epithelium and cause cell death.

MM5 329-330

148 **(C)** **Exotoxin that causes unregulated cyclic adenosine monophosphate levels.** The child has pertussis caused by *Bordetella pertussis.* This is a small, gram-negative rod that grows only on media supplemented with charcoal, starch, blood, or albumin to absorb the toxic substances present in agar. Nicotinamide is also required for growth. These growth requirements are present in Bordet-Gengou medium, charcoal-horse blood agar, or Regan-Lowe medium. *B. pertussis* produces a number of adhesions and toxins that are important for its virulence. Pertussis toxin is an A-B toxin consisting of a toxic subunit (S1) and five binding subunits (S2 to S5 with two S4 subunits). The S2 subunit binds to a glycolipid present on ciliated epithelial cells. The S3 subunit binds to receptors on phagocytic cells, initiating phagocytic uptake, where the intracellular bacteria can survive. The S1 subunit has adenosine diphosphate-ribosylating activity for the membrane surface G protein. This interaction causes cyclic adenosine monophosphate levels to be unregulated, resulting in increased respiratory secretions and mucus production characteristic of the paroxysmal stage of pertussis (stage of disease characterized by repetitive coughing with whoops during inspiration, vomiting, and leukocytosis).

MM5 377-378, 380-381

149 **(D)** **Organism normally found in the oropharynx.** Organisms responsible for otitis media normally originate in the oropharynx. They spread through the eustachian tube into the middle ear. The patient typically experiences a preceding or concurrent upper respiratory tract infection that causes congestion of the eustachian tube opening. Infections of the outer ear (otitis externa) can originate from the ear or adjacent skin surface (e.g., infections caused by *Staphylococcus aureus*) or by exposure to contaminated water ("swimmer's ear" caused by *Pseudomonas aeruginosa*).

MM5 483

150 **(C)** **Culture on selective media.** The laboratory diagnosis of *Legionella* infections is difficult. The bacteria were first observed in clinical specimens using the Dieterle silver stain. Although this stain is still commonly used in surgical pathology laboratories, it is insensitive and nonspecific. The direct fluorescent antibody stain detects *Legionella* using fluorescein-labeled monoclonal antibodies; however, this stain can detect only selected serotypes of *Legionella pneumophila* and *Legionella micdadei.* Cross-reactions with non-*Legionella* bacteria have also been reported. The current tests, such as EIA, to detect *Legionella* antigens are primarily restricted to *L. pneumophila* serogroup 1. Although this is the most commonly isolated strain of *Legionella,* many other serogroups and species are associated with disease. Serologic confirmation of *Legionella* infections is slow (e.g., seroconversion may take 3 or more weeks) and may not be observed if antibiotic treatment is initiated early in the course of disease. Antibodies may also persist for many weeks or months. Therefore the most sensitive and specific test for confirming the diagnosis is culture on selective media. *Legionella* requires growth on a medium supplemented with iron salts and L-cysteine. The most commonly used medium is BCYE agar. Antibiotics are also added to the medium to suppress the growth of rapidly growing contaminating organisms.

MM5 391, 394-395

151 **(D)** *Listeria monocytogenes.* All of the bacteria listed in the answers to this question are gram-positive. *L. monocytogenes* organisms typically appear as gram-positive coccobacilli arranged in pairs or singularly. The positive catalase and motility reactions are consistent with *Listeria.* Pregnant women are at increased risk of infection, with most infections either presenting as asymptomatic or as a mild influenza-like illness. *B. anthracis,* the etiologic agent of anthrax, is a nonmotile, catalase-positive spore-forming rod that produces nonhemolytic colonies. *B. cereus* is a motile, catalase-positive spore-forming rod that produces strongly beta-hemolytic colonies. *C. ulcerans* is a catalase-positive, coryneform rod that rarely causes human disease, although the diphtheria toxin gene may be carried by this organism. *Streptococcus agalactiae* (group B streptococcus) is an important pathogen in pregnant women and neonates. It is a gram-positive cocci that is weakly beta-hemolytic and nonmotile.

MM5 273-277

152 (C) *Salmonella enteritidis.* *Salmonella* binds to the M cells by specific fimbriae. *Salmonella*-secreted invasion proteins are then introduced into the cell, which leads to membrane rearrangement and engulfment of the bacteria. The bacteria then replicate with subsequent host cell death and spread to adjacent cells. Enteroinvasive *E. coli* and *S. sonnei* invade the colonic epithelium. Enterohemorrhagic *E. coli* disrupts colonic epithelium without invasion into the cells. *V. cholerae* produces a toxin-mediated hypersecretion of intestinal fluids without cell invasion.
MM5 330-331

153 (E) **The most important factor for recovering bacteria in blood cultures is to collect a large volume of blood.** Bacteremic patients typically have an organism count of less than 1/ml of blood. The success of detecting bacteria in blood is directly related to the volume of blood collected for culture. It is recommended that each culture should consist of 20 ml of blood for adults and proportionately less blood for children and infants. In contrast with bacteremic patients, most patients with untreated meningitis have a bacterial count of at least 10^5/ml of cerebrospinal fluid. Although cystitis was historically defined as the bacterial count of 10^5/ml of urine, it is now appreciated that the majority of patients with cystitis have fewer organisms (as few as 100/ml). Patients with intravascular infections (e.g., subacute bacterial endocarditis) have persistent bacteremia. All blood cultures should be positive if an adequate volume of blood is cultured. Patients with bacterial gastroenteritis typically have the largest number of pathogens in their intestine at the time the symptoms begin. The numbers of organisms will rapidly decrease with the frequent bowel movements. Therefore the best opportunity to detect the pathogen is to collect the stool specimen as early as possible in the course of the disease.
MM5 213-219

154 (D) *Nocardia brasiliensis.* Each of the organisms listed in the answers to this question can cause localized skin infections presenting as this patient's infection. *N. brasiliensis* infections are primary cutaneous infections with the organism introduced into the subcutaneous layer of the skin through trauma. The organism grows slowly (3 to 5 days are generally required before colonies are seen) and can grow on most nonselective laboratory media. The best growth of *Nocardia* species has been reported on BCYE agar. Trimethoprim/sulfamethoxazole has historically been the drug of choice for treating an *N. brasiliensis* infection, but other drugs such as ciprofloxacin and imipenem have good in vitro activity. *E. rhusiopathiae* causes a zoonotic infection, introduced following subcutaneous inoculation of the organism through an abrasion or pucture wound during handling of animal products or soil contaminated with the organism. *M. chelonae* is a rapidly growing mycobacteria that is ubiquitous in the environment. In contrast with *M. fortuitum* (another common rapidly growing mycobacterium), *M. chelonae* is generally resistant to trimethoprim/sulfamethoxazole, ciprofloxacin, and imipenem. *M. marinum* infections are

associated with exposure to contaminated water from aquariums or marine sources. *S. schenckii* is a dimorphic fungus that produces cutaneous infections after exposure to contaminated soil, such as an infection following a puncture with a contaminated rose bush. *Sporothrix* produces darkly pigmented colonies and is not susceptible to antibacterial antibiotics.
MM5 290-291

155 (A) **Antibiotic resistance.** Although *Enterococcus* species are relatively avirulent, antibiotic resistance is a primary factor that permits these organisms to produce disease. These organisms are resistant to all cephalosporins, oxacillin and related penicillin, and many other antibiotics, including vancomycin and the aminoglycosides. Endotoxin is produced by gram-positive but not gram-negative bacteria. Exfoliative toxin is produced by *Staphylococcus aureus.* Exotoxins and phospholipase C are produced by a number of organisms but not *Enterococcus.*
MM5 259-260, 262

156 (A) **Deregulation of adenylate cyclase in host cells.** The patient's symptoms are consistent with the diagnosis of pertussis or whooping cough. This disease is caused by *Bordetella pertussis,* a bacterium that produces several toxins, including pertussis toxin, a cytotoxin, and extracytoplasmic adenylate cyclase. The pertussis toxin activates the guanosine diphosphate-binding proteins to promote the action of adenylate cylcase. This activity interferes with chemotaxis, phagocytosis, and other cellular functions.
MM5 377-378

157 (B) **Ciprofloxacin.** The selection of a prophylactic antibiotic for exposure to *N. meningitidis* is controversial. Historically, a sulfonamide, such as sulfadiazine, was recommended. Resistance to sulfa drugs have become widespread, however, and these drugs are not recommended now unless there is evidence that the epidemic strain of *N. meningitidis* is susceptible. Although penicillin can be used to treat infections, this antibiotic is not effective in eradicating carriage. Resistance to chloramphenicol and rifampin have been observed, although rifampin can be selected as an alternative to ciprofloxacin. Minocycline can also be considered for prophylaxis, but toxic side effects have limited the use of this antibiotic. Ciprofloxacin appears highly active and effective in eliminating the organism in carriers and has not been associated with significant side effects; this drug is recommended for chemoprophylaxis, although these recommendations are subject to change.
MM5 319-320

158 (A) **Blocks peptide elongation by inhibiting peptidyltransferase.** Clindamycin is a bacteriostatic antibiotic in the family of lincosamide antibiotics. Similar to chloramphenicol and the macrolides, clindamycin blocks peptide elongation by binding to the 50S ribosome. It inhibits peptidyltransferase by interfering with the binding of the aminoacyl-tRNA complex.
MM5 210

159 **(D)** *Nocardia.* Of the five organisms listed in the answers to this question, only *Actinomyces* and *Nocardia* form filamentous, branching rods. These organisms can be differentiated by the acid-fast stain. *Actinomyces* is not acid-fast, and *Nocardia* is weakly acid-fast. *Mycobacterium* and *Rhodococcus* are acid-fast; however, *Mycobacterium* does not form filaments, and *Rhodococcus* is a weakly acid-fast coccobacillus. One species of *Legionella*, *L. micdadei*, is acid-fast when initially observed in the clinical specimen but loses this property when isolated in culture. This organism is eliminated because it is a gram-negative rod.
MM5 287-292

160 **(E)** **Routine bacterial culture.** The presence of squamous epithelial cells in expectorated sputum indicates the specimen has been contaminated with oral secretions. Because most bacterial infections of the lower respiratory tract are preceded by colonization of the oropharynx, contaminated specimens submitted for routine bacterial culture should not be processed. Anaerobe cultures should only be performed with respiratory specimens collected in a manner to avoid any oral contamination (e.g., lung aspirate or biopsy). Fungal cultures and Nocardia cultures can be performed using a contaminated respiratory specimen because selective media are used to eliminate the contaminating oral flora, and the fungal pathogens (e.g., *Cryptococcus*, dimorphic fungi) and Nocardia are not normal residents of the oropharynx. Respiratory specimens processed for mycobacteria are decontaminated to eliminate the oral contaminants before the specimen is cultured.
MM5 217

161 **(A)** *Capnocytophaga canimorsus.* *C. canimorsus* (formerly called *Capnocytophaga* group DF-2) is an organism that is normally found in the mouths of canines and is associated with bite wound infections. Infections are particularly serious for alcoholics, individuals who are functionally asplenic, and patients receiving immunosuppressive drugs. The organism is a slow-growing, facultative anaerobic, filamentous gram-negative rod that requires carbon dioxide for growth (capnophilic). *C. canimorsus* is separated from other species in this genus by the

positive catalase and oxidase reactions. *E. corrodens* is associated with human bites, not dog bites, and is catalase-negative. *P. multocida* has been associated with dog bites, although *Pasteurella canis* is the more common isolate from dogs. *P. multocida* is oxidase-positive and catalase-positive but does not require carbon dioxide for growth. *S. minus* is an agent of rat bite fever and has not been associated with dog bites. *V. vulnificus* produces wound infections and systemic illnesses associated with exposure to contaminated marine waters.
MM5 399

162 **(D)** **Positive acid-fast stain.** Leprosy can be subdivided into two forms of the disease: tuberculoid and lepromatous. Tuberculoid leprosy is characterized by a vigorous immune response to the infection. Thus, patients with the tuberculoid form of leprosy have relatively few acid-fast organisms in their tissues, have a low level of infectivity, and are reactive in the skin test to lepromin. These patients also have few erythematous or hypopigmented skin lesions. In contrast, patients with the lepromatous form of leprosy have a specific defect in their cellular response to infection and are hypergammaglobulinemic. Thus, they have a large number of bacteria in their tissues (acid-fast organisms that make the stain positive), are infectious, and are characterized clinically by the presence of many erythematous macules, papules, or nodules. These patients have extensive tissue destruction and diffuse nerve involvement.
MM5 301-303

163 **(A)** *Corynebacterium diphtheriae.* The *C. diphtheriae* toxin is inactivated by formalin treatment and administered to children in combination with vaccines prepared against pertussis and tetanus antigens (DPT vaccine). The capsular antigens from *N. meningitidis* and *S. pneumoniae* are used in the vaccines for these two organisms. The whole killed cell is used to prepare vaccines against *V. cholerae* and *Y. pestis*. A live attenuated vaccine has also been developed against *V. cholerae*.
MM5 160-162, 282-283

164 **(D)** **Group B** *Streptococcus agalactiae.* This baby girl has evidence of early onset neonatal disease. The three cardinal features of this disease are sepsis, pulmonary symptoms, and meningitis. Blood and CSF should be collected for the diagnosis. Although the number of organisms present in the blood is below the limit of detection by microscopy, microscopic examination of CSF is indicated for a rapid diagnosis of the etiologic agent (as was demonstrated in this patient). The two most common organisms responsible for early onset disease are group B *S. agalactiae* and *Escherichia coli*. Less commonly, *L. monocytogenes*, a gram-positive rod, causes early onset disease. The Gram stain result for this patient is more consistent with group B *Streptococcus*. Meningitis can be caused by all of the organisms listed in the answers to this question; however, the clinical history should narrow the differential diagnosis. *S. aureus* is an uncommon cause of meningitis in the absence of a neurosurgical procedure. *S. pneumoniae* is a common cause of meningitis but is not

typically seen in neonates. The gram-stain morphology of *S. pneumoniae*, gram-positive cocci in pairs, is not consistent with the Gram stain in this patient. *N. meningitidis* is a gram-negative diplococci. Penicillin is the most active antibiotic for treating infections with this organism.
MM5 247-250

165 (E) *Propionibacterium.* All of the organisms in the answers to this question are anaerobic gram-positive rods and would be expected to grow on anaerobic blood agar plates. *Propionibacterium* is the correct answer because organisms that reside on the skin's surface (e.g., coagulase-negative *Staphylococcus*, *Corynebacterium*, *Propionibacterium*) cause most shunt infections. The other organisms listed in this question are not found on the skin's surface and have not been associated with shunt infections.
MM5 419

166 (C) **Modification of PBPs.** Oxacillin and related penicillins (e.g., methicillin, nafcillin, dicloxacillin) are resistant to beta-lactamase hydrolysis. Resistance to this class of penicillins is mediated by acquisition of a gene, *mec*A, that codes for a novel penicillin-binding protein, PBP 2′. The penicillins and other beta-lactam antibiotics kill bacteria by their ability to bind to PBPs, which are enzymes responsible for construction of the cell wall peptidoglycan. PBP 2′ is not bound by penicillins but retains its enzymatic activity.
MM5 204-207

167 (D) **Culture on selective agar incubated in a micro-aerophilic atmosphere.** Growth of *Campylobacter* requires the use of a selective medium incubated in a microaerophilic atmosphere (decreased oxygen and increase carbon dioxide) and at an elevated temperature. The selective media that have been used for the recovery of *Campylobacter* must contain blood or charcoal to remove toxic oxygen radicals, and antibiotics are added to inhibit the growth of contaminating organisms. Blood agar is a nonselective medium and is not useful for stool cultures except to determine if there is a disruption of the normal balance of enteric bacteria. *Campylobacter* does not grow on MacConkey or sorbitol/MacConkey agar. Sorbitol/MacConkey agar is used for the detection of enterohemorrhagic *Escherichia coli*. Toxins such as Shiga toxin and *Clostridium difficile* toxins are detected by immunoassays.
MM5 337, 350, 411-413

168 (D) *Clostridium perfringens:* **food poisoning associated with meat products.** *C. perfringens* food poisoning is associated with contaminated meat products, particularly gravy. *C. difficile*, not *C. perfringens*, causes antibiotic-associated colitis. *C. botulinum* blocks release of the neurotransmitter acetylcholine, whereas *C. tetani* blocks neurotransmitters (e.g., GABA) for inhibitory synapses. *C. difficile* is not associated with a flaccid form of paralysis.
MM5 405-406

169 (A) *Bacillus cereus.* Both *B. cereus* and *C. perfringens* are found in nature, can cause rapidly progressive diseases, and can produce beta-hemolytic colonies on blood agar plates. This organism, however, grows aerobically, which would exclude *C. perfringens*. *C. jeikeium* colonizes the skin surfaces and, although it could be isolated in an eye specimen, it would not be associated with this type of infection. *E. rhusiopathiae* colonizes the intestinal tract of wild and domestic animals and is associated with cutaneous and disseminated diseases (but not eye infections). *P. aeruginosa* is a gram-negative rod that is found in nature and causes opportunistic infections, including eye infections.
MM5 269-270

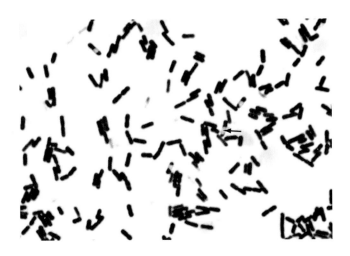

170 (D) **Stimulates increased adenylate cyclase activity.** *V. cholerae* toxin is an A-B toxin. A ring of five identical B subunits binds to the ganglioside G_{M1} receptors on the intestinal epithelial cells. The toxic A subunit is internalized and interacts with G proteins that control adenylate cyclase, leading to the catabolic conversion of ATP to cyclic AMP. This results in a hypersecretion of water and electrolytes.
MM5 196-198

171 (B) **Person-to-person contact.** Shigellosis is a human disease, transmitted by the fecal-to-oral route, primarily by contact with people who have contaminated hands and less commonly by drinking or eating contaminated water or food. This disease is most commonly seen in young children (e.g., in daycare centers, nurseries, custodial institutions) and in male homosexuals. Contaminated water can be the source of a number of enteric pathogens, including *Cryptosporidium*; steamed rice is associated with *Bacillus cereus* infections; undercooked chicken is associated with *Salmonella* and *Campylobacter* infections; and undercooked hamburger is associated with *Escherichia coli* O157 infections.
MM5 332-333

172 (C) **Exfoliative toxins A and B.** Two exfoliative toxins have been described, each of which can mediate scalded skin syndrome in babies. These are serine proteases that split the

intercellular bridges in the stratum granulosum epidermis. Cytolysis and inflammation are not present in the involved skin, so Gram stains and culture are not useful. Toxins A and B have also been associated with a severe form of pulmonary disease. *Staphylococcus aureus* produces a variety of other toxins that mediate disease. Alpha-toxin is an example of a cytotoxic toxin produced by this organism. This toxin is an important mediator of tissue damage and is toxic for many cells (e.g., erythrocytes, leukocytes, platelets), but it does not produce the clinical pictures described for this patient. Leukocidin is also a cytotoxic toxin. Enterotoxin A is one of eight serologically distinct, heat-stable enterotoxins described for *S. aureus*. Enterotoxin A is the toxin most commonly associated with staphylococcal food poisoning. Because this disease is mediated by ingestion of preformed toxin, the incubation period after ingestion of the contaminated food is only a few hours, and the duration of disease is less than 24 h. TSST-1 was originally described as an enterotoxin (enterotoxin F) and is still associated with diarrhea. Multiorgan dysfunction, skin desquamation, shock, and death are characteristic of toxic shock syndrome.
MM5 224-226

173 **(E) Susceptibility to bacitracin.** The organism responsible for this infection is *Streptococcus pyogenes* (group A *Streptococcus*). *S. pyogenes* is catalase-negative, like all streptococci, so the catalase test would not identify the organism. This species is susceptible to bacitracin and also produces L-pyrrolidonyl-arylamidase (PYR), properties unique to this *Streptococcus* species. Production of coagulase is used to differentiate *Staphylococcus aureus* from the other staphylococcal species. Susceptibility to optochin and solubility in bile are tests used to identify *Streptococcus pneumoniae*.
MM5 246-247

174 **(D) Rickettsial pox.** *Rickettsia akari*, a member of the spotted fever group of Rickettsia, is the etiologic agent of rickettsial pox. Infections with *R. akari* are maintained in the rodent population through the bite of mites and in mites by transovarian transmission. Humans become accidental hosts when bitten by infected mites.
MM5 453

175 **(A) Chlamydia trachomatis.** The patient has lymphogranuloma venereum (LGV) caused by *C. trachomatis*. The infection is endemic in Africa, Asia, and South America and is sporadically reported in North America, Australia, and Europe. The disease is caused by four specific serotypes of *C. trachomatis*: serotypes L_1, L_2, L_{2a}, and L_3. Adenopathy ("bubo") with ulcer formation is characteristic of the disease. Herpes simplex virus produces a painful ulcer at the site of initial infection. The swollen, ulcerating lymph nodes seen in LGV are not characteristic of herpes infections. *K. granulomatis* is not culturable. *N. gonorrhoeae* can be cultured on chocolate agar and specialized media (e.g., Thayer-Martin) but does not present as described in this patient's infection. *T. pallidum*, etiologic agent of syphilis,

produces a painful ulcer and is not characterized by ulcerating lymph nodes.
MM5 464-469

176 **(D) Staphylococcus aureus.** Enteric pathogens that are most commonly associated with intoxications (i.e., disease produced by preformed toxins) are *S. aureus*, *Bacillus cereus*, *Clostridium botulinum*, and *Clostridium perfringens*. Examples of enteric pathogens that require replication of the organism in the host before they express their virulence factors are *Salmonella*, *Shigella*, *Yersinia*, and *Vibrio*. Intoxications are characterized by a short incubation period after consumption of the contaminated food product (generally 2 to 6 h) and brief duration (generally less than 24 hours, except for *C. botulinum* where the toxin is tightly bound to the host receptor).
MM5 225-226, 229-230

177 **(C) Modified Thayer-Martin (MTM) agar.** The organism responsible for this infection is *Neisseria gonorrhoeae*, which is a fastidious organism that requires complex media, such as modified Thayer-Martin agar, for growth. Soluble starch is added to medium to neutralize the toxic effects of fatty acids and trace metals present in the peptone hydrolysates and agar common in most laboratory media. Antibiotics are also present in the medium to suppress the growth of other organisms that colonize the urethra. Optimum growth of *N. gonorrhoeae* also requires incubation at 37° C in an atmosphere enriched with CO_2. BCYE is used for the recovery of *Legionella*, and Bordet-Gengou agar is used for the recovery of *Bordetella pertussis*. Mueller-Hinton agar was developed originally for the growth of *N. gonorrhoeae* but is nonselective, allowing the growth of other organisms that can obscure the colonies of *N. gonorrhoeae*. Mueller-Hinton agar is now only used for the performance of antimicrobial susceptibility tests. Nutrient agar is a minimal growth medium; failure to grow on nutrient agar is one test that is used to identify *N. gonorrhoeae*.
MM5 317-319

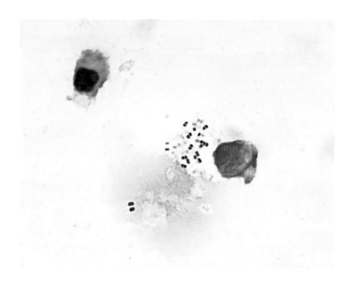

178 **(C)** *Mycobacterium haemophilum.* M. *haemophilum* is a slow-growing organism that is iron dependent and has an optimal growth temperature between 30° and 32°C. This organism grows either very poorly or not at all at 37°C. The most common clinical presentation of *M. haemophilum* disease is cutaneous and subcutaneous lesions, consistent with the observation that the organism grows best at cooler body sites. Therefore it is important to clearly describe the source of clinical material submitted to the laboratory so that appropriate incubation conditions can be used. In addition, the specimens should be inoculated onto media supplemented with iron compounds (e.g., chocolate agar or a medium with ferric ammonium citrate, hemin, Fildes supplement, or lysed horse blood). None of the other mycobacterial species listed in this question requires iron products for growth. *M. avium* has an optimum growth temperature of 38° to 40°C; *M. fortuitum* grows in a broad range of temperatures; *M. marinum* grows best at 30° to 32°C; and *M. leprae* has not been grown in vitro.

MM5 305, 307

179 **(E) Exotoxin A.** The organism responsible for this woman's infection is *Pseudomonas aeruginosa.* Infections are associated with localized trauma, in this case caused by the irritation of unclean contact lens that abraded the surface of the cornea. Infections typically start as a localized ulcer that rapidly progress to destroy the eye. The toxin primarily responsible for this destructive infection is exotoxin A. Exotoxin A inhibits protein synthesis by inactivating EF-2, a factor required for the movement of peptide chains on the ribosomes. This toxin is identical in action to diphtheria toxin. A variety of other organisms can produce keratitis and corneal ulcers. These include *Staphylococcus aureus* (alpha-toxin), *Clostridium perfringens* (alphatoxin, beta-toxin), *Bacillus cereus* (cereolysin and phospholipase C), and other gram-negative rods (e.g., *Proteus mirabilis*). The Gram stain morphology and biochemical properties of this patient's organism differentiate *P. aeruginosa* from other possible pathogens.

MM5 357-362

180 **(D) Pyrogenic exotoxin.** The children's symptoms are a description of the classic rash seen in scarlet fever caused by *Streptococcus pyogenes.* The rash is mediated by one of three immunologically distinct, heat-labile pyrogenic exotoxins.

MM5 241-243

181 **(E) Clinical diagnosis of erythema migrans.** The first sign of Lyme disease is the presence of a characterized rash, called erythema migrans. At the time the rash develops, culture is insensitive and antibodies may or may not be present; less than half of patients have a history of a recent tick bite. *Borrelia* organisms that are responsible for a relapsing fever will be detected in Giemsa-stained blood; however, *B. burgdorferi* is not detected by this method.

MM5 435-437

182 **(C)** *Moraxella catarrhalis.* M. *catarrhalis* can cause sinusitis and bronchopneumonia. *B. pertussis* is responsible for whooping cough. *C. diphtheriae* is the cause of diphtheria. *M. pneumoniae* causes atypical pneumonia. *N. gonorrhoeae* can lead to gonococcal pharyngitis.

MM5 217, 365

183 **(B)** *Bifidobacterium.* The human colon is the most densely populated organ in the body, with a bacterial count of more than 10^{11}/g of feces. Anaerobes are the most numerous bacteria, outnumbering aerobic bacteria by 1000-fold. Each of the bacteria listed in the answers to this question (*Bacteroides, Bifidobacterium, Enterococcus, Escherichia,* and *Pseudomonas*) is found in the colon. The most common genera are *Bifidobacterium* and *Eubacterium,* neither of which is commonly associated with disease. In contrast, the other genera are all significant enteric pathogens.

MM5 84-85

184 **(B) Ocular infection: corneal scraping.** The appropriate specimen for a disease is the one that samples the site of infection and avoids contamination with the patient's normal microbial flora. A swab or scraping of the cornea is the appropriate specimen for an ocular infection. Deep intraocular infections may also require aspiration of the ocular fluids. The diagnosis of cystitis requires collection of midstream urine, which avoids the bacteria that colonize the urethra. Diagnosis of pneumonia requires collection of lower airway secretions (i.e., sputum) with the avoidance of contamination with saliva. The diagnosis of sinusitis requires aspiration of the involved sinus. A wound should be cultured after the superficial drainage and surrounding surfaces are cleaned and disinfected.

MM5 217

185 **(A) Dipicolinic acid.** Some bacteria, such as *Bacillus* and *Clostridium,* can form endospores (spores) under the adverse conditions of a low level of nutrients, high heat, or drying. These structures are extremely stable and can survive in the environment for months to years. This ability is due to the unique structure of the spore. Under adverse conditions, the nuclear material divides into two with a septum formed to separate the genetic material. Other layers then develop in the endospore—an inner membrane, a cortex layer consisting of two peptidoglycan layers, and an outer keratin-like protein coat. The cortex layer is stabilized by a high concentration of calcium bound to dipicolinic acid. Lipid A, lipoteichoic acid, O antigen, and peptidoglycan are found in many vegetative forms of bacteria and are not unique to spores.

MM5 22-24

186 **(C) Endotoxin.** This female college student has meningitis caused by *Neisseria meningitidis.* Characteristic of this disease are diffuse vascular changes, including endothelial damage, inflammation of vessel walls, thrombosis, and disseminated intravascular coagulation. These symptoms are attributed to the action of the LOS endotoxin present in the outer membrane of cells. The polysaccharide capsule protects the bacteria from antibody-mediated phagocytosis. Meningococci can be serologically classifed into 13 serogroups based on antigenic differences in the capsule, and they can also be categorized into multiple serotypes based on the antigenic variations in the outer membrane proteins and oligosaccharide component of LOS. Some serotypes are more commonly associated with disseminated disease, presumably because these strains are more resistant to serum killing. Pili bind to specific receptors in the nasopharynx and are responsible for colonization. No A-B type exotoxin has been associated with *N. meningitidis*.

MM5 314-317

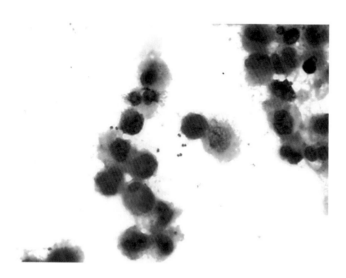

187   (B) Ability to bind complement (C3b). Replication of *Legionella* in macrophages is initiated by binding complement to an outer membrane porin protein. This permits the organism to bind to C3b receptors on the surface of macrophages and is followed by endocytosis. The bacteria are not killed in their intracellular location because fusion of the phagosome and lysosome that contain toxic superoxide, hydrogen peroxide, and hydroxyl radical is inhibited. The bacteria proliferate in the vacuole, produce a variety of hydrolytic enzymes, and kill the host cell when the phagosome membrane is lysed.

MM5 391-393

188   (D) Fluorescent treponemal antibody-absorption (FTA-ABS) test. *Treponema pallidum*, the organism responsible for syphilis, has not been grown in culture and is too thin to be seen by Giemsa stain. Although darkfield examination is very sensitive for confirming the diagnosis of primary and secondary syphilis, relatively few bacteria are present in the tissues of patients with tertiary or late syphilis. The nontreponemal VDRL test is positive for only approximately 70% to 75% of the infected patients. In contrast, the treponemal FTA-ABS tests have very high sensitivity (greater than 95%) for late or tertiary syphilis.

MM5 430-432

189   (A) ASO test: *S. pyogenes*. The ASO antibody test, spelled out as the antistreptolysin O antibody test, is used to identify recent infections with *S. pyogenes* (group A *Streptococcus*). Streptolysin O is an oxygen-labile hemolysin that lyses a variety of blood cells. Patients with pharyngitis develop antibodies against streptolysin O, so this test is a useful marker for recent *S. pyogenes* infections in patients who develop the nonsuppurative complications of rheumatic fever or acute glomerulonephritis. Streptolysin O is bound to cholesterol in skin lipids, so the ASO test is negative in cutaneous infections. Identification of *S. pyogenes* in culture is confirmed by susceptibility to bacitracin and the presence of PYR. *S. pyogenes* is the only *Streptococcus* species that produces this enzyme. Susceptibility to optochin is used to identify *S. pneumoniae*. Colonies of *S. pneumoniae* are also dissolved when exposed to a drop of bile (e.g., sodium desoxycholate, bile solubility test). *S. anginosus*, an important species in the viridans group of streptococci, is resistant to optochin. The CAMP test is positive for *S. agalactiae* (group B *Streptococcus*). This organism is also able to hydrolyze hippurate.

MM5 246-247

190   (B) *Burkholderia pseudomallei*. *B. pseudomallei* is responsible for the melioidosis disease, which can appear as an acute suppurative disease or present as described in this question, as a chronic pulmonary disease resembling tuberculosis. This organism has acquired renewed interest in the late twentieth and early twenty-first centuries because it has been identified as an organism that could be used by bioterrorists. *B. pseudomallei* is listed on the Select Agent and Toxin List of organisms of biological concern. *A. baumannii* is oxidase-negative; *C. hominis* is fermentative; *P. aeruginosa* is resistant to trimethoprim/sulfamethoxazole; and *S. maltophilia* is oxidase-negative. All of the organisms listed in the answers to this question, with the exception of *B. pseudomallei*, are readily isolated in this country.

MM5 363-364

191   (A) *Bacteroides fragilis*. Metronidazole is active against protozoa (e.g., *Trichomonas*, *Entamoeba*, *Giardia*) and strict anaerobes (e.g., *B. fragilis*). This drug has no significant activity against aerobic or facultatively anaerobic bacteria (e.g., *Helicobacter pylori*, *Staphylococcus aureus*, *Streptococcus pyogenes*, *Yersinia enterocolitica*). The antimicrobial properties of metronidazole stem from the reduction of its nitro group by bacterial nitroreductase, thereby producing cytotoxic compounds that disrupt the host DNA.

MM5 211, 426

192   (B) Culture on MacConkey agar. Isolation of enteric pathogens is a difficult and expensive process for the clinical laboratory. Growth of the many bacterial species normally present in the intestines must be suppressed, so selective culture media (and not the nonselective blood agar media) are commonly used. *Shigella* can be detected as a nonlactose fermenting bacteria that grows well on MacConkey agar. Sorbitol/MacConkey agar is a special formulation of MacConkey agar that is used for the detection of enterohemorrhagic *Escherichia coli*. Incubation in a microaerophilic atmosphere is used for the specific detection of *Campylobacter* species. The toxin produced by *Shigella* is Shiga toxin. This toxin can be detected with a specific immunoassay. Toxins A and B are two toxins produced by *Clostridium difficile*. This organism produces a spectrum of diseases ranging from antibiotic-associated diarrhea to pseudomembranous colitis. These two toxins are most commonly detected by specific immunoassays.

MM5 337

193 **(E) Pyruvate.** Bacteria require energy for survival. This energy is derived from the breakdown (catabolism) of various organic substrates (e.g., carbohydrates, lipids, and proteins) and then synthesis (anabolism) of cellular constituents (e.g., cell walls, proteins, fatty acids, nucleic acids). Various metabolic pathways accomplish the conversion of the catabolic product into cellular constituents. The first stage of this conversion involves production of pyruvate, which is then channeled toward energy production or synthesis of new carbohydrates, amino acids, lipids, and nucleic acids. Acetaldehyde, acetyl-coenzyme A, and lactate are intermediate fermentation by-products of pyruvate. Glucose is converted into pyruvate in the Embden-Meyerhof-Parnas glycolytic pathway.

MM5 25-30

194 **(A) Endocarditis.** Continuous bacteremia is associated with intravascular infections, such as endocarditis (infection of the lining of the heart), septic thrombophlebitis (infection of the lumen of a blood vessel), and intravascular catheter infections. The other infections listed in the answers to this question (e.g., meningitis, osteomyelitis, peritonitis, and septic arthritis) are associated with intermittent bacteremia: the infection is in a localized space that periodically spills organisms into the blood. The concept of continuous versus discontinuous bacteremia is important because most or all blood cultures will be positive in a patient with an intravascular infection but not in a patient with a discontinuous bacteremia.

MM5 213-216

195 **(C) Lactobacillus.** *Lactobacillus* species are preferentially found in acidic areas, such as in the stomach, upper small intestine, and genitourinary tract. *Bacteroides* and *Escherichia* species are primarily restricted to the intestines; *Malassezia* is a lipophilic fungus that is found in areas of the body that are rich in sebaceous glands, such as the skin; and viridans streptococci are found primarily in the upper respiratory tract.

MM5 84-86, 420

196 **(E) Rhodococcus.** Each of the organisms listed in the answers to this question will stain with the modified acid-fast stain (for the *Legionella* species, only *Legionella micdadei*). Only *Rhodococcus*, however, will initially appear as cocci or coccobacilli. With prolonged incubation, *Rhodococcus equi*, the most

common species causing human disease, will appear more rod-like and develop a salmon-pink color. *Gordonia* and *Legionella* are true rods and are not pigmented. *Mycobacteria* are not salmon colored, and most species that cause pulmonary disease will require prolonged incubation before the culture is positive. *Nocardia* appear as branching filamentous rods, so even though they are frequently pigmented, they would not be mistaken for *Rhodococcus*. *Rhodococcus* is also catalase-positive, is slowly urease-positive, and fails to ferment carbohydrates. This species is most commonly recovered from immunocompromised patients, such as those with malignancies, transplants, or HIV infections. The most common presentation is invasive pulmonary disease with abscess formation and dissemination to distal organs (e.g., meninges, pericardium, skin).

MM5 292-293

197 **(C) Proteus mirabilis.** This woman has a urinary tract infection complicated with pyelonephritis. The organism that was recovered is a gram-negative rod because it grew on both blood and MacConkey agars. All of the organisms listed in the answers to this question are gram-negative rods, so this information does not help select the correct organism. The organism was colorless on MacConkey agar, which indicates the organism is unable to ferment lactose. *E. coli* and *K. pneumoniae* are lactose–fermenters, so these organisms can be eliminated. Strong production of urease is characteristic of *P. mirabilis*. This property results in production of ammonia with an increase in the urine pH and subsequent formation of renal stones. *S. typhi* does not hydrolyze urea, and only about half of the *P. aeruginosa* strains do. The spreading growth of *P. mirabilis* (commonly called "swarming") on blood agar is characteristic of this organism and differentiates it from all other bacteria listed. Indeed, an accurate preliminary identification of *P. mirabilis* can be made simply by noting that swarming bacteria do not ferment lactose in MacConkey agar and have a rapidly positive urease reaction.

MM5 336

198 **(A) Escherichia coli.** An opportunistic pathogen is a microbe that is normally nonpathogenic except when introduced into normally sterile sites (e.g., deep tissues, normally sterile body fluids) or in patients that are less competent in resisting infections (e.g., immunocompromised patients). *E. coli* is part of the normal flora of bacteria living in the human intestine. When this organism, however, is introduced into a normally sterile location, disease can occur (e.g., organisms in the peritoneal cavity cause peritonitis; organisms in the lungs cause pneumonia; organisms in cerebrospinal fluid are associated with meningitis). Strict pathogens are microbes that always cause human disease. The other organisms listed in the answers to this question are strict pathogens: *F. tularensis* causes tularemia; *M. tuberculosis* causes tuberculosis; *N. gonorrhoeae* causes gonorrhea; and *S. typhi* causes typhoid fever.

MM5 83

199 **(D) Penicillin plus gentamicin.** *Lactobacillus* endocarditis is very difficult to treat because the organism is not susceptible to killing by any one antibiotic. Combination therapy with penicillin and an aminoglycoside (e.g., gentamicin) is recommended for serious infections such as endocarditis. Other antibiotics (e.g., ampicillin) may inhibit the growth of the organism but will not kill *Lactobacillus*. Most strains of *Lactobacillus* are resistant to vancomycin.
MM5 420

200 **(D) Production of the *mecA* gene product.** Resistance to oxacillin in *Staphylococcus* is most commonly mediated by acquisition of the *mecA* gene. This gene codes for a novel PBP2′. The beta-lactam antibiotics are able to kill bacteria by binding to proteins (the penicillin-binding proteins or PBPs) that catalyze construction of the peptidoglycan layer of the cell wall. PBP2′ is not bound by oxacillin or any other beta-lactam antibiotic, and this protein is thus able to function in cell wall synthesis.
MM5 234-235

201 **(E) Urine.** Pathogenic organisms present in blood, cerebrospinal fluid, and stool specimens would be considered significant regardless of the number of organisms present. Determination of the significance of a pathogen in a respiratory specimen is accomplished by noting the quality of the specimen (i.e., whether the lower respiratory secretions are contaminated with upper respiratory secretions), clinical presentation of the patient, and the organism isolated. In contrast, urine specimens are frequently contaminated with a small number of organisms present in the urethra. Because these organisms may be uropathogens (i.e., organisms capable of producing urinary tract infections), the number of organisms present in urine are quantitated. Large numbers of organisms are typically associated with infection if the specimen is properly collected.
MM5 217-218

202 **(D) Late manifestations of disseminated disease include arthritis, cardiac abnormalities, and neurologic disease.** Late manifestations of Lyme disease develop in the majority of patients who are not treated. These develop in two phases. The first involves neurologic symptoms (i.e., meningitis, encephalitis, peripheral nerve neuropathy) and cardiac dysfunction (heart block, myopericarditis, congestive heart failure). These symptoms develop in 10% to 15% of patients and can last for days to months. The second phase is characterized by arthralgias and arthritis. These complications can persist for months to years. The other answers listed for this question are incorrect because Lyme disease is transmitted by ticks and not fleas; whitefooted mice and white-tail deer are reservoirs for the disease but ground squirrels are not; the disease is common to all age groups with exposure to ticks (generally not the very young or old); and, finally, microscopy and culture are very insensitive laboratory tests.
MM5 436-437

203 **(E) Subacute endocarditis.** The viridans group of *Streptococcus* consists of more than 20 species of streptococci that colonize the oropharynx, gastrointestinal tract, and genitourinary tract. Most members of this group are organisms with relatively low virulence potential (the exception is *S. pneumoniae*); however, some species are able to adhere to damaged heart valves and produce a subacute form of endocarditis. Most infected patients either have poor oral hygiene or develop disease following a dental procedure.
MM5 251-252

204 **(B) Formaldehyde.** Mycobacteria and spores are the bacteria most resistant to chemical killing.; only formaldehyde and glutaraldehyde can reliably kill these organisms. Hydrogen peroxide and chlorine compounds can kill mycobacteria and some spores. Alcohol and phenolics have poor activity against spores; iodophors and quaternary ammonium compounds are not active against spores and have little or no activity against mycobacteria.
MM5 89-91

205 **(D) Polyribitol phosphate.** The major virulence factor in *H. influenzae* type B is the antiphagocytic polysaccharide capsule that contains ribose, ribitol, and phosphate (commonly referred to as polyribitol phosphate or PRP). Antibodies directed against the capsule greatly stimulate phagocytosis and complement-mediated bactericidal activity. The use of PRP-based vaccines has virtually eliminated meningitis, epiglottitis, and cellulitis diseases in children. The first vaccines were ineffective in children younger than 18 months because the immune response to polysaccharide antigens is immature in very young children. By conjugating the PRP to a protein carrier, however, the vaccine was effective in children as young as 2 months.
MM5 367-369

206 **(A) Chicken.** More than half of all *Campylobacter* infections are caused by consumption of improperly cooked chicken. Chicken and other fowl are important reservoirs for these bacteria.
MM5 350

207 **(A) *Borrelia burgdorferi*.** This woman's symptoms are a classic description of erythema migrans, a rash that develops in the primary stage of Lyme disease. The rash initially develops at the site of the tick bite. The rash will disappear after a few weeks, and other transient lesions may subsequently appear. It is common to have no history of a tick bite at the time of presentation because the most common stage of the hard tick is the nymph stage where the tick vector is the size of a poppy seed. A spider bite would have a more aggressive stage of development with localized necrosis. *L. interrogans* infections may be associated with a disseminated rash but not with a localized skin lesion as in the patient. *S. schenckii* infections are characterized by subcutaneous nodules that develop along the lymphatics with

subsequent necrosis and ulcer formation of the overlying skin. *T. mentagrophyte* infections may present with similar symptoms, but the systemic symptoms would be absent.
MM5 198-201

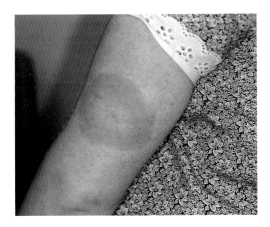

208 (B) Inhibition of phagosome/lysosome fusion. An important virulence factor in *Neisseria gonorrhoeae* is a family of outer membrane proteins (Por proteins) that form pores or channels for nutrients to pass into the cell and waste products to exit. One of the proteins, PorB, is also important for the intracellular survival of *N. gonorrhoeae*. PorB proteins interfere with degranulation of neutrophils by preventing phagosome/lysosome fusion.
MM5 198-201

209 (A) *Bartonella henselae*. The presentation of this infection is consistent with cutaneous bacillary angiomatosis caused by either *B. henselae* or *B. quintana*. The differential diagnosis includes Kaposi's sarcoma and pyogenic granuloma. The definitive diagnosis is confirmed with the results of the Gram stain and culture.
MM5 397-398

210 (B) Erythromycin. Erythromycin belongs to the macrolide class of antibiotics. They exert their antibacterial effect by binding to the 50S ribosome and blocking polypeptide elongation. Tetracycline also inhibits protein synthesis by binding to the 30S ribosomal subunit, which interferes with peptide chain elongation. Ciprofloxacin disrupts DNA replication; imipenem interferes with synthesis of the peptidoglycan layer of the cell wall; and rifampin inhibits the initiation of RNA synthesis.
MM5 210

211 (B) *Corynebacterium diphtheriae*. This patient's disease is respiratory diphtheria, which is characterized by an abrupt onset of malaise, a sore throat, exudative pharyngitis, and a low-grade fever. A firm, adherent pseudomembrane consisting of bacteria, lymphocytes, plasma cells, and fibrin will develop over the tonsils and adjacent structure. *B. pertussis*, *N. gonorrhoeae*, and *S. pyogenes* can produce pharyngitis, but none of these organisms are associated with pseudomembrane formation. *S. aureus* is not a common cause of pharyngitis.
MM5 282

212 (E) Outer membrane. The cell wall structure of gram-negative bacteria differs from the structure of gram-positive bacteria. For gram-negative bacteria, the peptidoglycan layer is thin and is surrounded by an outer membrane. Pores in the outer membrane regulate the transport of nutrients, metabolites, and other factors into and out of the bacterial cell. Both gram-positive and gram-negative bacteria have a cytoplasmic membrane. The endoplasmic reticulum, Golgi apparatus, and nuclear membrane (surrounding a defined nucleus structure) are found only in eukaryotic cells and not in bacterial prokaryotic cells.
MM5 13-17

213 (D) Erythromycin. Erythromycin has been demonstrated to reduce infectivity and symptoms in infected patients and to protect those who have immediate contact with active cases. Ampicillin has in vitro activity against *B. pertussis* but is ineffective in vitro. Likewise, in vitro data indicate that *B. pertussis* is susceptible to ciprofloxacin, but no clinical data have been collected. Doxycycline has been used with limited success to treat pertussis, but no data exist for the use of this drug for prophylaxis. Vancomycin is ineffective in vitro or in vivo against *Bordetella*.
MM5 381

214 (E) *Streptococcus mutans*. This patient most likely has subacute bacterial endocarditis, which is characterized by an indolent onset and vague symptoms of poor health developing over weeks to months. *S. mutans* is a member of the viridans group of streptococci and is a normal resident of the upper respiratory tract. It has the ability to adhere to the surface of teeth, as well as damaged heart valves. It is recognized that patients with preexisting damaged heart valves (e.g., rheumatic heart disease) are at significant risk for developing valvular infections unless prophylactic antibiotics are administered before dental procedures. The other organisms listed in the answers to this question are members of the upper respiratory tract and could theoretically be responsible for endocarditis. However, *C. albicans* is an uncommon cause of endocarditis; *S. aureus* is more commonly associated with a rapidly developing course of disease (i.e., acute endocarditis); *S. epidermidis* is associated with subacute diseases but those typically involving a surgical cardiac procedure; and *S. pneumoniae* is an uncommon cause of endocarditis and almost always presents in an acute form.
MM5 251-252

215 (B) Inhibition of phagosome/lysosome fusion. *M. tuberculosis* is an intracellular pathogen. In contrast with most phagocytized bacteria, *M. tuberculosis* prevents fusion of phagosomes with lysosomes by blocking the specific bridging molecule (early endosomal autoantigen 1 or EEA1). At the same time, the phagosome is able to fuse with other intracellular vesicles,

permitting access to nutrients and facilitating intravacuole replication. Other bacteria that inhibit phagolysosome fusion include *Legionella* and *Chlamydia*.
MM5 198-201

216 **(E) No antibiotic.** The most likely cause of this food poisoning is *Staphylococcus aureus*. Staphylococcal food poisoning is produced by preformed toxins present in food. Viable bacteria may not be in the food at the time it is consumed because reheating the food after preparation can kill the staphylococci without affecting the heat-stable toxin or its activity. For this reason, antibiotic therapy would not alter the clinical course of this condition and is not recommended.
MM5 229-230

217 **(B) Erythromycin.** This child has inclusion conjunctivitis caused by *Chlamydia trachomatis*. The infection is acquired at birth during passage through an infected birth canal. After a 2- to 3-week incubation period, the infant develops symptoms as described in this case. Pneumonitis may also develop. *C. trachomatis* lacks a peptidoglycan layer in the cell wall, so beta-lactam antibiotics (e.g., penicillin, imipenem) are ineffective in treating infections caused by this organism. Erythromycin and newer macrolide antibiotics (e.g., azithromycin) are the drugs of choice for treating this infection. Tetracyclines are not recommended for infants, and resistance has been found against this antibiotic, as well as against the fluoroquinolones (e.g., ciprofloxacin).
MM5 467, 469-470

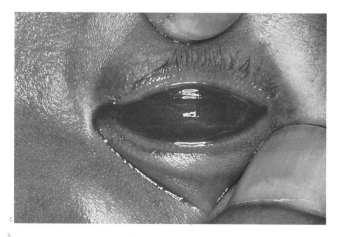

From Morse S et al: *Atlas of sexually transmitted diseases and AIDS*, ed 3, St Louis, 2003, Mosby.

218 **(B) Inhibition of phagosome/lysosome fusion.** *L. pneumophila* organisms are facultative intracellular pathogens that can multiply in alveolar macrophages and monocytes. After phagocytosis, fusion with lysosomes is inhibited. The bacteria replicate in the phagosomes, produce proteolytic enzymes, phosphatase, lipase, and nuclease, which eventually kill the host cell when the vacuole is lysed.
MM5 198-201

219 **(E) Nasopharyngeal aspirate.** *Bordetella pertussis* is a labile organism that is susceptible to drying or delays in processing the specimen for culture. The organism also is fastidious and requires media that are supplemented with charcoal, starch, blood, or albumin to absorb toxic fatty acids; with nicotinamide; and with antibiotics to inhibit organisms normally present in the upper respiratory tract. The nasopharynx is moist and relatively devoid of normal flora compared with the oropharynx. Comparative studies have shown that a washing of the nasopharynx is the best specimen for recovery of *B. pertussis*. Cough plates were used historically, but these are insensitive and a potentially hazardous method for specimen collection. Expectorated and induced sputa are also insensitive because *B. pertussis* is confined to the ciliated cells of the upper airways. Dissemination of *Bordetella* in the blood does not occur, so blood cultures are not useful for this diagnosis.
MM5 380-381

220 **(B) *Escherichia coli*.** The baby has early onset meningitis (i.e., disease developing within 7 days of birth), and the two most common organisms responsible for this disease are group B *Streptococcus* and *Escherichia coli*. The organism's hemolytic properties and ability to ferment lactose in MacConkey agar are consistent with *E. coli*. The most common *E. coli* strains responsible for neonatal meningitis possess the K1 capsular antigen. This serogroup is also present in the gastrointestinal tract of many pregnant women. *E. cloaceae* and *K. pneumoniae* are both lactose-fermenting gram-negative rods; however, neither organism is a common cause of meningitis. *S. typhi* is a member of the family Enterobacteriaceae (as are *E. coli*, *E. aerogenes*, and *K. pneumoniae*) but fails to ferment lactose. Therefore, *S. typhi* organisms will appear as colorless colonies on MacConkey agar. *P. aeruginosa* is a nonfermentative organism in the family Pseudomondaceae, and organisms will also appear as colorless colonies on MacConkey agar.
MM5 327-328, 337

221 **(A) Spore formation is an important feature of these organisms.** The ability to form spores allows *Clostridium* organisms to survive in the environment under the harshest of conditions. Botulinum toxin prevents the release of the neurotransmitter acetylcholine, leading to a flaccid form of paralysis (in contrast with tetanospasm that blocks release of neurotransmitters for inhibitory synapses, leading to spastic paralysis). Human disease has been associated with four of the seven types of botulinum toxin, so multiple episodes of botulism can occur. *C. perfringens* has not been associated with tetanus, and metronidazole or vancomycin should be used to treat *C. difficile* infections. Clindamycin is associated with the development of *C. difficile* disease.
MM5 401

222 **(C) *Clostridium botulinum*.** This case describes a somewhat unusual outbreak of infant botulism because none of the children had a history of ingestion of honey or other contaminated food products. They lived in an area where construction was underway, however, and they were exposed to dust

contaminated with *C. botulinum* spores. The diagnostic clue in these cases was the clinical presentation of the infants. Botulism should be suspected in infants that are less than 1 year of age and who are constipated and have weakness in sucking, swallowing, or crying. Progressive muscle weakness and respiratory failure are symptoms of advanced disease. All of these infants' symptoms were effects of the botulinum toxin that blocks neurotransmission at peripheral cholinergic synapses by preventing release of the neurotransmitter acetylcholine.
MM5 409-410

223 **(C) Culture in tissue culture cells.** This infant has pneumonitis caused by *Chlamydia trachomatis*. Although infected at the time of birth, infants generally develop signs and symptoms of disease 1 to 2 months later. Characteristic of this infection is the "staccato pattern" of the cough. A history of infection in the mother would also be helpful in developing the differential diagnosis. *Chlamydia* is an intracellular pathogen, restricting growth in nonciliated columnar, cuboidal, or transitional epithelial cells found on mucous membranes of the urethra, endocervix, endometrium, fallopian tubes, anorectum, respiratory tract, and conjunctiva. A variety of in vitro grown tissue culture cells will support the growth of this pathogen (e.g., Hela, McCoy, BHK-21, buffalo green monkey kidney cell), but the organisms will not grow on cell-free media (e.g., blood, chocolate, or Thayer-Martin [medium for *Neisseria gonorrhoeae*] agars). The organism lacks the peptidoglycan layer, so Gram stains of discharge or infected tissues would not be helpful. The serological response would develop in an adult but not an infant. No urine antigen test has been developed to date. Direct immunofluorescent (DFA) tests and enzyme-linked immunoassays (ELISAs) have been developed but are generally less sensitive than culture.
MM5 467-469

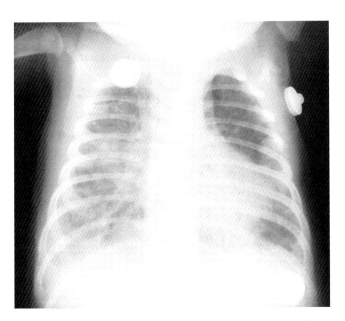

From Morse S et al: *Atlas of sexually transmitted diseases and AIDS*, St Louis, 2003, Mosby.

224 **(A) Use of exogenous thymidine.** The sulfonamides are antimetabolites that compete with p-aminobenzoic acid (PABA), thereby preventing the synthesis of the folic acid required by some organisms. This inhibition blocks the formation of thymidine, some purines, methionine, and glycine. The enterococci are able to use exogenous thymidine and are therefore intrinsically resistant to the sulfonamides.
MM5 211-212

225 **(C) Louse.** These soldiers have louse-borne relapsing fever caused by *Borrelia recurrentis*. This disease is spread person-to-person by infected lice, with humans the only reservoirs. The louse ingests the *B. recurrentis* during a blood meal, and the bacteria multiply in the hemolymph of the parasite. Infection is transmitted when the louse is crushed on the skin surface (bacteria are not present in the saliva or feces of the lice). Fleas, mites, and mosquitos are not infected with *B. recurrentis*. Soft ticks are the vectors of endemic relapsing fever, and hard ticks are the vectors of Lyme disease.
MM5 435-436

226 **(A) Ampicillin.** Ampicillin used either alone or combined with gentamicin is the treatment of choice for *Listeria* infections. Resistance has been reported for the other antibiotics listed in the answers to this question.
MM5 276

227 **(B)** *Pseudomonas aeruginosa*. This patient has malignant otitis externa. External ear infections caused by *P. aeruginosa* have two dramatically different presentations: swimmer's ear and malignant otitis externa. Swimmer's ear occurs in a moist setting (e.g., associated with swimming or a humid environment) and is characterized by an itchy or painful ear with discharge. This is generally treated with agents to dry the ear and antibiotic-containing otic solutions. Malignant otitis externa is a much more serious progression of swimmer's ear, with extension and destruction of the underlying bony structures. This is a condition seen most commonly in the elderly with diabetes. The other organisms listed in the answers to this question are associated with middle ear infections but not the progressively destructive infection described in this question.
MM5 360-362

228 **(C) Clinical clues of anaerobic infections include a wound with foul odor, gas in the tissue, and presence of a sinus tract with sulfur granules.** *B. fragilis* colonizes the colon but not the pharynx. Specimens submitted for anaerobic culture should not be contaminated with the patient's normal flora; therefore midstream urine sample is not an acceptable specimen for anaerobic culture. *Peptostreptoccous* and other anaerobic gram-positive cocci are always susceptible to penicillin. *Actinomyces* is a gram-positive, non–spore-forming rod.
MM5 421

229 **(D)** *Mycoplasma pneumoniae*. M. pneumoniae will not grow on the routine media used for blood and sputum cultures

because it requires sterols (present in serum), nucleic acid precursors (present in yeast extract), and glucose. The negative Gram stain is consistent with the diagnosis because this bacterium lacks a cell wall. *C. pneumoniae* is a strict intracellular pathogen that can only grow in cell cultures. *K. pneumoniae* and *S. pneumoniae* are typically recovered in blood cultures and can grow on the media used for sputum cultures. *L. pneumoniae* grows only on media supplemented with L-cysteine and iron (e.g., BCYE agar) and would not be recovered on the medium used for growing *M. pneumoniae*.
MM5 443-447

230   (D) *Mobiluncus.* Bacterial vaginosis is a polymicrobic infection. A key organism observed in specimens collected from infected women is *Mobiluncus*. The organism is a curved grampositive rod that typically stains gram-negative or gram-variable. *Actinomyces* is a gram-positive rod that can cause pelvic actinomycosis but not vaginosis. *Bacteroides* and, less commonly, *Prevotella* can cause pelvic abscesses but not vaginosis. *Lactobacillus* is normally present in the vagina. When the bacterial flora is disrupted as in vaginosis, these bacteria decrease in numbers.
MM5 419

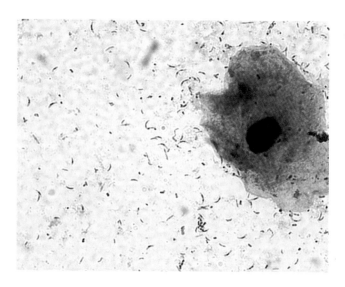

231   (A) *Bacteroides fragilis.* This patient has septic thrombophlebitis caused by *B. fragilis*. The organism was introduced most likely at the time the catheter was inserted and was able to grow in the blood vessel wall. Keys to the identification of the organism are that this is a strict anaerobe (does not grow aerobically) and typically appears as a pleomorphic rod. *F. nucleatum* is also an anaerobic gram-negative rod, but it typically appears as a thin, fusiform-shaped rod. *C. fetus* is microaerophilic (requires an atmosphere with a low concentration of oxygen and carbon dioxide). *C. fetus* can cause septic thrombophebitis. *E. cloacae* is a facultative anaerobe; *P. aeruginosa* is a strict aerobic bacterium. Both *E. cloacae* and *P. aeruginosa* can cause septic thrombophlebitis, but both would grow aerobically.
MM5 423-425

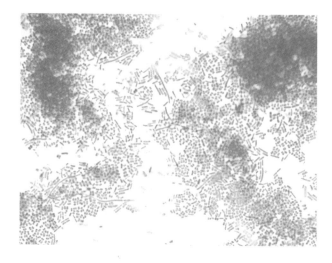

232   (D) *Staphylococcus epidermidis.* *S. epidermidis* and other bacteria living on the skin can colonize the surface of the eyes. Generally, the bacteria are in small quantities and produce no pathology. Trauma to the eye or the presence of a foreign body, however, can introduce the bacteria into the deeper eye tissues and progress to disease. The other bacteria listed in this question (*E. coli*, *P. aeruginosa*, *S. aureus*, and *S. pneumoniae*) can occasionally colonize the eye surface transiently but are more commonly associated with significant eye disease. Recovery of these organisms in a culture of the eye should be considered significant.
MM5 84

233   (B) *Campylobacter fetus.* Most species of *Campylobacter* have been recovered in blood cultures, but this type of culture is the most common source for *C. fetus*. In contrast with the other *Campylobacter* species, *C. fetus* is an uncommon cause of gastroenteritis. Diseases associated with *C. fetus* include bacteremia, endocarditis, and septic thrombophlebitis. *C. fetus* infections are most common in debilitated and immunocompromised patients, such as those with liver disease, diabetes mellitus, chronic alcoholism, or malignancies. With the exception of *C. fetus*, all of the *Campylobacter* species listed in this question are thermophilic; that is, they prefer to grow at 42°C.
MM5 347-351

234   (C) *Mycobacterium haemophilum.* All of the organisms listed in the answers to this question are acid-fast and have been associated with infections in AIDS patients. *M. chelonae*, *N. asteroides*, and *R. equi* all should grow within the first week of incubation on both bacterial and mycobacterial media. *M. avium* is a more slow-growing organism, but growth should also be observed within the first month of incubation. *M. haemophilum* can grow only on media supplemented with hemin and prefers incubation at cooler temperatures; hence these are the reasons the nodules were superficial.
MM5 307

235 (E) *Pasteurella multocida.* *P. multocida* is normally present in the mouths of cats and dogs. Human infections result from getting a deep bite or scratch, developing superficial contamination of an open wound, or sharing food with animals. Human disease can present as described in this girl's case or can be manifest as exacerbation of a chronic respiratory infection or as a systemic infection in an immunocompromised patient. The properties that are somewhat unique for this gram-negative bacterium is the poor growth on MacConkey agar and the susceptibility to penicillin. *B. melitensis, F. tularensis,* and *H. influenzae* will not grow on blood agar, and *E. coli* will grow on MacConkey agar.

MM5 374-375

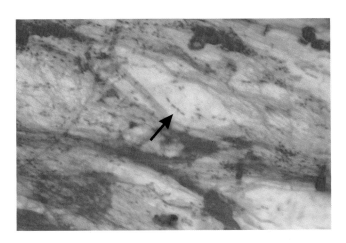

236 (B) **Lipid A.** One of the most important virulence factors in gram-negative bacteria is endotoxin activity in lipopolysaccharide (LPS), which is localized in the outer membrane of the cell wall. LPS consists of polysaccharides covalently bound to a phosphorylated glucosamine disaccharide backbone with attached fatty acids (referred to as lipid A). Lipid A is the component of LPS that mediates endotoxin activities, including induction of fever and release of cytokines, such as tumor necrosis factor alpha (TNF-α), interleukin-1 (IL-1), and IL-6. Although LPS is found in most gram-negative bacteria, it is not present in gram-positive organisms. The core polysaccharide and O antigens are the polysaccharide components of LPS. These serve as antigenic markers for gram-negative bacteria but do not have endotoxin activity. Lipoteichoic acids are polymers of chemically modified ribose or gylcerol connected by phosphates. These molecules are anchored in the cytoplasmic membrane. The peptidoglycan layer is the major structural component of the bacterial cell wall. Both lipoteichoic acids and peptidoglycans can be released from the bacterial cell wall and stimulate toxin-like pyrogenic responses, but these activities are distinct from the activity of endotoxin.

MM5 16-22

237 (C) *Eikenella.* The organisms listed in the answers to this question are referred to as the HACEK bacteria, after the first letters of the genus names. All are normal residents of the human oropharynx and can cause subacute bacterial endocarditis. The clinical presentation of disease caused by each organism is similar, so blood cultures are required to make a definitive diagnosis. *Eikenella* is a facultative anaerobe and is capable of growth on blood and chocolate agars but does not grow well on MacConkey agar. The organism is able to pit or corrode agars and produces a characteristic bleach-like odor.

MM5 320-321

238 (B) **Resistance to aztreonam, cephalothin, ceftazidime, and piperacillin; susceptibility to cefoxitin, imipenem, and piperacillin-tazobactam.** Strains of gram-negative rods, particularly *Klebsiella* and *Escherichia,* that have ESBLs have an altered beta-lactamase with an extended spectrum. These beta-lactamases are able to inactivate all penicillins, cephalosporins, and aztreonam. Beta-lactam antibiotics that are not inactivated by these beta-lactamases include cephamycins (e.g., cefoxitin), carbapenems (e.g., imipenem), and combinations of penicillins with beta-lactamase inhibitors (piperacillin-tazobactam).

MM5 204-206

239 (D) **Filtration through a 0.45-mm filter.** *Campylobacter* organisms are thin bacteria (0.3 to 0.6 µm in diameter) and are difficult to detect by microscopy. Although *Campylobacter fetus* was originally isolated in blood, the enteric *Campylobacter* species were discovered when stool specimens were processed for enteric viruses. The specimens were filtered through bacteriologic filters and then cultured on monolayers of cells. After overnight incubation, the bacteria were observed. This technique is still used for some selected strains of *Campylobacter* species that fail to grow on common isolation media for these enteric pathogens. Once these bacteria were isolated, special culture media were developed for their isolation. It was also appreciated that these bacteria are microaerophilic and that some of the more important species grow best at 42°C. BCYE medium was originally developed for *Legionella* and is now used for a variety of fastidious bacteria (but not for *Campylobacter*). McCoy cells are primarily used for the isolation of *Chlamydia.* Thioglycolate broth is an enrichment broth used for the recovery of anaerobes. Differential centrifugation has not been used for processing microbiology specimens.

MM5 347-350

240 (A) *Enterococcus faecalis.* Although *Staphylococcus* is the most common cause of surgical wound infections, the Gram stain and negative catalase reaction are inconsistent with this diagnosis (staphylococci are catalase-positive, gram-positive cocci arranged in clusters). *S. pyogenes* can cause wound infections, but these organisms typically appear as long chains of gram-positive cocci. Both *S. pneumoniae* and *E. faecalis* appear as gram-positive cocci in pairs and short chains; however, *S. pneumoniae* is not a likely cause of surgical wound infections. The proximity of the surgical site to the perianal area is also consistent with contamination of the wound with *E. faecalis.*

MM5 259-262

241 **(D) Streptomycin.** This patient is infected with *Yersinia pestis* and has a classical presentation of bubonic plague. *Y. pestis* is a zoonotic infection with humans as the accidental host. The disease is maintained in squirrels, rabbits, rats, and domestic cats, with fleas serving as the vector. When the natural reservoir dies, the infected fleas will bite either other reservoir hosts or humans. The bacterium in humans travels to the regional lymph nodes and replicates, producing the enlarged lymph node or bubos characteristic of this infection. Plague is characterized by a rapid onset of symptoms, extremely painful bubos, and high mortality unless appropriately treated. The drug of choice remains streptomycin, although alternative treatment includes administration of tetracycline, chloramphenicol, or trimethoprim/sulfamethoxazole.

MM5 334-335

242 **(A) Antibiotic resistance.** Enterococci have a limited potential for causing disease. They do not possess potent toxins, and the importance of their hydrolytic enzymes (e.g., cytolysins, gelatinase) is not well defined. The most important factor that affects their virulence is their resistance to many antibiotics. This is particularly true for *Enterococcus faecium*, which is resistant to most beta-lactam antibiotics and commonly resistant to vancomycin.

MM5 259-262

243 **(E) Staphylococci that are resistant to oxacillin are resistant to all penicillins, cephalosporins, and carbapenems.** Resistance to oxacillin is mediated by alterations in the PBPs in the bacterial cell wall. This change also renders the bacteria resistant to all penicillins, cephalosporins, and carbapenems. The other answers to this question are incorrect because the enterotoxin is heat-stable; clostridia are responsible for gas gangrene; staphylococcal scalded skin syndrome is primarily seen in neonates; and coagulase-negative staphylococcal infections are typically slow to develop and have a chronic course.

MM5 234-235

244 **(C) *Haemophilus influenzae*.** Many of the *Haemophilus* species are opportunistic pathogens. The identity of this *H. influenze* organism is determined by the inability to grow on blood agar and the requirement for both X (hematin) and V (NAD) factors. *H. parainfluenzae* and *H. aphrophilus* do not require X factor, and *H. aphrophilus* and *H. ducreyi* do not require V factor. Although X and V factors are present in intact erythrocytes, the blood cells must be lysed ("chocolatized") to release the factors and inactivate the inhibitors of V factor present in the blood agar. *M. catarrhalis* can cause exacerbations of COPD but would appear as gram-negative diplococci on Gram stain and grow on both blood and chocolate agars.

MM5 367-369, 372-375

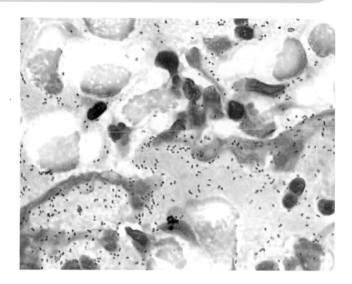

245 **(C) Lung aspirate.** Because most anaerobic infections are endogenous, care must be used to avoid contamination of the clinical material with a patient's endogenous bacterial flora. For that reason, certain specimens are unacceptable for anaerobic culture. Catheterized urines and urethral swabs can be contaminated with the bacteria in the urethra, expectorated sputum with bacteria in the oropharaynx, and rectal swabs with bacteria in the intestines. A lung aspirate that avoids oral contamination is the specimen of choice for the diagnosis of an anaerobic pleuropulmonary infection.

MM5 483

246 **(C) P1 adhesin protein.** *Mycoplasma pneumoniae* adheres to the respiratory epithelium by means of a specialized terminal protein attachment factor called P1. This adhesin protein binds specifically with glycoprotein receptors at the base of cilia on the epithelial cell surface, producing ciliostasis and then causing destruction of the ciliated epithelium. The organism also acts as a superantigen, stimulating inflammatory cells to migrate to the respiratory tree and release cytokines. Endotoxin is found only in gram-negative bacteria. Exotoxin A is an important virulence factor in *Pseudomonas* and is responsible for blocking protein synthesis. Phospholipase C is present in many virulent bacteria. This enzyme breaks down lipids and lecithin, leading to tissue destruction. Tracheal cytotoxin is produced by *Bordetella pertussis*. It is a peptidoglycan fragment that acts like the P1 adhesin, binding to ciliated epithelial cells, which leads to their death.

MM5 443-447

247 **(E) Tetracycline.** Tetracyclines inhibit protein synthesis by binding to the 30S ribosomal subunits, thus blocking the binding of aminoacyl-tRNA to the 30S ribosome/mRNA complex. Ciprofloxacin disrupts DNA replication by binding to the alpha subunit of DNA gyrase. Erythromycin binds to the 50S ribosomal subunit and blocks polypeptide elongation. Imipenem disrupts synthesis of the peptidoglycan layer in the bacterial cell

wall. Rifampin binds to DNA-dependent RNA polymerase and inhibits the initiation of RNA synthesis.
MM5 209-210

248 (E) Peptostreptococcus. *Peptostreptococcus*, as well as other gram-positive cocci and *Propionibacterium*, are found on the skin's surface, but the other genera listed in the answers to this question do not survive on the skin. *Actinomyces* is primarily found in the oropharynx, intestines, and genitourinary tract. *Bacteroides* and *Bifidobacterium* are primarily found in the colon. *Fusobacterium* is found in the oropharynx and intestines.
MM5 415-416

249 (A) Endocarditis: blood culture. Endocarditis is an infection of the inner surface of the heart. As such, the involved area is continuously washed with blood, so it is expected that infected patients would be persistently bacteremic. Food poisoning is an intoxication with a toxin that was produced in a food product before consumption. The organism may be present in the food but is typically not found in stool specimens. If *S. aureus* were present in a stool specimen, it would not be known if its presence represents previous colonization of the patient with this organism or a more significant finding. Impetigo is a localized cutaneous infection. Although bacteremia could be present, the diagnostic test of choice is culture of the involved cutaneous site. Scalded skin syndrome and toxic shock syndrome are both mediated by toxins that spread in the blood to distal sites. The diagnostic test for these two infections would be to culture the site where the infection is localized, such as a wound (which might appear minor) or the vagina.
MM5 228-233

250 (A) Borrelia burgdorferi. *I. scapularis* is a hard tick responsible for transmitting *Borrelia burgdorferi*, the agent responsible for Lyme disease, as well as transmitting organisms responsible for babesiosis and relapsing fever. Hard ticks have three periods of feeding: larva, nymph, and adult phases. Most infections in humans are caused by the nymph stage that is small and rarely observed during the feeding stage. Transmission of the other bacteria listed in the answers to this question is by direct contact with the bacterium (*L. interrogans*), with a flea (*Y. pestis*), with a body louse (*R. prowazekii*), and with a mosquito (*P. falciparum*).
MM5 433-437

251 (D) Lactobacillus. This immunocompromised man is bacteremic with *Lactobacillus*, a normal resident in the stomach and upper small intestine. Infections with this organism have been reported with increasing frequency since 1990. Patients most susceptible to infections with this organism include women who have just given birth, immunocompromised patients (particularly those with disruption of the lining of their gastrointestinal tract), and patients with a preexisting heart disease. *Lactobacillus* strains are either strictly anaerobic or facultatively anaerobic and are commonly resistant to vancomycin. The

vancomycin resistance differentiates *Lactobacillus* from the other organisms listed in the answers to this question.
MM5 420

252 (E) Streptobacillus. This patient has rat-bite fever caused by *Streptobacillus moniliformis*. The clinical picture of fevers, myalgias, and arthralgias is consistent with this diagnosis. In addition, *S. moniliformi* is a poorly staining, pleomorphic gram-negative rod that characteristically forms bulbous swellings at the ends of the rods. The organism can grow slowly in conventional blood cultures and from joint fluid if the fluid is cultured on media supplemented with 15% blood, 20% horse or calf serum, or 5% ascites fluid (not commonly used for most bacterial cultures). *Spirillum minus* can also cause rat-bite fever; however, the organism has not been grown in culture. Diagnosis of *Spirillum* infections is made by darkfield examination of blood, ulcer exudates, or lymph node aspirates. Blood smears can also be stained with Giemsa or Wright stains. *Leptospira* infections can result from exposure to infectious rat urine (in a contaminated standing pool of water). Isolation of *Leptospira* requires culture of the patient's blood or urine on specially enriched broth media (i.e., Fletcher, EMJH, or Tween 80-albumin), and the organism is not detected in routine blood cultures. *Capnocytophaga* and *Eikenella* infections have not been associated with rat bites. Moreover, both of these organisms would grow on conventional nonselective laboratory media.
MM5 399-400

253 (D) Slime layer. The slime layer is a loose lay[er] saccharides, peptides, and proteins that allow stap[ ] adhere to synthetic surfaces such as catheters, shu[ ] thetic devices. This layer is the major virulence fa[ ] coagulase-negative staphylococci. The other vir[ ] listed in the answers to this question (i.e., cyto[ ] toxins, protein A, and TSST-1) are primarily fou[nd in] *coccus aureus*.
MM5 222-223

254 (A) Azithromycin. Resistance in *N. go[ ]* [ ]en reported for penicillin, ciprofloxacin, and ery[ ] [ ]ra-

chomatis is resistant to all cell wall active antibiotics, including ceftriaxone and penicillin. Thus the macrolide azithromycin remains the most active antibiotic against these two agents of sexually transmitted diseases.
MM5 319-320

255   (E) Polysaccharide capsule. The polysaccharide capsule of *B. fragilis* protects the organism from phagocytosis and stimulates abscess formation. Cytotoxins and enterotoxins are not prominent in this organism, the LPS molecule does not have endotoxin activity (in contrast with aerobic gram-negative rods), and metronidazole resistance has not been reported for *Bacteroides*.
MM5 421-423

256   (C) *Erysipelothrix rhusiopathiae*. The man's skin lesion is typical of that caused by *E. rhusiopathiae*. The Gram stain confirms the presence of this organism by showing gram-positive rods that appear decolorized, which is typical of *E. rhusiopathiae*. *B. fragilis* is a strict anaerobic organism and would not grow in the aerobic culture. *P. aeruginosa* is a strict aerobic organism and would not grow in the anaerobic culture. *E. faecalis* and *S. pyogenes* are gram-positive cocci and would not be mistaken for *E. rhusiopathiae* on the Gram stain. *B. fragilis*, *P. aeruginosa*, and *S. pyogenes* can all cause purulent wound infections.
MM5 276-277

257   (C) Inactivates EF-2 and prevents protein synthesis. Diphtheria toxin is a classic A-B exotoxin. A receptor-binding region and a translocation region reside on the B subunit, and a catalytic region is on the A subunit. The receptor for the toxin is the heparin-binding epidermal growth factor that is present on the surface of many cells. Attachment and translocation is mediated by the B subunit. The A subunit moves into the cytosol and terminates host protein synthesis by inactivating EF-2, a factor required for the movement of peptide chains on ribosomes.
MM5 196-197

258   (D) Polysaccharide capsule. The primary virulence factor found in *S. pneumoniae* is the polysaccharide capsule. This capsule protects the organism from phagocytosis.
MM5 252-254

259   (E) Urease production. Urinary tract pathogens must be able to bind to the surface of the bladder and replicate. This binding is mediated by specific pili. Dissemination from this site is facilitated by other virulence factors, such as resistance to serum killing and resistance to antibiotic killing. Endotoxin production is also an important virulence factor for gram-negative bacteria but is not present in gram-positive bacteria. A variety of organisms can produce infections in the kidneys (i.e., pyelonephritis), and a subset of these organisms can cause stone (calculi) formation. These include *Proteus mirabilis*, *Morganella morganii*, *Klebsiella pneumoniae*, *Corynebacterium*

urealyticum, *Staphylococcus saprophyticus*, and *Ureaplasma urealyticum*. One property these bacteria have in common is production of urease. This enzyme is able to hydrolyze urea and produce ammonia. The increased alkalinity facilitates formation of stones.
MM5 193-201

260   (B) *Leptospira interrogans*. Leptospirosis is typically an asymptomatic infection. For patients who develop clinically apparent disease, the onset of symptoms generally develops 1 to 2 weeks after exposure to the bacteria. The initial presentation is a flu-like illness with fever and myalgias. These may remit after 1 week or progress to a more advanced disease, such as meningitis or a generalized illness with headache, rash, vascular collapse, thrombocytopenia, hemorrhage, and hepatic and renal dysfunction. The reservoirs for *Leptospira* infections in humans are rodents, particularly rats, dogs, and farm animals. The bacteria can colonize the renal tubules of infected animals and be shed in urine. Human infections are most commonly acquired by contact with contaminated water (e.g., standing water, lakes).
MM5 438-441

261   (B) Enterotoxin A. Enterotoxin A is one of eight serologically distinct, heat-stable enterotoxins described for *Staphylococcus aureus*. Enterotoxin A is most commonly associated with staphylococcal food poisoning. Because this disease is mediated by ingestion of a preformed toxin, the incubation period after ingestion of the contaminated food is only a few hours, and the duration of disease is less than 24 h. *S. aureus* produces a variety of other toxins that mediate disease. Alpha-toxin is an example of a cytotoxic toxin produced by this organism. This toxin is an important mediator of tissue damage and is toxic for many cells (e.g., erythrocytes, leukocytes, platelets), but it does not produce the clinical pictures described here. Leukocidin is also a cytotoxic toxin. TSST-1 was originally described as an enterotoxin (enterotoxin F) and is associated with diarrhea. Toxic shock syndrome is characterized by multiorgan dysfunction, skin desquamation, shock, and death. Two exfoliative toxins (A and B) have been described, each of which can mediate scalded skin syndrome in babies. These are serine proteases that split the intercellular bridges in the stratum granulosum epidermis. Neither cytolysis nor inflammation is present in the involved skin, so Gram stains and culture are not useful.
MM5 223-226

262   (D) Peptidoglycan. A major component of the cell wall of gram-positive and gram-negative bacteria is the peptidoglycan layer. This layer consists of linear polysaccharide chains made up of repeating disaccharides of N-acetylglucosamine and N-acetylmuramic acid. These polysaccharide chains are cross-linked with peptide bridges (hence the origin of the term *peptidoglycan*). The peptidoglycan of gram-positive bacteria is many layers thick; gram-negative bacteria have a much thinner peptidoglycan layer. Eukaryotic cells, such as fungi and protozoa, do not have a peptidoglycan layer in their cell wall but do contain

mitochondria, Golgi bodies, and an endoplasmic reticulum in their cytoplasm. These structures are absent in prokaryotic cells. In addition, the ribosomal structure differs in these two groups of organisms. The eukaryotic cell ribosome is 80S (composed of 40S and 60S subunits), and the prokaryotic cell ribosome is 70S (composed of 30S and 50S subunits).
MM5 13-15

263 (B) Inhalation. *C. burnetii* is found in a variety of animals, as well as ticks. Ticks are important vectors for animal infections but much less commonly implicated in human infections. Most human disease is initiated by inhalation of the bacteria. *C. burnetii* is extremely stable, surviving in adverse conditions for many weeks to years. Human disease can follow inhalation of the bacteria from dried feces, urine, or placentas left on the ground after parturition. Infections with this bacterium can also be acquired by consumption of contaminated, unpasteurized milk, although this is uncommon in the United States. Mosquitos have not been implicated in transmission of this bacterium, and *C. burnetii* is not able to directly penetrate unbroken skin.
MM5 460-462

264 (E) Giemsa stain of the ulcer exudate. This patient has granuloma inguinale, a granulomatous disease affecting the genitalia and inguinal area. The organism responsible for this infection is *Klebsiella* (formerly *Calymmatobacterium*) *granulomatis*. The organism has not been grown in cell-free cultures, so the diagnostic test of choice is microscopic examination of exudates stained with Giemsa stain. The organism appears as small rods in the cytoplasm of histiocytes, polymorphonuclear leukocytes, and plasma cells. A prominent capsule surrounds the individual rods. Thayer-Martin medium is used for the isolation of *Neisseria gonorrhoeae;* McCoy cells are used for the recovery of *Chlamydia;* MacConkey agar is a selective, differential medium for enteric bacteria; and darkfield examination is used to detect *Treponema pallidum.*
MM5 335-336

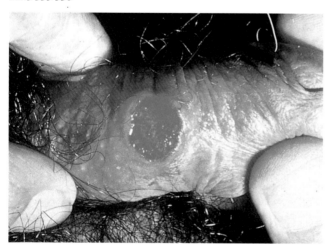

From Morse SA et al: *Atlas of sexually transmitted diseases and AIDS,* ed 3, 2003, Mosby.

265 (E) Serology. Laboratory confirmation of leptospirosis is difficult. The organism is thin and cannot be seen on Gram stain. Darkfield examination of clinical specimens is very helpful for a rapid diagnosis, but the test is insensitive and nonspecific (e.g., cell membrane fragments can be misdiagnosed as bacteria). Culture of blood and cerebrospinal fluid can be positive during the first week of clinical illness; however, special selective media (e.g., Fletcher, EMJH, Tween 80-albumin broths) must be inoculated and held for up to 4 weeks. Culture of urine can be positive after the first week, and the bacteria can persist for weeks in this specimen. This culture, however, is also insensitive and time consuming. Most clinical infections are confirmed using serology testing (i.e., indirect hemagglutination test, enzyme-linked immunosorbent assay, microscopic agglutination test). These tests are both sensitive and specific, with detectable antibodies developing in the second week of illness (although some patients may not mount a serologic response for weeks into the illness).
MM5 438-441

266 (E) Peptidoglycan. The peptidoglycan is degraded by the action of lysozyme on the glycan backbone. Without the peptidoglycan, the bacteria are osmotically unstable and lyse. Lysozyme is an enzyme present in human tears and mucus, so it forms a natural line of defense against bacterial infections. The enzyme has no effect on capsules (composed of either polysaccharides or proteins), on the cytoplasmic (inner) membrane or DNA present in all bacteria, or on the outer membrane present only in gram-negative bacteria.
MM5 13-15

267 (B) Fitz-Hugh-Curtis syndrome. This patient has pelvic inflammatory disease (PID) and clinical signs and symptoms of perihepatitis. Teenage girls are at increased risk for PID, and this risk is further increased by the use of douching. Acute perihepatitis, Fitz-Hugh-Curtis syndrome, is characterized by the abdominal pain, hepatic tenderness, and right upper quadrant pain. This condition results from the direct extension of the bacteria from the fallopian tubes to the liver and peritoneum, where adhesions form. This diagnosis can be confirmed by laparoscopy. Hepatic involvement is confined primarily to the surface of the liver and does not involve hepatic abscess formation. High levels of endotoxin may be found in systemic *N. gonorrhoeae* infections, but this endotoxin is not responsible for the localized symptoms reported for this patient. Reiter's syndrome is an immune-mediated reactive arthritis that has been associated with urethritis caused by *Chlamydia trachomatis.* Toxic shock syndrome is a multiorgan systemic disease primarily caused by toxin produced by *Staphylococcus aureus.*
MM5 315-316

268 (D) Blocks release of the neurotransmitter acetylcholine. The botulinum toxin is similar in structure and function to the tetanus toxin, differing only in the target neural cell. Botulinum toxin is specific for cholinergic nerves, blocking the release of acetylcholine at the peripheral cholinergic synapses.

This leads to the symptoms described in the question and can progress to bilateral descending weakness of the peripheral muscles with flaccid paralysis and then death attributed to respiratory paralysis.
MM5 409

269 **(B) Culture on anaerobic blood agar.** This man has cervicofacial actinomycosis caused by *Actinomyces*, which is an anaerobic gram-positive rod. Although some strains may grow slowly on aerobic media, anaerobic incubation is required for reliable recovery of this organism. BCYE agar is used for the recovery of *Nocardia*, as well as of *Legionella*. *Nocardia* can resemble *Actinomyces* morphologically but is not associated with a disease presenting like the one described for this man. Tests for *Cryptococcus* and *Histoplasma* would also not be indicated here.
MM5 418

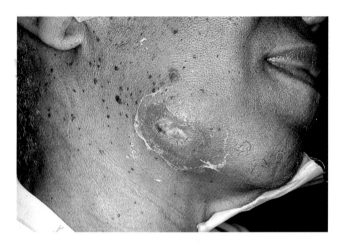

270 **(B) *Bacteroides*.** Metronidazole is an agent that is primarily active against gram-negative anaerobes. The only anaerobic gram-negative bacterium listed in this question is *Bacteroides*. *Actinomyces*, *Clostridium*, and *Peptostreptococcus* are resistant to metronidazole. *Mobiluncus* is also resistant to metronidazole, although this organism is associated with bacterial vaginosis, a disease routinely treated with metronidazole.
MM5 211, 426

271 **(A) *Anaplasma phagocytophilum*.** *A. phagocytophilum*, formerly *Ehrlichia phagocytophila*, is the etiologic agent of human anaplasmosis (previously called human granulocytic ehrlichiosis). Clinically, it is difficult to differentiate *A. phagocytophilum* infections from *Rickettsia rickettsii* infections, although a rash is less commonly seen in *A. phagocytophila* infections. In addition, ticks are the vectors for *A. phagocytophilum* and *R. rickettsii*, the etiologic agent of Rocky Mountain spotted fever. The observation of intracellular bacteria (i.e., morula) in peripheral blood granulocytes is useful for distinguishing between these two organisms. Infected blood cells are observed more frequently with human anaplasmosis than with monocytic ehrlichiosis. Despite this positive result, the diagnostic tests of choice for anaplasmo-

sis are nucleic acid amplification and serology. *C. burnetii* is a related intracellular organism that causes infections most commonly by the airborne route (although ticks can be responsible for some infections). *B. microti* and *P. vivax* cause blood infections but infect erythrocytes.
MM5 458-459

272 **(C) Measurement of anti-DNase B antibodies.** Acute glomerulonephritis is an immunologically based reaction to *S. pyogenes* infection of the pharynx or skin. Antibodies develop 3 to 4 weeks after the initial infection. An elevated antibody titer to streptolysin O (ASO) is observed in patients with a pharyngeal infection but not in patients with a primary skin infection. Streptolysin O is bound by cholesterol in the skin lipids, so it does not stimulate an immune response in pyoderma. For these patients, an antibodies against DNase B (anti-DNase B) test should be performed. Two forms of streptokinase are produced by *S. pyogenes*, but this does not appear to be a sensitive or specific marker for glomerulonephritis. Because the disease is an immunologic reaction to strains producing pharyngitis or pyoderma, culture of blood or urine is not helpful.
MM5 246-247

273 **(B) *Rhodococcus*.** Bacteria with medium- to long-chain mycolic acids are able to stain with acid-fast stains. The length of the mycolic acid chains influences the staining ability. For example, mycobacteria have 60 to 90 carbon atoms in their mycolic acid chains and typically stain with all acid-fast stains; *Gordonia*, *Nocardia*, *Rhodococcus*, and *Tsukamurella* have shorter chains (e.g., 34 to 78 carbon atoms) and typically stain acid-fast only when weak acid/alcohol solutions are used (i.e., stain only with modified acid-fast stains). *Actinomyces* and *Streptomyces* form filamentous rods and are commonly confused with *Nocardia*. In contrast with *Nocardia*, both of these organisms do not retain acid-fast stains. *Rothia* and *Tropheryma* (the etiologic agent of Whipple disease) are gram-positive rods or coccobacilli. These organisms do not have mycolic acids in their cell walls and do not retain the acid-fast stain.
MM5 292-293

274 **(C) Cell wall proteins.** The composition of the mycobacterial cell wall is extremely complex. This property renders the organisms resistant to most commonly used antibacterial antibiotics and disinfectants and is responsible for the unique staining properties of the organisms (i.e., the acid-fast property). The basic structure of the cell wall is typical of gram-positive bacteria; that is, the innermost layer is the cytoplasmic membrane, overlaid with the thick peptidoglycan layer, and the absence of the outer membrane found in gram-negative bacteria. The peptidoglycan layer consists of repeating subunits of N-acetylglucosamine and N-acetylmuramic acid, cross-linked with a tetrapeptide bridge containing D-alanine, L-alanine, D-glutamic acid, and M-diaminopimelic acid. The extent of cross-linkage determines the stability of the bacterial cell wall. Over the peptidoglycan layer is the arabinogalactan/mycolate layer, consisting

of D-arabinose, D-galactose, and mycolic acids. Finally, the outermost layer contains free polypeptides and a hydrophobic layer of mycolic acids consisting of free lipids, glycolipids, and peptidoglycolipids. These lipids constitute 60% of the dry weight of the cell wall. The peptide chains in the outermost layer constitute 15% of the cell wall weight and are biologically important antigens, stimulating the patient's cellular immune response to infection. Extracted, species-specific, purified proteins are used as skin test antigens in the purified protein derivatives (PPD) test.
MM5 297-298

275   (D) _Clostridium septicum._ All of the organisms listed in the answers to this question are gram-positive rods; however, _E. rhusiopathiae_ is not a genus that forms spores. _B. anthracis_ and _B. cereus_ have not been associated with rapidly progressive myonecrosis, so they should be excluded. Both _C. perfringens_ and _C. septicum_ can produce a disease as seen in this patient; however, _C. perfringens_ can be excluded because it rarely produces spores in clinical samples and in culture. In addition, _C. septicum_ sepsis has been associated with colon cancer, acute leukemia, and diabetes.
MM5 413

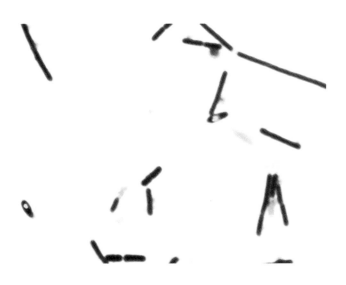

276   (C) _Nocardia._ Of the organisms listed, _Actinomyces_ and _Streptomyces_ can be excluded because they are not acid-fast or partially acid-fast. _Actinomyces_ is also an anaerobic organism (some strains are aerotolerant), so it would not be expected to grow on bacterial (blood agar), fungal (Sabouraud), or mycobacterial (Middlebrook) media. The rapidly growing mycobacteria can grow in 4 days in the three media in which this organism was recovered; however, the mycobacteria do not develop an orange color or aerial hyphae (filamentous growth extending above the surface of the colony). The presence of aerial hyphae also is not observed with _Rhodococcus._ This organism can also be excluded because rhodococci appear as cocci or coccobacilli, not branching filamentous rods. Nocardiae are the only partially acid-fast organisms that produce aerial hyphae. They are not fastidious organisms and can grow on most nonselective laboratory

media. The difficulty in recovering these organisms arises in their slow growth, and they may not be visible on media at the time the culture is discontinued. It is important to alert the laboratory that _Nocardia_ is considered in the clinical differential, so the incubation of the culture can be extended to 5 to 7 days. Most infections with _Nocardia_ begin as a localized disease in the lungs; however, dissemination can occur, most commonly to the central nervous system or cutaneous sites.
MM5 287-292

277   (B) _Brucella canis._ _B. canis_ is antigenically distinct from the other _Brucella_ species. _B. abortus_ has the highest concentration of A antigen, and _B. melitensis_ has the highest concentration of M antigen. The antigen used in the _Brucella_ agglutination test is from _B. abortus._ Antibodies directed against _B. melitensis_ or _B. suis_ cross-react with this antigen; however, there is no cross-reactivity with _B. canis._ Specific _B. canis_ antigen must be used to diagnose infections with this organism.
MM5 383-386

278   (B) Pilin protein. _N. gonorrhoeae_ organisms have pili that extend from the cytoplasmic membrane through the outer membrane. The pili are composed of pilin proteins. These proteins have a conserved region that attaches to the cytoplasmic membrane and a highly variable region that is exposed. The lack of immunity to reinfection results partially from the antigenic variation among pilin proteins and partially from the phase variation in pilin expression. Por proteins are porin proteins that render _N. gonorrhoeae_ resistant to serum killing and promote intracellular survival. Opa proteins mediate binding to epithelial cells. Rmp (reduction-modifiable proteins) stimulate antibodies that block serum bactericidal activity. The transferrin-binding protein is one of three iron binding proteins present in _N. gonorrhoeae._
MM5 311-315

279   (D) _Mycobacterium kansasii._ Mycobacterial infections in HIV-infected patients are a significant cause of morbidity and mortality. In countries where both tuberculosis and HIV are common (e.g., Africa), tuberculosis is the most common cause of death in HIV-infected patients. Tuberculosis is a less common complication in HIV-infected patients in the United States because of the relatively low incidence of tuberculosis. However, infections with nontuberculosis mycobacteria are particularly common. The two most frequent mycobacterial isolates are _M. avium_ complex and _M. kansasii._ _M. kansasii_ is a photochromogenic mycobacteria. That is, the organism produces intensely yellow carotenoid pigments only after exposure to light. _M. avium_ can appear pale yellow, but this coloration is not induced by light exposure and is not as intense as that seen in the chromogenic mycobacteria. _M. haemophilum_ is not pigmented and will not grow on Lowenstein-Jensen medium or Middlebrook broth unless the media are supplemented with hemin.
MM5 297-298, 305

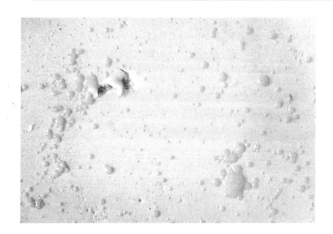

From Baron EJ, Peterson LR, Finegold SM: *Bailey and Scott's diagnostic microbiology* ed 9, St Louis, 1994, Mosby.

280 **(A) Capsule.** This patient's infection is caused by *Bacteroides fragilis*. Rapid tests that can be used for the preliminary identification of this organism include demonstration of resistance to kanamycin, vancomycin, and colistin (performed by subculturing the colony onto anaerobic blood agar and placing the antibiotic disks on the plate) and demonstrating enhanced growth on media supplemented with bile. *B. fragilis* produces a variety of virulence factors. The most important virulence factor is the polysaccharide capsule, which is antiphagocytic. Purified capsular polysaccharides can produce abscesses in experimental animals. The organism does not have endotoxin because, in contrast with aerobic gram-negative rods, the *Bacteroides* glycolipid that resides in the cell wall lipopolysaccharide has little or no endotoxin activity. Fimbria is an important adhesion factor, and superoxide dismutase helps protect the *Bacteriodes* bacteria from oxygen toxicity. Phospholipase C is not found in *Bacteroides*.
MM5 421-426

281 **(B) Blocks release of GABA.** *C. tetani* neurotoxin (tetanospasmin) is an A-B toxin. The B subunit binds to specific sialic acid receptors (e.g., polysialogangliosides) and adjacent glycoproteins on the surface of motor neurons. The intact toxin is internalized in endosomal vesicles and transported in the neuron axon to motor neuron soma located in the spinal cord. In this location, the endosome becomes acidified, leading to a conformation change in the toxin, which allows transport of the A subunit from the endosome to the cell cytosol. The A subunit is an endopeptidase that cleaves core proteins involved in the release of inhibitory neurotransmitters, specifically GABA.
MM5 196, 406-407

282 **(C) *Streptococcus pneumoniae*.** The most common organisms responsible for middle ear infections are *S. pneumoniae* and *Haemophilus influenzae* (typically nontypable strains). *S. aureus* is a less common cause of middle ear infections and typically has a more acute presentation. *P. aeruginosa* is responsible for otitis externa (swimmer's ear), as well as a more fulminant, destructive ear infection called malignant otitis externa. *S.*

pyogenes is an unknown cause of middle ear infections and *S. salivarius*, a member of the viridans group of *Streptococcus*, is relatively avirulent and is not associated with otitis media.
MM5 255-256

283 **(E) Production of metallo beta-lactamase.** Carbapenem antibiotics (e.g., imipenem, meropenem, ergopenem) are potent antibiotics that are active against virtually all groups of organisms, with only a few exceptions (e.g., resistance has been reported for all oxacillin-resistant staphylococci, selected Enterobacteriaceae and *Pseudomonas*, as well as some other gram-negative rods). Resistance to this class of antibiotics is most commonly caused by production of metallo beta-lactamases.
MM5 207

284 **(B) Darkfield examination.** The patient presents with a classic picture of primary syphilis. The genital ulcer is typically painless unless a secondary bacterial infection is present. At this stage of disease, the exudate from the ulcer is teaming with spirochetes. Although darkfield examination is not commonly done in clinical laboratories, this is the most sensitive test for detecting the bacteria (sensitivity approaches 100%). The reason the test is not commonly performed is because primary syphilis is relatively uncommon, and technologists have lost the skill in interpreting the stains. The organism has not been cultured, so a culture would not be useful. Likewise, the organism is too thin to be seen on Gram stain, so this test should not be used. The VDRL is a nonspecific (nontreponemal) test for syphilis. Although the test is very sensitive for secondary syphilis, the sensitivity for primary syphilis is 75% to 80%. The FTA-ABS test is a specific treponemal test that has a sensitivity of approximately 85% for primary syphilis. This test also has a sensitivity of almost 100% for secondary and late syphilis.
MM5 430-433

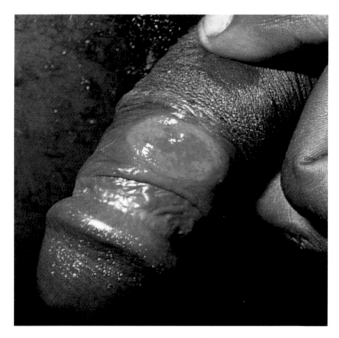

From Morse S et al: *Atlas of sexually transmitted diseases and AIDS*, ed 3, St Louis, 2003, Mosby.

285 **(A) Culture in Middlebrook broth at 30°C.** This infection is caused by *Mycobacterium marinum.* The optimum temperature for growing this organism in culture is 30° to 33°C. Any mycobacterial medium (e.g., Lowenstein-Jensen, Middlebrook agar, Middlebrook broth) will support the growth of this organism. It is important that the laboratory be notified that the infection is from a superficial site and that this specific mycobacterium is in the differential diagnosis because *M. marinum* grows very slowly or not at all at 37°C. *Nocardia* (which grows best on BCYE agar) can cause an infection with this presentation, but contaminated soil and not water would be the most likely source. *Sporothrix* can also cause an infection such as the one in this woman's case, but that pathogen is most commonly associated with trauma from contaminated garden soil rich in organic material. *Mycobacteria* do not stain with the Gram stain, so this stain would be an unreliable diagnostic tool.

MM5 305-308

286 **(B) Cysteine-tellurite agar.** Although *C. diphtheriae* can grow on a variety of laboratory media (including sheep blood), the reliance on nonselective media is not recommended because the bacteria that are found normally in the oropharynx will obscure *C. diphtheriae.* The best medium for the selective isolation of this organism is cysteine-tellurite agar. Cysteine enhances growth of the organism, and *C. diphtheriae* reduces tellurite, forming dark gray colonies. *C. diphtheriae* does not grow on Bordet-Gengou agar (for *B. pertussis*), MacConkey agar (for gram-negative rods), or Thayer-Martin agar (used for the recovery of *N. gonorrhoeae*).

MM5 379-382

287 **(E) Penicillin is the drug of choice for treating infections caused by *Peptostreptococcus*.** Virtually all isolates are susceptible to penicillin. Most anaerobic infections are polymicrobic, involving a mixture of aerobic and anaerobic species. *Actinomyces* is associated with sinus tracks, and *Clostridium perfringens* is associated with gas gangrene. Anaerobes rarely cause UTIs.

MM5 415

288 **(C) The organism is capable of producing heat-stable enterotoxins.** An important toxin-mediated disease caused by *Staphylococcus* is food poisoning, which is caused by one of eight types of enterotoxins. The other answers to this question are incorrect because of the following explanations. Staphylococci are arranged in clusters, not in pairs and chains. *S. aureus* is coagulase-positive, a property that separates *S. aureus* from the other staphylococcal species. The toxin responsible for rheumatic fever does not have cytotoxic activity. PV leukocidin is associated with fulminant necrotizing pneumonia and wound infections. Exfoliative toxins are associated with scalded skin syndrome.

MM5 225-226, 229-230

289 **(A) *Abiotrophia*.** These organisms resemble streptococci by their morphology and the absence of catalase activity. Without growth supplements, these organisms fail to grow on blood agar media. The other organisms listed in the answers to this question are all catalase-negative and resemble streptococci in morphology; however, they all grow well on blood agar.

MM5 262

290 **(D) *Neisseria meningitidis*.** All of the organisms listed in the answers to this question can cause meningitis. The clinical picture, however, is consistent with bacterial meningitis, so it is unlikely that *C. neoformans* would cause meningitis in a previously healthy person. Furthermore, the Gram stain is inconsistent with *Cryptococcus* (a fungus). The most common causes of meningitis in college students are *N. meningitidis* and *S. pneumoniae. N. meningitidis* is a gram-negative diplococci with sides flattened against each cocci, and *S. pneumoniae* is a gram-positive diplococci with the cells arranged end-to-end. The Gram stain and clinical presentation for this patient is consistent with *N. meningitidis. H. influenzae* is a gram-negative rod that causes meningitis in unvaccinated children ages 3 months to 5 years. *L. monocytogenes* is a gram-positive rod that causes meningitis in the very young and the elderly.

MM5 216-217

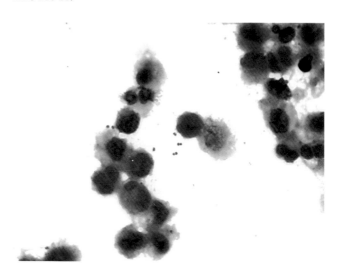

291 **(C) Modification of DNA gyrase.** Ciprofloxacin is a fluoroquinolone antibiotic. These antibiotics inhibit bacterial DNA gyrases or topoisomerases, which are required for DNA replication, recombination, and repair. Alteration of these enzymes is the principal mechanism of bacterial resistance, although decreased drug uptake has also been observed.

MM5 210-211

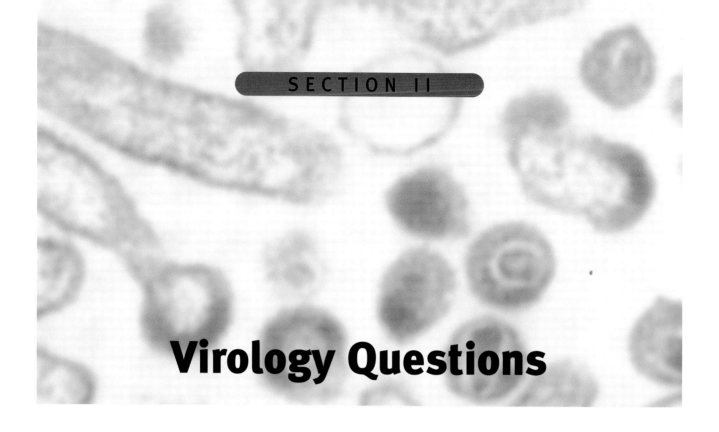

Virology Questions

1 At an office visit, a 38-year-old man complains of jaundice, dark urine, anorexia, abdominal pain, and malaise. Serologic tests are positive for both HB$_c$Ag and HB$_s$Ag. Which statement most accurately describes the virus responsible for these findings?

- ☐ (A) Its genome is a messenger RNA (mRNA) that encodes a polyprotein.
- ☐ (B) Its genome is linear double-stranded DNA.
- ☐ (C) Its genome is RNA, but it replicates through a DNA intermediate.
- ☐ (D) Its replication requires a helper virus.
- ☐ (E) Its replication requires an RNA-dependent DNA polymerase.

2 A 35-year-old Native American man is brought to the emergency department of a hospital in New Mexico suffering from pulmonary edema. He dies of respiratory failure. Which description characterizes this virus?

- ☐ (A) It is assayed by reverse transcriptase polymerase chain reaction (RT-PCR) technology.
- ☐ (B) It is an enveloped, single-stranded, positive-sense RNA virus.
- ☐ (C) It normally causes benign disease.
- ☐ (D) It is spread by mosquitoes.
- ☐ (E) Is susceptible to amantadine treatment if diagnosed early.

3 In December, many teachers in an elementary school begin to suffer from the common symptoms of influenza A, including sore throat, runny nose, cough, fever, headache, myalgia, and fatigue. The teachers who have not been vaccinated against this infection are offered prophylactic treatment with amantadine. What is the mechanism of action for this drug?

- ☐ (A) Blockade of nucleocapsid release into the cytoplasm
- ☐ (B) Blockade of viral glycoprotein synthesis
- ☐ (C) Blockade of viral protein synthesis
- ☐ (D) Inhibition of RNA-dependent DNA polymerase
- ☐ (E) Inhibition of RNA-dependent RNA polymerase

4 What is a target cell receptor for Epstein-Barr virus (EBV)?

- ☐ (A) C3d complement receptor on B lymphocytes
- ☐ (B) CD4 molecule and chemokine coreceptor on T lymphocytes
- ☐ (C) Immunoglobulin superfamily protein on epithelial cells
- ☐ (D) Acetylcholine receptor on neurons
- ☐ (E) Sialic acid receptor on epithelial cells

5 A 48-year-old man has been receiving blood products for hemophilia since childhood. He is now suffering from a low-grade fever, weight loss, thrush, serious bouts of diarrhea, and symptoms of pneumonia. A deficiency in the production of which substance would be most pronounced in this patient?

- ☐ (A) Complement components
- ☐ (B) Immunoglobulin G (IgG)
- ☐ (C) Interferon-alpha (IFN-α)
- ☐ (D) Interferon-gamma (IFN-γ)
- ☐ (E) Interleukin-1 (IL-1)

6 A 15-year-old boy develops conjunctivitis, pharyngitis, and an upper respiratory tract infection 3 days after swimming in a friend's pool. He has a mild fever but no rash. The suspected cause is an agent that can be isolated from a nasal wash and is able to rapidly kill African green monkey kidney cells. Which agent is the most likely the cause of this boy's condition?

- ❐ (A) Enveloped, double-stranded DNA virus
- ❐ (B) Gram-negative diplococcus
- ❐ (C) Gram-negative, oxidase-positive rod
- ❐ (D) Gram-positive diplococcus
- ❐ (E) Nonenveloped, double-stranded DNA virus with spikes at its vertices

7 A 65-year-old Japanese man has acute T cell lymphocytic leukemia. His leukemic cells are found to be producing a virus. The patient most likely acquired the viral infection via which route?

- ❐ (A) Blood transfusion
- ❐ (B) Contact with saliva
- ❐ (C) Fecal-oral route
- ❐ (D) Respiratory route
- ❐ (E) Vertical genetic transmission

8 A 60-year-old Japanese woman has acute T cell lymphocytic leukemia. Her T cells express the human T lymphotropic virus type I (HTLV-I) genome. What is the mechanism of leukemogenesis for this virus?

- ❐ (A) Activation of IFN-γ production
- ❐ (B) Activation of interleukin-2 (IL-2) receptor expression
- ❐ (C) Expression of a virus-encoded growth hormone receptor
- ❐ (D) Expression of a virus-encoded guanosine triphosphate binding protein
- ❐ (E) Expression of a virus-encoded tyrosine kinase

9 Cell culture of an isolate from a patient with epidemic keratoconjunctivitis (also called shipyard eye) contains cells with dark basophilic nuclear inclusion bodies. Which structure characterizes the virus responsible for this condition?

- ❐ (A) Enveloped, single-stranded, negative-sense RNA virus
- ❐ (B) Enveloped, single-stranded, positive-sense RNA virus
- ❐ (C) Nonenveloped, double-stranded, circular DNA virus
- ❐ (D) Nonenveloped, double-stranded DNA virus with penton fibers at its vertices
- ❐ (E) Nonenveloped, single-stranded, positive-sense RNA virus

10 A 56-year-old man complains of severe pain caused by a belt of vesicular lesions across the left side of his abdomen. What is the source of his infection?

- ❐ (A) Aerosolized droplets of the causative agent
- ❐ (B) Contaminated food or water
- ❐ (C) Endogenous reactivation of an earlier infection

- ❐ (D) Puncture with a contaminated object
- ❐ (E) Sexual activity

11 A newly developed compound is shown to have a broad range of antiviral activity and is capable of inhibiting numerous types of RNA and DNA viruses, including those with and without envelopes. When the compound is used in studies involving influenza B virus, no viral synthesis is detected, although viral mRNA is detected in low amounts. Which antiviral agent has a mode of action similar to this compound and would inhibit a similar step in replication?

- ❐ (A) Acyclovir
- ❐ (B) Amantadine
- ❐ (C) Azidothymidine
- ❐ (D) IFN-α
- ❐ (E) Ribavirin

12 The Centers for Disease Control and Prevention (CDC) is called to evaluate an outbreak of disease in passengers who are vacationing on a 7-day cruise. The symptoms last 2 days and include diarrhea, vomiting, abdominal cramps, nausea, and headache. A small, single-stranded, positive-sense RNA virus with an icosahedral capsid is isolated from the stool of several passengers. Which virus is most likely the cause of the disease?

- ❐ (A) Adenovirus
- ❐ (B) Coronavirus
- ❐ (C) Coxsackievirus
- ❐ (D) Norwalk virus
- ❐ (E) Rotavirus

13 A virus isolated from a patient with liver disease is detergent-sensitive, and its genome is infectious. Which virus do these findings describe?

- ❐ (A) Papillomavirus
- ❐ (B) Adenovirus
- ❐ (C) Hepatitis A virus (HAV)
- ❐ (D) Hepatitis E virus (HEV)
- ❐ (E) Yellow fever virus

14 A 6-month-old girl has been experiencing bouts of diarrhea and vomiting for 24 h. An enzyme-linked immunosorbent assay (ELISA) of a stool sample yields positive results for rotavirus. Which action would have been the best means for preventing the infant's infection?

- ❐ (A) Boiling the eating utensils
- ❐ (B) Breast-feeding the infant
- ❐ (C) Carefully washing the infant's hands prior to eating
- ❐ (D) Immunizing the infant with a killed vaccine
- ❐ (E) Treating the infant with amantadine

15 Which virus is characterized by nonenveloped RNA?

- ❐ (A) Herpes simplex virus (HSV)
- ❐ (B) Influenza virus
- ❐ (C) Lassa fever virus

❒ (D) Norwalk virus
❒ (E) Respiratory syncytial virus

16 A 32-year-old man with AIDS develops symptoms consistent with the diagnosis of cytomegalovirus (CMV) retinitis. Confirmation of the diagnosis could be obtained by which test result?

❒ (A) Atypical lymphocytes in blood sample
❒ (B) ELISA for antibody to CMV in serum sample
❒ (C) Epithelial cells with owl's eye inclusion bodies in urine sample
❒ (D) Immunofluorescence of tear-infected tissue culture fibroblasts
❒ (E) PCR analysis for viral DNA in blood sample

17 Primary monkey kidney cells are coinfected with an influenza A isolate from 1991 (A/Texas/91-like H1N1) and an isolate from 1989 (A/Beijing/89-like H3N2). Genetic analysis of the two parental viruses and a virus isolated from the resultant infection shows the data in the figure. Which designation is correct for the progeny virus of this coinfection?

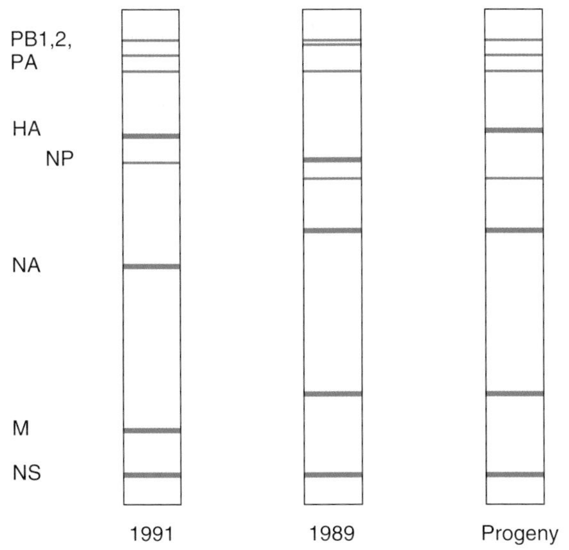

PB1,2, PA

HA

NP

NA

M

NS

1991   1989   Progeny

❒ (A) H1N1
❒ (B) H1N2
❒ (C) H3N1
❒ (D) H3N2
❒ (E) None of the above

18 A 30-year-old African woman has lost approximately 20 lb during the past 3 months and complains of fever, chills, and a bad cough. She is found to be suffering from multiple infections, including tuberculosis and a severe oral yeast infection. Which viral protein is important for causing the patient's disease but is not essential for replication?

❒ (A) gag
❒ (B) gp120
❒ (C) Integrase

❒ (D) nef
❒ (E) Protease

19 A 6-year-old girl is brought to the emergency department because she has had a fever for 4 days, has begun vomiting after meals, and is suffering from a severe headache, irritability, and fatigue. Examination shows nuchal rigidity but no rash or conjunctivitis. A cerebrospinal fluid (CSF) sample is somewhat cloudy and has a white blood cell (WBC) count of $4/mm^3$, with a predominance of lymphocytes. The CSF glucose level is slightly low (60 mg), and the protein level is high (84 mg). A Gram stain is negative. An infection with echovirus 11 is suspected, and the child recovers within 8 days without antibiotic treatment. Transmission from person to person of echovirus is facilitated by which viral characteristic?

❒ (A) Envelope
❒ (B) Hemagglutinin (HA)
❒ (C) Icosahedral capsid
❒ (D) Neuraminidase (NA)
❒ (E) Spike protein

20 A 57-year-old man from southern Japan has acute leukemia. PCR analysis of T cells from the patient indicates the presence of retroviral DNA. Which scenario is consistent with these data?

❒ (A) Environmental factors in Japan may have promoted the development of HTLV-I leukemia.
❒ (B) An oncogene from HTLV-I may have triggered the development of leukemia.
❒ (C) Presence of retroviral DNA may be due to an endogenous virus.
❒ (D) Recent infection with human immunodeficiency virus (HIV) may have promoted the development of leukemia.
❒ (E) Recent infection with HTLV-I may have promoted the development of leukemia.

21 Lassa fever is suspected in an African patient who died after suffering from fever, coagulopathy, petechiae, severe heart and liver damage, and shock. A nurse who cared for the patient presents with the prodrome of pharyngitis, diarrhea, and vomiting. Treatment with which agent would be most appropriate for the nurse?

❒ (A) Acyclovir
❒ (B) Amantadine
❒ (C) Azidothymidine
❒ (D) Foscarnet
❒ (E) Ribavirin

22 A new drug is being tested to determine its ability to inhibit the replication of herpes simplex virus. If the drug is given before exposure to the virus or is given 1, 3, or 5 h after exposure, 100% inhibition occurs. Only 20% inhibition occurs, however, if the drug is given 8 h after exposure.

Which step in viral replication is the likely target for this new drug?

❏   (A) Assembly
❏   (B) Binding
❏   (C) DNA synthesis
❏   (D) Penetration
❏   (E) Protein synthesis

23   Which property is associated with an inactivated vaccine?

❏   (A) A single dose may be administered.
❏   (B) IgG and IgA response to the vaccine.
❏   (C) There is a good cellular immune response.
❏   (D) The vaccine is usually administered with an adjuvant.
❏   (E) The duration of immunity is lifelong.

24   Which vaccine is available in a live, attenuated form, as well as a killed form?

❏   (A) Hepatitis B vaccine
❏   (B) Influenza vaccine
❏   (C) Lyme disease vaccine
❏   (D) Polio vaccine
❏   (E) Varicella vaccine

25   A wrestler has a vesicular lesion on his shoulder. One of his teammates has a similar lesion on his wrist, and another has a crusted lesion at the vermillion border of his lips. Which enzyme is encoded by the virus responsible for these lesions?

❏   (A) Integrase
❏   (B) 5N-methyl capping enzyme
❏   (C) Neuraminidase
❏   (D) RNA-dependent RNA polymerase
❏   (E) Thymidine kinase

26   A Pap-stained cervical smear from a sexually active 36-year-old woman with cervical dysplasia shows cells with enlarged nuclei and cytoplasmic vacuoles (koilocytotic cells), indicating a viral infection. Which technique would be useful to confirm the diagnosis of the agent most likely to be present in these cells?

❏   (A) ELISA for antiviral antibody in serum
❏   (B) Hemadsorption to the cells in the cervical smear
❏   (C) Immunofluorescent analysis of cells from the cervical smear
❏   (D) In situ DNA hybridization analysis of cells from the cervical smear
❏   (E) Virus isolation in HeLa cell cultures

27   A 28-year-old man is taken to the emergency department during the winter; he is suffering from a fever, headaches, seizures, speech and behavioral problems, and other symptoms of encephalitis. He dies within hours of arriving at the hospital.

Which finding in brain tissue would confirm that HSV was the causative agent?

❏   (A) Cowdry type A inclusion bodies
❏   (B) Downey cells
❏   (C) HA
❏   (D) Negri bodies
❏   (E) Owl's eye inclusion bodies

28   Which virus is a single-stranded DNA virus?

❏   (A) Adenovirus
❏   (B) Epstein-Barr virus
❏   (C) Papillomavirus
❏   (D) Parvovirus B19
❏   (E) Poliovirus

29   A 26-year-old man who died of AIDS suffered from numerous infections and progressively lost his speech, vision, coordination, and cognitive ability. The autopsy reveals foci of demyelination in the brain that are surrounded by oligodendrocytes and appear as glioblastomas. A PCR probe for T antigen-specific sequences confirms the identity of the virus responsible for these findings. Which genome structure best characterizes this virus?

❏   (A) Circular double-stranded DNA
❏   (B) Linear double-stranded DNA
❏   (C) Linear single-stranded negative RNA
❏   (D) Linear single-stranded positive RNA
❏   (E) Partially double-stranded DNA

30   An attenuated vaccine is used to prevent infections caused by which virus?

❏   (A) HAV
❏   (B) Hepatitis B virus (HBV)
❏   (C) Influenza virus
❏   (D) Rabies virus
❏   (E) Varicella-zoster virus (VZV)

31   A 47-year-old Japanese man has a rash and nodules on his skin. A biopsy of a nodule shows a T cell lymphoma and the presence of CD4 T cells that carry HTLV-I. Which answer is characteristic of this disease?

❏   (A) Disease is preventable by use of a vaccine.
❏   (B) Disease is sexually transmitted.
❏   (C) HTLV-I infection rapidly promotes lymphomagenesis.
❏   (D) Lymphoma is susceptible to azidothymidine treatment.
❏   (E) RNA-dependent RNA polymerase is present in the lymphoma cells.

32   HSV infection is reported as the cause of a neonate's death, and the parents wish to file a lawsuit. To determine the source of infection, a virus isolate is obtained at autopsy and compared with isolates obtained from the parents, health care professionals, and others who came into contact with the neonate. Which test would be sufficient to determine whether two samples had the same source of infection?

❑ (A) Cytopathologic examination of tissue cultures
❑ (B) Immunofluorescence of infected cells
❑ (C) In situ DNA hybridization
❑ (D) Restriction fragment length polymorphism (RFLP) techniques
❑ (E) Western blot analysis of serum samples

33 A 4-year-old boy with sickle cell disease is taken to his pediatrician's office because he is pale and is suffering from fatigue and flu-like symptoms. A blood test shows that the peripheral hemoglobin concentration is considerably lower than normal, with no change in the WBC or platelet counts. The pediatrician suspects that the patient is suffering from aplastic crisis. Which description is relevant to the findings of anemia in this patient?

❑ (A) Sickle cell trait decreases the patient's resistance to the virus infection.
❑ (B) Sickle cell trait promotes infection of erythrocytes by the virus.
❑ (C) Virus infection activates malaria and causes the aplastic crisis.
❑ (D) Virus infection promotes IFN production.
❑ (E) Virus infection targets erythrocyte precursor cells.

34 Which property is associated with HSV?

❑ (A) Can be spread easily on fomites (e.g., utensils) or via hand-to-hand contact
❑ (B) Modifies the host cell membrane during replication
❑ (C) Is released from infected cells by cell-to-cell fusion
❑ (D) Appears stable to drying
❑ (E) Is stable to exposure to detergents

35 Vaccinia virus was used as a vaccine against smallpox and is now being used as a vector for the genes of antigens of other viruses. Vaccinia virus is useful as a vector because of which fact?

❑ (A) The population has already been immunized against vaccinia.
❑ (B) The viral genome contains many nonessential genes.
❑ (C) The virus does not spread readily to other hosts.
❑ (D) The virus has a broad range of hosts.
❑ (E) The virus is cytolytic.

36 Which step in viral replication is inhibited by amantadine?

❑ (A) Attachment
❑ (B) Uncoating
❑ (C) Transcription
❑ (D) Replication
❑ (E) Viral assembly

37 Which vaccine can be given safely to a child who is being treated for leukemia?

❑ (A) Influenza vaccine
❑ (B) Measles vaccine
❑ (C) Mumps vaccine
❑ (D) Oral polio vaccine
❑ (E) Varicella vaccine

38 Effective vaccine programs have been established to prevent smallpox (caused by variola virus) and rubella (caused by rubella virus). Although the agents of these diseases share several characteristics that facilitate disease prevention, which characteristic of rubella virus distinguishes it from variola virus and limits the possibility of eliminating rubella?

❑ (A) Rubella virus causes asymptomatic infection.
❑ (B) Rubella virus causes viremia.
❑ (C) Rubella virus has only one serotype.
❑ (D) The host range for rubella virus is limited to humans.
❑ (E) The rubella vaccine is a live vaccine.

39 The herpesviruses are able to evade the host's immune response by which mechanism?

❑ (A) Block IFN production
❑ (B) Block IL-1 and tumor necrosis factor (TNF)-mediated inflammation
❑ (C) Cause genetic change after infection
❑ (D) Establish latent infections
❑ (E) Prevent CD8 T cell killing

40 A 25-year-old man complains of intermittent fever, chills, headache, and severe myalgia approximately 10 days after returning from a hiking trip in the western United States. The physician suspects he has Colorado tick fever. Which property of the viral agent of this disease enables its transmission from mammals to ticks?

❑ (A) Capsid protein located at the vertex that binds to tick cells
❑ (B) Double capsid that withstands rigorous environments
❑ (C) Efficient replication of virions in the tick salivary gland
❑ (D) Persistence in erythrocytes that establishes prolonged viremia
❑ (E) Segmented genome that can reassort segments from viruses of different species

41 A gynecologist discovers vesicular lesions on his thumb that he attributes to contact with an infectious agent while examining a patient. The lesions have an erythematous base and contain clear fluid. A smear of the cells can be stained with hematoxylin and eosin stains. Which finding would also be expected?

❑ (A) Cowdry type A inclusion bodies
❑ (B) Downey cells

❑   (C) Koilocytotic cells
❑   (D) Negri bodies
❑   (E) Owl's eye inclusion bodies

42   The skin on the face and neck of an 18-month-old boy suddenly begins to appear red. Approximately 2 days later, other parts of his body are affected. Large blisters begin to appear, and superficial layers start to rub off like peach skin. When the boy is taken to his pediatrician, he has a mild fever but no other signs of serious illness. The agent responsible for this disease would have which type of genetic material?

❑   (A) Circular double-stranded DNA
❑   (B) Linear double-stranded DNA with protein attached to the 5N ends
❑   (C) Multiple linear diploid DNA strands
❑   (D) Negative-sense single-stranded RNA
❑   (E) Positive-sense single-stranded RNA

43   An inactivated vaccine is used to prevent infections caused by which virus?

❑   (A) HBV
❑   (B) Influenza virus
❑   (C) Rubella virus
❑   (D) Smallpox virus
❑   (E) VZV

44   A 7-year-old girl with leukemia is exposed to VZV. Her physician prescribes varicella-zoster immune globulin as therapy. Although HSV and VZV are both herpesviruses, the immune globulin is effective only against VZV. Which property distinguishes the two viruses and accounts for this difference in the action of the immune globulin?

❑   (A) HSV can produce syncytia.
❑   (B) HSV is a neurotropic virus.
❑   (C) VZV encodes thymidine kinase.
❑   (D) VZV establishes viremia.
❑   (E) VZV is transmitted by the respiratory route.

45   A 15-year-old boy complains of extreme fatigue and is found to have swollen glands, hepatomegaly, splenomegaly, and positive results in the test for heterophile antibody. Which activity is associated with the agent responsible for these findings?

❑   (A) Activation of unrelated antibody production
❑   (B) Binding of erythrocytes to infected cell surfaces
❑   (C) Continued release of surface antigen
❑   (D) Expression of characteristic inclusion bodies
❑   (E) Integration of cDNA into host chromatin

46   A 27-year-old woman who is infected with HIV develops CMV retinitis, and ganciclovir is prescribed. A mutation in which enzyme would confer resistance to this drug?

❑   (A) DNA-dependent DNA polymerase
❑   (B) Neuraminidase
❑   (C) Ribonucleotide reductase
❑   (D) RNA-dependent DNA polymerase
❑   (E) Thymidine kinase

47   Human immune globulin is available for treating patients who have been recently exposed to which disease?

❑   (A) Diphtheria
❑   (B) Rabies
❑   (C) Streptococcal necrotizing fasciitis
❑   (D) Toxic shock syndrome
❑   (E) Typhoid fever

48   The agent shown in the electron micrograph (see figure) is an RNA virus that causes deadly outbreaks of hemorrhagic disease in Africa. Which virus is most likely the cause of these outbreaks?

❑   (A) Dengue virus
❑   (B) Ebola virus
❑   (C) Hantavirus
❑   (D) Lassa virus
❑   (E) Rift Valley fever virus

49   A 16-year-old boy has a sore throat, swollen cervical lymph nodes, fever, malaise, and hepatosplenomegaly. Serum samples from the patient are found to agglutinate sheep erythrocytes but not guinea pig erythrocytes. Which serologic profile would most likely be obtained at this time? Answers A through E are presented horizontally in the table.

	IgM Anti-VCA	IgG Anti-VCA	Anti-MA	Anti-EBNA
A.	+	−	−	−
B.	+	+	−	+
C.	−	+	−	+
D.	−	+	+	+
E.	+	+	+	+

VCA, viral capsid antigens; MA, monoclonal antibodies; EBNA, Epstein-Barr nuclear antigen; +, present; −, absent.

50 An 80-year-old man in a nursing home is exposed to a visitor with influenza A virus infection. Which immediate course of action would be most appropriate for this patient?

- ❐ (A) Immunization with influenza vaccine
- ❐ (B) Treatment with acyclovir
- ❐ (C) Treatment with immune globulin
- ❐ (D) Treatment with rimantadine
- ❐ (E) Waiting and watching

51 A 42-year-old man is suffering from fatigue and has a headache. The next day, he awakens with a fever and stabbing pains in the chest and abdomen. The symptoms last for 6 days. Bornholm disease (pleurodynia) is suspected. A stool sample shows a small icosahedral virus. Which statement best describes this virus?

- ❐ (A) Viral genome is produced in the cytoplasm; virus is encapsulated in the cytoplasm.
- ❐ (B) Viral genome is produced in the cytoplasm; virus is enveloped at the plasma membrane.
- ❐ (C) Viral genome is produced in the nucleus; virus is encapsulated in the nucleus.
- ❐ (D) Viral genome is produced in the nucleus; virus is enveloped at the nuclear membrane.
- ❐ (E) Viral genome is produced in the nucleus; virus is enveloped at the plasma membrane.

52 An 11-year-old boy has a benign growth on his foot that is characterized by hyperplasia of the prickle cells and koilocytosis (vacuolated squamous epithelial cells). What is the most likely cause of the growth?

- ❐ (A) Fungus that exhibits septate hyphae and is not thermally dimorphic
- ❐ (B) Fungus that metabolizes keratin
- ❐ (C) Large, enveloped, linear double-stranded DNA virus
- ❐ (D) Virus that replicates in most tissue culture cells
- ❐ (E) Virus whose replication is dependent on the epithelial cell differentiation stage

53 In August, a 26-year-old man sees his family physician with complaints of a low-grade fever and severe headaches. The patient states that 1-week earlier, he·developed blisters at the back of his throat and base of his tongue. His headaches began shortly after the blisters appeared and increased in severity for 5 days. The man is transferred to a local hospital, where a lumbar puncture is performed. He has 177 cells with 81% lymphocytes, a normal glucose (54 mg/dl), and elevated protein (60 mg/dl). CSF is collected for microbiology stains and cultures. No organisms are observed on Gram stain, and bacterial, fungal, and viral cultures are negative after 5 days of incubation. After 2 weeks, the patient's headaches gradually decrease in frequency and intensity. The most likely cause of this patient's symptoms is which organism?

- ❐ (A) *Cryptococcus neoformans*
- ❐ (B) Coxsackievirus A

- ❐ (C) HSV
- ❐ (D) *Naegleria fowleri*
- ❐ (E) *Streptococcus pneumoniae*

54 An outbreak of influenza in Hong Kong forces authorities to collect and eliminate all the chickens in the region. Which explanation best justifies the action of the authorities?

- ❐ (A) Chicken feathers harbor influenza viruses and can readily spread influenza.
- ❐ (B) Chickens are a reservoir and mosquitoes are a vector for influenza viruses.
- ❐ (C) Chickens are the incubators for new strains of influenza virus.
- ❐ (D) Influenza viruses can contaminate the meat supply.
- ❐ (E) Partial immunity induced by the chicken virus exacerbates human influenza disease.

55 In July, a mother brings her 3-year-old boy to the emergency department because he is suffering from severe headaches, irritability, and drowsiness. The mother states that the toddler recently began vomiting after his meals. He has a temperature of 40°C, and a physical examination shows nuchal rigidity. A CSF sample is cloudy and has a normal glucose concentration, an elevated protein concentration, and a WBC of 350/mm³, consisting of 70% mononuclear cells and 30% polymorphonuclear leukocytes. A Gram stain is negative for bacteria. RT-PCR analysis of the CSF generates a genome-length cDNA product that encodes a polymerase gene. The patient recovers completely within 48 h and is released from the hospital. Which agent is likely to have caused the patient's disease?

- ❐ (A) *Cryptococcus neoformans*
- ❐ (B) Echovirus 11
- ❐ (C) *Escherichia coli*
- ❐ (D) HSV
- ❐ (E) *Streptococcus pneumoniae*

56 The 35-year-old father of a 3-year-old girl experiences the sudden onset of fever, fatigue, nausea, stomach pain, and loss of appetite. Jaundice is observed 5 days later. The diagnosis of hepatitis A is made on the basis of the clinical data. Which piece of information from this patient's history is key to differentiating infection with HAV from infection with other hepatitis viruses?

- ❐ (A) 5-day delay of jaundice
- ❐ (B) Presence of fever, fatigue, nausea, stomach pain, and loss of appetite
- ❐ (C) Presence of jaundice
- ❐ (D) Sexual contact with a carrier
- ❐ (E) Sudden onset of symptoms

57 Which virus has enveloped, double-stranded DNA?

- ❐ (A) Hepatitis C virus (HCV)
- ❐ (B) Papillomavirus

❐   (C) Respiratory syncytial virus

❐   (D) Smallpox virus

❐   (E) West Nile virus

58   A 22-year-old man has multiple nodular lesions in the genital area. Each lesion is dome-shaped, is 2 to 10 mm in diameter, and has a central caseous plug. The virus causing the lesions cannot be isolated in tissue culture. Which virus is in the same family?

❐   (A) Coxsackievirus A

❐   (B) Human papillomavirus (HPV) type 11

❐   (C) Mumps virus

❐   (D) Smallpox virus

❐   (E) VZV

59   A pharyngeal isolate from a 20-year-old man with pharyngitis is inoculated into tissue culture cells. Findings include syncytia, margination of the chromatin, and nuclear inclusion bodies. Which agent best fits this description?

❐   (A) Adenovirus

❐   (B) Epstein-Barr virus

❐   (C) HSV

❐   (D) Influenza virus

❐   (E) Measles virus

60   An 8-year-old boy who has been attending summer camp develops flu-like symptoms that progress to encephalitis. The physician suspects infection with St. Louis encephalitis virus or California encephalitis virus. Which characteristic would distinguish this virus from the others?

❐   (A) Broad range of hosts

❐   (B) Envelope

❐   (C) Genome consisting of RNA

❐   (D) Genome that is infectious

❐   (E) Transmission via mosquitoes

61   A 65-year-old man suffers from severe headaches, memory loss, confusion, and a constant tremor of the left hand. Approximately 4 months after these symptoms appear, he lapses into a coma. Spontaneous clonic twitching of the arms and legs is noted. The patient subsequently dies, and an autopsy is performed. The presence of extensive vacuolation and degeneration of neurons in the brain confirms the diagnosis. Which answer best describes the structural components of the agent of this disease?

❐   (A) Glycoproteins and lipids

❐   (B) Protein

❐   (C) Proteins and glycoproteins

❐   (D) Proteins and lipids

❐   (E) Proteins, glycoproteins, and lipids

62   What is a target cell receptor for rabies virus?

❐   (A) C3d complement receptor on B lymphocytes

❐   (B) CD4 molecule and chemokine coreceptor on T lymphocytes

❐   (C) Immunoglobulin superfamily protein on epithelial cells

❐   (D) Acetylcholine receptor on neurons

❐   (E) Sialic acid receptor on epithelial cells

63   Premalignant cells are seen in a Pap smear from a 40-year-old woman. Which agent is most likely to be present in these cells?

❐   (A) Adenovirus type 2

❐   (B) *Chlamydia trachomatis*

❐   (C) HSV type 2

❐   (D) HPV type 16

❐   (E) Parvovirus B19

64   A 23-year-old mother of two young children is exposed to rubella during the first trimester of her third pregnancy. The woman's medical records show that she was vaccinated against measles, mumps, and rubella when she was a child. Which description is most accurate for the expected outcome of this pregnancy?

❐   (A) The infant will have cataract, deafness, and mental retardation.

❐   (B) The infant will have mental retardation and microcephaly.

❐   (C) The infant will have vesicular lesions and disseminated disease, leading to fatal encephalitis.

❐   (D) The infant will be blind.

❐   (E) The infant will be healthy.

65   A 23-year-old man has a fever, rash, and swollen glands. He had unprotected sex with a male partner 2 weeks before the onset of these symptoms and has just learned that the partner is positive for HIV infection. At this time, which test would be appropriate for confirming an HIV diagnosis?

❐   (A) Cell culture isolation of the virus

❐   (B) ELISA for antibodies to gp120

❐   (C) ELISA for p24 antigen

❐   (D) Latex agglutination test for antibodies to gp41

❐   (E) Western blot test

66   A 6-month-old girl is taken to the emergency department in January because she has had a low-grade fever and has been suffering for the past 2 days from bouts of vomiting and watery diarrhea. The girl appears dehydrated. Immunoelectron microscopic examination of a stool sample indicates the presence of enveloped virions. Which virus is the most likely cause of the patient's symptoms?

❐   (A) Adenovirus

❐   (B) Coronavirus

❐   (C) Norwalk virus

❐   (D) Reovirus

❐   (E) Rotavirus

67 Which step in viral replication is inhibited by IFN-α?

❏ (A) Attachment

❏ (B) Uncoating

❏ (C) Translation

❏ (D) Replication

❏ (E) Viral assembly

68 Some herpesvirus infections are sensitive to acyclovir and foscarnet. Which target distinguishes these two drugs?

❏ (A) DNA-dependent DNA polymerase

❏ (B) DNA-dependent RNA polymerase

❏ (C) Protease

❏ (D) RNA-dependent DNA polymerase

❏ (E) Thymidine kinase

69 A 26-year-old woman received a blood transfusion during the second trimester of her pregnancy. At birth, her infant is small and appears to have a disproportionately small head. Within 2 days, the infant develops jaundice, hepatosplenomegaly, and a petechial rash. Urine samples are found to contain cells with owl's eye inclusion bodies. An x-ray of the infant's head at 1 week of age shows intracranial calcifications. The infant becomes increasingly lethargic and begins to experience respiratory distress and seizures. The infant eventually dies. The findings suggest a congenital infection with which agent?

❏ (A) CMV

❏ (B) HSV

❏ (C) Rubella virus

❏ (D) *Streptococcus*

❏ (E) *Toxoplasma*

70 A 36-year-old man is bitten when he picks up a baby raccoon near his home. The man receives a series of therapeutic immunizations because of the risk of developing rabies. Which composition of these immunizations is correct?

❏ (A) Attenuated rabies virus

❏ (B) Formalin-treated, rabies virus-infected cells

❏ (C) Heat-inactivated purified rabies virus

❏ (D) Rabies subunit vaccine

❏ (E) Vaccinia virus containing the G protein of rabies virus

71 A medical student on a pediatric rotation is concerned about contagion from his patients. His medical records show that he received routine childhood immunizations and that he had chickenpox when he was 5 years old. Which virus poses the greatest risk for a nosocomial infection?

❏ (A) California encephalitis virus

❏ (B) Influenza virus

❏ (C) Rubella virus

❏ (D) VZV

❏ (E) Variola virus

72 Epithelial cells are obtained from a 55-year-old man and then infected with either influenza A H3N2 or influenza A H1N1. T lymphocytes and antibody are taken from the same man and are tested for their cytotoxic activity against the infected cells. The antibody reaction includes complement. The results are shown in the table.

	Cell Lysis			
	Cells	No treatment	T cells	Antibody and complement
Uninfected	5%	5%	2%	—
H3N2-infected	—	4%	45%	55%
H1N1-infected	—	2%	35%	5%

Which explanation is consistent with the data shown in the table?

❏ (A) The H1N1-infected cells inactivate complement.

❏ (B) The H3N2 virus causes greater cytopathology than the H1N1 virus.

❏ (C) The man has a history of infection with both H3N2 and H1N1 viruses.

❏ (D) The man recently recovered from infection with H3N2 virus.

❏ (E) The T cells react with an antigen other than hemagglutinin.

73 Which virus has enveloped, single-stranded RNA?

❏ (A) Adenovirus

❏ (B) Norwalk virus

❏ (C) Parainfluenza virus

❏ (D) Rotavirus

❏ (E) VZV

74 A child with numerous vesicular lesions around the crimson border of the mouth requires treatment. The drug of choice acts by which mechanism?

❏ (A) Blockade of peptidoglycan cross-linkage

❏ (B) Blockade of uncoating and entry of the causative agent

❏ (C) Inhibition of DNA polymerase

❏ (D) Inhibition of 70S ribosome

❏ (E) Inhibition of topoisomerase

75 A 19-year-old college student visits the student health center suffering from a sore throat and is treated with ampicillin. She subsequently returns with complaints of fatigue and a persisting sore throat. Physical examination shows swollen glands, a copper-colored rash on the trunk, and a temperature of 39.4°C. A blood smear shows 10% atypical lymphocytes and an elevated WBC count. Confirmation of the patient's diagnosis can be made by detection of antibody to which factor?

❑ (A) Cardiolipin
❑ (B) DNA
❑ (C) EBV capsid antigen
❑ (D) EBNA
❑ (E) Sheep erythrocytes

76 During an influenza epidemic, a 45-year-old woman suffers for 3 days from fever, headache, myalgia, malaise, and cough. The next day, she experiences increasing shortness of breath and goes to the emergency department. Sputum examination shows numerous leukocytes and gram-positive cocci. Which factor predisposes an influenza patient to bacterial lung infections?

❑ (A) Change in the pharyngeal microflora
❑ (B) Destruction of ciliated columnar epithelial cells
❑ (C) Loss of alveolar macrophages
❑ (D) Patient's inability to mount a delayed-type hypersensitivity reaction
❑ (E) Patient's inability to produce antibodies

77 A 32-year-old woman sees her family physician with a 5-day history of fevers, headaches, retro-orbital pain, myalgias, and a rash. The symptoms began 3 days after she returned from a 1-month trip to Thailand. The rash developed initially on her face and then spread over her trunk and extremities. Before her travels, she received all the appropriate vaccinations and maintained malaria prophylaxis during her trip. Physical examination shows diffuse erythroderma with blanching erythema and petechial formation resulting from pressure applied to her skin. Bilateral conjunctival suffusion is noted. Laboratory tests reveal leukopenia and thrombocytopenia. Which organism is most likely responsible for this infection?

❑ (A) Dengue virus
❑ (B) HAV
❑ (C) *Leptospira interrogans*
❑ (D) *Plasmodium falciparum*
❑ (E) *Salmonella typhi*

78 Which virus can exchange genetic material with a different strain of a related virus by reassortment of segmented genomes?

❑ (A) Ebola virus
❑ (B) Coxsackievirus
❑ (C) Dengue virus
❑ (D) Influenza virus
❑ (E) Parainfluenza virus

79 Yellow fever virus can initiate an urban cycle (human-to-mosquito-to-human) of infection. In contrast, Venezuelan equine encephalitis (VEE) virus has a sylvan cycle of infection, with humans serving as a dead-end host. Which description explains why humans are a dead-end host for VEE virus?

❑ (A) VEE virus and yellow fever virus are transmitted by different genera of mosquitoes.
❑ (B) VEE virus encodes only one glycoprotein.
❑ (C) VEE virus infection causes only limited viremia in humans.
❑ (D) VEE virus infection causes only mild disease in humans.
❑ (E) VEE virus replicates in mosquito salivary glands.

80 A medical student who suffers from common cold symptoms, including a runny nose, sore throat, sneezing, and a headache, asks her professor to explain why a vaccine has not been developed to prevent this disease. Which explanation is the best one?

❑ (A) A cytolytic T cell response would be required.
❑ (B) The agent does not cause significant disease.
❑ (C) The agent has the potential to establish chronic or transforming infections.
❑ (D) The disease does not affect a significant portion of the population.
❑ (E) There are too many agents that cause this disease.

81 Which step in viral replication is inhibited by protease inhibitors?

❑ (A) Penetration
❑ (B) Uncoating
❑ (C) Transcription
❑ (D) Replication
❑ (E) Viral assembly

82 A Pap smear of a 50-year-old woman shows cervical dysplasia. Which method would be most useful in detecting the presence of HPV 18?

❑ (A) ELISA
❑ (B) Immunofluorescence testing
❑ (C) In situ DNA hybridization
❑ (D) Tissue culture
❑ (E) Western blot assay

83 A 5-year-old girl is bitten by a baby racoon that is thought to be rabid. The girl is vaccinated in time to prevent the onset of rabies. Without the vaccination, an immune response would be undetectable until the final stages of disease and would therefore fail to protect the infected girl from disease and death. Which property of the rabies virus is responsible for the delay?

❑ (A) Antigenic shift
❑ (B) Infection of T cells
❑ (C) Production of an IgA protease
❑ (D) Production of Fc receptors on the infected cells
❑ (E) Replication in a privileged site

84 A 42-year-old man has malaise, anorexia, abdominal pain, jaundice, and dark-colored urine. Serologic results are positive for HB$_s$Ag, HB$_e$Ag, and anti-HAV; they are negative for anti-HB$_x$. Which viral enzyme would be a good target for drugs against this infection?

- ☐ (A) DNA-dependent DNA polymerase
- ☐ (B) DNA-dependent RNA polymerase
- ☐ (C) RNA-dependent DNA polymerase
- ☐ (D) RNA-dependent RNA polymerase
- ☐ (E) Thymidine kinase

85 A 5-year-old boy has a viral disease that causes mild flu-like symptoms. He subsequently develops myalgia and a rash that covers the cheeks but spares the mouth, giving him a "slapped cheek" look. The viral disease eventually resolves without treatment. Which condition would predispose the patient to a severe disease by this virus?

- ☐ (A) Chédiak-Higashi syndrome
- ☐ (B) Chronic granulomatous disease
- ☐ (C) Chronic hemolytic anemia
- ☐ (D) Cystic fibrosis
- ☐ (E) Diabetes mellitus

86 A 23-year-old man has been suffering from a fever, pharyngitis, arthralgia, and myalgia for approximately 1 week. Throat examination shows white exudate on enlarged tonsils. Other findings include cervical lymphadenopathy, hepatomegaly, and splenomegaly. Which analysis would be most useful for confirming the diagnosis?

- ☐ (A) Evaluation for antibody to CMV
- ☐ (B) Evaluation for HIV viremia
- ☐ (C) Monospot test to screen for EBV infection
- ☐ (D) Rapid plasmin reagin (RPR) test to screen for syphilis
- ☐ (E) Throat swab to screen for *Streptococcus pyogenes* infection

87 The agent shown in the electron micrograph (see figure) is a zoonotic virus that is transmitted in saliva. Which structure is characteristic of this virus?

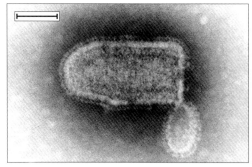

From Hart CA, Shears P: *Color atlas of medical microbiology,* ed 2, St Louis, 2004, Mosby.

- ☐ (A) Enveloped, double-stranded DNA virus
- ☐ (B) Enveloped, single-stranded, negative-sense DNA virus
- ☐ (C) Enveloped, single-stranded, negative-sense RNA virus
- ☐ (D) Enveloped, single-stranded, positive-sense RNA virus
- ☐ (E) Nonenveloped, double-stranded DNA virus

88 A 23-year-old woman is concerned because 1 week ago she had sexual contact with a man infected with HIV. She thinks she might have contracted the infection, but the standard serologic methods for evaluation yield negative results. The woman should be counseled that the test result is inconclusive for which reason?

- ☐ (A) The antibody to HIV has not risen to detectable levels.
- ☐ (B) ELISA is not sensitive enough to detect the virus.
- ☐ (C) Isolation of the virus in tissue culture is inconclusive.
- ☐ (D) Virus replication has not yet started.
- ☐ (E) Western blot analysis is not sensitive enough to detect the virus.

89 A 58-year-old man receiving immunosuppressive therapy after undergoing a kidney transplant begins to suffer from multifocal neurologic symptoms, including memory loss, difficulty speaking, coordination problems, and loss of some use of his right arm. PCR analysis of a CSF sample is performed using viral sequences from simian virus 40 (SV40). The results indicate the presence of a related virus. Which virus is the most likely the cause of this man's condition?

- ☐ (A) Echovirus 11
- ☐ (B) HSV
- ☐ (C) JC virus
- ☐ (D) Measles virus
- ☐ (E) Western equine encephalitis (WEE) virus

90 Which statement is correct?

- ☐ (A) Most RNA viruses replicate in the nucleus.
- ☐ (B) Most RNA viruses produce persistent, latent infections.
- ☐ (C) RNA viruses must encode an RNA polymerase.
- ☐ (D) DNA viruses do not require host transcriptional enzymes.
- ☐ (E) Viral DNA is labile.

91 A 3-year-old boy is undergoing treatment for leukemia. His older sibling develops a cough, conjunctivitis, coryza, and photophobia and subsequently develops a rash. Exposure to the agent responsible for the older sibling's disease would place the 3-year-old at risk for which condition?

- ☐ (A) Exanthema subitum
- ☐ (B) Giant cell pneumonia
- ☐ (C) Hemorrhagic pulmonary syndrome
- ☐ (D) Orchitis
- ☐ (E) Progressive multifocal leukoencephalopathy

92 A 16-year-old boy has a severe sore throat, swollen cervical lymph nodes, fever, malaise, and hepatosplenomegaly. When ampicillin is administered for his sore throat, he develops a generalized maculopapular rash. Laboratory tests show atypical lymphocytes and heterophil antibodies in the blood. Which property is associated with the agent causing this disease?

- ❑ (A) Binding of C3d receptors on B lymphocytes
- ❑ (B) Infection of CD8 T cells
- ❑ (C) Killing of CD4 T cells
- ❑ (D) Susceptibility to acyclovir treatment
- ❑ (E) Tumor promotion in keratinocytes

93 Poxvirus is able to evade the host's immune response by which mechanism?

- ❑ (A) Blocking IFN production
- ❑ (B) Blocking IL-1 and TNF-mediated inflammation
- ❑ (C) Causing genetic change after infection
- ❑ (D) Causing latent infection
- ❑ (E) Preventing CD8 T cell killing

94 A 25-year-old woman is exposed to a virus during the first trimester of pregnancy. The woman gives birth to an infant who is deaf and has cataracts, a heart murmur, and microcephaly. If present, which immune function would have protected the infant from the viral disease?

- ❑ (A) Inhibition of viral replication by IFN
- ❑ (B) Inhibition of viremic spread by antibodies
- ❑ (C) Killing of virus-infected cells by cytotoxic T cells
- ❑ (D) Killing of virus-infected cells by natural killer cells
- ❑ (E) Uptake and neutralization of the virus by macrophages

95 A 56-year-old man has a belt of blister-like lesions distributed in a band across his abdomen. He complains of severe pain. Which virus is most similar to the virus causing the patient's disease?

- ❑ (A) Coxsackievirus A
- ❑ (B) HSV
- ❑ (C) Measles virus
- ❑ (D) Parvovirus B19
- ❑ (E) Rubella virus

96 A Pap smear from a sexually active 32-year-old woman is being evaluated for the presence of HPV 16. Which procedure would provide the best evidence of this virus?

- ❑ (A) Hemadsorption
- ❑ (B) Immunofluorescence testing for viral glycoprotein
- ❑ (C) In situ hybridization
- ❑ (D) Microscopic examination for owl's eye inclusion bodies
- ❑ (E) RT-PCR methods

97 A 32-year-old man with AIDS has been undergoing monotherapy with zidovudine for 7 years. He becomes resistant to this treatment, so alternative drugs must be considered. Resistance to which drug would be expected because of its similarity to zidovudine in terms of structure or target?

- ❑ (A) Nelfinavir
- ❑ (B) Nevirapine
- ❑ (C) Ritonavir
- ❑ (D) Stavudine
- ❑ (E) Zovirax

98 An 8-year-old girl is bitten on the face by a rabid dog. The disease progresses in an uncharacteristically rapid manner, and the patient dies. What is the most likely explanation for the rapid progression of rabies in this case?

- ❑ (A) The amount of rabies virus transmitted via the bite was large.
- ❑ (B) The disease progresses faster in children than in adults.
- ❑ (C) The infection site was close to the brain.
- ❑ (D) The patient did not receive her childhood rabies vaccination.
- ❑ (E) The strain of rabies virus was extremely virulent.

99 HIV infection is suspected in a 28-year-old man who has recently lost weight, complains of intermittent fever and chills, and is suffering from pneumonia and oral thrush. Detection of which enzyme in the patient's blood would be diagnostic of this infection?

- ❑ (A) DNA-dependent DNA polymerase
- ❑ (B) DNA-dependent RNA polymerase
- ❑ (C) RNA-dependent DNA polymerase
- ❑ (D) RNA-dependent RNA polymerase
- ❑ (E) Thymidine kinase

100 A 4-year-old girl is brought to the emergency department because of a continuous, loud, barking cough and difficulty catching her breath. Her breathing improves in the presence of humidified air. A virus is isolated from a nasal wash. The virus causes hemagglutination and promotes syncytia formation in cell culture. Which virus is most likely the cause of this patient's condition?

- ❑ (A) Influenza virus
- ❑ (B) Parainfluenza virus
- ❑ (C) Parvovirus
- ❑ (D) Reovirus
- ❑ (E) Rhinovirus

101 HIV is able to evade the host's immune response by which mechanism?

- ❑ (A) Blocks IFN production
- ❑ (B) Blocks IL-1 and TNF-mediated inflammation
- ❑ (C) Genetic change after infection
- ❑ (D) Latent infection
- ❑ (E) Prevents CD8 T cell killing

102 A neonate is born with a small head, intracerebral calcification, rash, and swollen liver and spleen. Cells with characteristic histology (see figure of photomicrograph) are obtained from the patient's urine. Which condition describes the most prevalent consequence of adult infection with this agent?

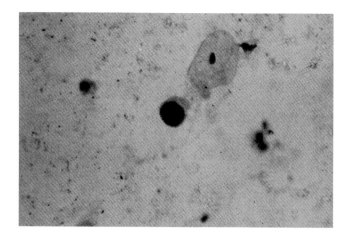

- ❑ (A) Immunosuppression and susceptibility to opportunistic diseases
- ❑ (B) Mild arthritic condition with a fine lacy rash
- ❑ (C) Mononucleosis with production of antibody to sheep red blood cells
- ❑ (D) No serious, definable disease symptoms
- ❑ (E) Pharyngoconjunctivitis

103 A 26-year-old woman in her second trimester of pregnancy develops arthritic symptoms and a maculopapular rash on her trunk. Serologic tests are negative for IgM antibodies to parvovirus B19 and measles virus, but the tests are positive for IgM antibodies to rubella virus and for IgG antibodies to measles and rubella viruses. The infant is at highest risk for having which condition?

- ❑ (A) Cerebral calcification
- ❑ (B) Chorioretinitis
- ❑ (C) Deafness
- ❑ (D) Hydrops fetalis
- ❑ (E) Keratoconjunctivitis

104 A new approach to immunization is to incorporate the gene from a pathogen (e.g., HIV) into the genome of a poxvirus (e.g., vaccinia virus or canarypox virus). Poxviruses are appropriate for this purpose because of which option?

- ❑ (A) Poxviruses assemble in the cytoplasm.
- ❑ (B) Poxviruses have a large genome and encode many accessory genes.
- ❑ (C) Poxviruses replicate in the cytoplasm.
- ❑ (D) Smallpox was eliminated in 1980.
- ❑ (E) Symptoms of vaccinia virus infection are visible.

105 Pleconaril is a new antiviral drug that inhibits viral replication by inserting itself in the viral capsid and preventing uncoating. The drug is effective against rhinoviruses and many other members of the same viral family. Which disease will most likely be inhibited by this drug?

- ❑ (A) Echovirus meningitis
- ❑ (B) HSV encephalitis
- ❑ (C) Influenza A virus pneumonia
- ❑ (D) Measles virus encephalitis
- ❑ (E) Respiratory syncytial virus (RSV) pneumonia

106 A 5-year-old boy who recently visited the tropics begins to experience mild flu-like symptoms. Approximately 4 days later, he develops jaundice and black vomitus. The physician suspects yellow fever. Which description best refers to the agent causing this disease?

- ❑ (A) Enveloped, negative-sense, single-stranded RNA virus without a matrix protein
- ❑ (B) Enveloped, negative-sense, single-stranded, segmented RNA virus
- ❑ (C) Enveloped, positive-sense, single-stranded RNA virus that makes a polyprotein
- ❑ (D) Enveloped, positive-sense, single-stranded RNA virus that makes early and late proteins from RNA of different sizes
- ❑ (E) Nonenveloped, double-stranded, segmented RNA virus with a double capsid

107 For the past 3 months, a 28-year-old man has experienced weight loss and intermittent fever and chills. He recently developed pneumonia and thrush. This combination of clinical manifestations indicates infection with which virus?

- ❑ (A) Adenovirus
- ❑ (B) *Coccidioides immitis*
- ❑ (C) HIV
- ❑ (D) HTLV
- ❑ (E) *Streptococcus pneumoniae*

108 A 4-year-old girl is brought to the emergency department because of a continuous, loud, barking cough and difficulty catching her breath. Her breathing improves in the presence of humidified air. A virus is isolated from a nasal wash. The virus causes hemagglutination and promotes syncytia formation in cell culture. Which description identifies the genome of this virus?

- ❑ (A) Double-stranded RNA
- ❑ (B) Nonsegmented, single-stranded, negative-sense RNA
- ❑ (C) Segmented, single-stranded, negative-sense RNA
- ❑ (D) Single-stranded DNA
- ❑ (E) Single-stranded, positive-sense RNA

109 A monoclonal IgG antibody directed against the hemagglutinin of influenza A virus acts to neutralize the binding of the virus to the target cells. A second monoclonal IgG antibody is made against the idiotype region of the first antibody, and it inhibits viral infection. Which factor is most likely recognized by the IgG anti-idiotype antibody?

- ❏ (A) HA
- ❏ (B) Matrix (M1) protein
- ❏ (C) Membrane (M2) protein
- ❏ (D) NA
- ❏ (E) Sialic acid

110 A 38-year-old man complains of jaundice, dark urine, anorexia, abdominal pain, and malaise. Serologic tests indicate that he is positive for anti-HB$_s$ and negative for anti-HB$_c$. Which interpretation for these findings is most likely?

- ❏ (A) The patient has acute HBV infection.
- ❏ (B) The patient has chronic HBV infection.
- ❏ (C) The patient has fulminant HBV infection.
- ❏ (D) The patient has the prodrome of HBV infection.
- ❏ (E) The patient is not infected with HBV.

111 What is the course of events in the immune response to primary varicella-zoster infection?

- ❏ (A) CD4 T cell activation, interferon-beta (IFN-β) production, natural killer (NK) cell activation, and IgG production
- ❏ (B) IFN-β production, NK cell activation, CD4 T cell activation, and IgG production
- ❏ (C) IFN-β production, NK cell activation, CD8 T cell activation, and IgM production
- ❏ (D) IFN-γ production, NK cell activation, CD4 T cell activation, and IgM production
- ❏ (E) NK cell activation, CD4 T cell activation, IFN-β production, and IgG production

112 A 28-year-old man is suffering from a low-grade fever, weight loss, thrush, serious bouts of diarrhea, and symptoms of pneumonia. He has a history of heroin addiction and admits to sharing needles at a "shooting gallery." Which combination antiviral therapy for this patient would be appropriate?

- ❏ (A) One inhibitor of DNA polymerase and one inhibitor of thymidine kinase (TK)
- ❏ (B) One inhibitor of reverse transcriptase (RT) and two inhibitors of integrase
- ❏ (C) Two inhibitors of RT and one inhibitor of protease
- ❏ (D) Two inhibitors of RT and one inhibitor of the *src* gene
- ❏ (E) Two inhibitors of RT and one inhibitor of TK

113 An infant who was infected with a virus in utero has ocular manifestations of the viral disease (see figure). The infant's mother was not vaccinated against the virus when she was a child. Which vaccine would be relevant for the infant?

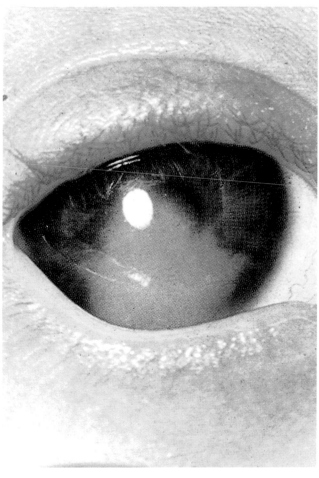

From Emond et al: *Colour atlas of infectious diseases*, St Louis, 2004, Mosby.

- ❏ (A) A vaccine consisting of a carbohydrate attached to a carrier protein
- ❏ (B) A vaccine consisting of formalin-inactivated whole virus
- ❏ (C) A vaccine consisting of subunits of the viral glycoprotein
- ❏ (D) A vaccine administered on the same schedule as the mumps vaccine
- ❏ (E) A vaccine administered on the same schedule as the polio vaccine

114 A nasal wash is obtained from a patient with a fever, sore throat, headache, and myalgia. Which procedure would be most effective in identifying the agent responsible for these symptoms?

- ❏ (A) Complement fixation test
- ❏ (B) Hemadsorption test
- ❏ (C) Hemagglutination inhibition (HAI) test
- ❏ (D) Ouchterlony test
- ❏ (E) Tissue culture growth

115   A 3-year-old boy has a temperature of 40°C for 4 days. After a day without fever, he develops a generalized rash. The rash lasts for 2 days. At which time is the child contagious?

☐   (A) Before the onset of fever
☐   (B) During the break in the fever
☐   (C) During the fever
☐   (D) During the rash
☐   (E) Never

116   Ribavirin is used to treat a 28-year-old Peace Corps volunteer who has been working in the Congo and has a fever and hemorrhagic disease believed to be caused by Lassa virus. Which virus is also treated with ribavirin?

☐   (A) California encephalitis virus
☐   (B) CMV
☐   (C) Ebola virus
☐   (D) Influenza virus
☐   (E) RSV

117   A 20-year-old woman who works in a pediatric unit begins to suffer from fatigue, sneezing, and a runny nose. She has no fever, but she soon develops a mild sore throat, headache, and stuffy nose. Her symptoms subside within 3 to 4 days. Which virus is the most likely cause of these symptoms?

☐   (A) EBV
☐   (B) Influenza virus
☐   (C) Norwalk virus
☐   (D) Parvovirus B19
☐   (E) Rhinovirus

118   Two brothers, ages 2 and 6 years, are brought to the pediatrician's office because of sore throats. The 6-year-old also has conjunctivitis. The pediatrician assures the mother that the symptoms in both boys will subside after 3 to 5 days. Which agent is the most likely cause of their symptoms?

☐   (A) Adenovirus
☐   (B) HSV
☐   (C) Measles virus
☐   (D) Rhinovirus
☐   (E) *Streptococcus pyogenes*

119   A 37-year-old man complains of night sweats, fever, unintentional weight loss, and severe fatigue. Other findings suggest HIV infection. Which procedure would provide useful information about the patient's immune function and progression toward AIDS?

☐   (A) Heterophil antibody test
☐   (B) Measurement of IgG antibody to measles virus
☐   (C) Measurement of IgM antibody to HIV
☐   (D) Measurement of serum levels of IL-1
☐   (E) Tetanus toxoid skin test

120   A 23-year-old woman who works in a daycare center experiences the sudden onset of fever, fatigue, nausea, stomach pain, and loss of appetite. Jaundice is observed 5 days later, and the diagnosis of hepatitis is made. Transmission of the virus causing these clinical manifestations is facilitated by which viral characteristics?

☐   (A) Ability to be secreted in saliva and be transmitted via eating utensils
☐   (B) Ability to cause viremia and be transmitted via blood products
☐   (C) Ability to cause viremia and be transmitted via mosquitoes
☐   (D) Ability to reach and replicate in the lung and be transmitted via aerosols
☐   (E) Ability to withstand acids and detergents and be transmitted via the fecal-oral route

121   A 5-year-old girl develops a mild sore throat, flu-like symptoms, and a high fever. Approximately 8 days later, her cheeks become red and have the appearance of being slapped. The patient's brother has a history of sickle cell anemia, and infection with the agent causing his sister's illness would put him at risk for an aplastic crisis. Which agent is most likely to cause this disease?

☐   (A) Encapsulated dimorphic yeast
☐   (B) Enveloped virus with a segmented genome
☐   (C) Gram-negative diplococcus
☐   (D) Gram-positive diplococcus with a capsule
☐   (E) Nonenveloped virus with a single-stranded DNA genome

122   A 20-year-old man has recurrent episodes in which vesicular lesions appear on the edge of his lip. In this case, why does the infection recur?

☐   (A) The causative agent cannot produce DNA polymerase during the initial infection of neurons.
☐   (B) The causative agent fails to activate T cell control mechanisms.
☐   (C) The causative agent has variable major proteins (VMPs) on its outer membranes.
☐   (D) The causative agent produces integrase.
☐   (E) The causative agent produces RNA polymerase during the initial infection of neurons.

123   Croup is suspected in a 2-year-old girl who has a fever and coughs with a seal-like bark. The most likely viral cause of this infection is an agent with which feature?

☐   (A) Expresses an F (fusion) protein
☐   (B) Grows optimally at 33°C
☐   (C) Has a genome that is infectious
☐   (D) Is susceptible to a killed vaccine
☐   (E) Is susceptible to acyclovir

124   A 27-year-old man complains of a sore throat, fatigue, difficulty breathing, night sweats, and fever. He has recently lost weight without dieting. His mouth and throat are covered with white patchy lesions. A radiograph of his lungs shows a lacy infiltrate in the upper lobes. Which CD4 or CD8 count would correlate with these findings?

- ❏ (A) CD4 count < 200/µl
- ❏ (B) CD4 count = 400/µl
- ❏ (C) CD4 count > 500/µl
- ❏ (D) CD8 count = 400/µl
- ❏ (E) CD8 count > 500/µl

125 A 25-year-old intern who is seronegative for VZV is exposed to a patient with chickenpox. The intern is concerned because he is undergoing chemotherapy for Hodgkin's disease. Which treatment would be the most appropriate to prevent VZV disease in the intern?

- ❏ (A) Bolus of amantadine
- ❏ (B) Bolus of pentamidine
- ❏ (C) Prophylactic dose of a beta-lactamase antibiotic
- ❏ (D) Varicella vaccine
- ❏ (E) Varicella-zoster immune globulin

126 A 37-year-old man with chronic hepatitis B is given combination therapy. Which indicator suggests successful therapy?

- ❏ (A) Absence of HB_eAg
- ❏ (B) Decrease in jaundice
- ❏ (C) Decrease in the anti-HB_s titer
- ❏ (D) Increase in the anti-HB_c titer
- ❏ (E) Increase in the serum alanine aminotransferase level

127 A 55-year-old man experiences sudden onset of fever, runny nose, sore throat, malaise, and myalgia. A serum sample is obtained 1 day after the onset of symptoms. Another sample is obtained 3 weeks after convalescence. An HAI test is performed to determine whether the patient had been infected with influenza virus strain H3N2, the currently prevalent strain. The results are shown in the figure.

| ○ No hemagglutination | ● Hemagglutination |

Acute ○ ○ ○ ○ ○ ○ ○ ● ● ● ● ● ● ●
Chronic ○ ○ ○ ○ ○ ○ ○ ● ● ● ● ● ●

2 4 8 16 32 64 128 256 512 1024 2048

Which epidemiologically useful conclusion can be drawn from the results?

- ❏ (A) The patient was never infected with the H3N2 strain.
- ❏ (B) The patient was not recently infected with a strain containing H3 but was infected with it earlier in life.
- ❏ (C) The patient was recently infected with a strain containing H3.
- ❏ (D) The patient was recently infected with a strain containing N2.
- ❏ (E) The patient was recently infected with the H3N2 strain.

128 What is a target cell receptor for parvovirus B19?

- ❏ (A) C3d complement receptor on B lymphocytes
- ❏ (B) CD4 molecule and chemokine coreceptor on T lymphocytes
- ❏ (C) Immunoglobulin superfamily protein on epithelial cells
- ❏ (D) Erythrocyte P antigen
- ❏ (E) Sialic acid receptor on epithelial cells

129 Vaccination with an inactivated polio vaccine elicits which protective mechanism?

- ❏ (A) Development of a delayed-type hypersensitivity (DTH) response to prevent transmission of virus from skin to nerve
- ❏ (B) Development of an antibody response that blocks viremia
- ❏ (C) Development of an antibody response that targets infected cells
- ❏ (D) Formation of an antibody that blocks neuronal spread of the virus
- ❏ (E) Initiation of CD8 T cell immunity to kill infected cells

130 A horse trainer keeps his horses in facilities that are clean but located near a marsh. A newly purchased horse becomes infected with the Western equine encephalitis (WEE) virus. The veterinarian assures the trainer that he and his other horses are not at risk of acquiring WEE infection from the sick horse. Which explanation best describes this assurance?

- ❏ (A) Standard vaccination procedures protect trainers and their horses.
- ❏ (B) Viremia in a horse is not sufficient to promote transmission.
- ❏ (C) WEE virus does not infect humans.
- ❏ (D) WEE virus is inactivated in marsh water.
- ❏ (E) WEE virus is a sexually transmitted virus.

131 A 23-year-old woman from Minnesota experiences the sudden onset of fever, jaundice, nausea, abdominal discomfort, and loss of appetite. She has antibodies to HB_sAg. What is the most likely diagnosis?

- ❏ (A) Hepatitis A
- ❏ (B) Hepatitis B
- ❏ (C) Hepatitis C
- ❏ (D) Hepatitis D
- ❏ (E) Hepatitis E

132 A 6-month-old girl is taken to the emergency department in January suffering from watery diarrhea and vomiting. She has had a low-grade fever for 48 h and appears to be dehydrated. The suspected cause of the diarrhea is an icosahedral virus that has a double capsid and a double-stranded RNA genome. Which virus caused this infection?

- ❏ (A) Adenovirus
- ❏ (B) Coronavirus

❑ (C) Coxsackievirus A
❑ (D) Norwalk virus
❑ (E) Rotavirus

133 A WEE virus strain isolated from an infected horse is grown in chicken embryo fibroblast tissue culture cells more than 50 times. The virus isolated after the 50th passage will replicate in horse cells but not in mosquito cells. Which mutation would be consistent with this result?

❑ (A) Change in horse cell receptor for the virus
❑ (B) Change in mosquito cell receptor for the virus
❑ (C) Change in viral capsid protein
❑ (D) Change in viral glycoprotein
❑ (E) Change in viral lipid composition

134 HIV and HTLV share many structural characteristics. Which characteristic accounts for the difference in the nature of the diseases they induce?

❑ (A) HIV causes a lytic infection of T cells.
❑ (B) HIV produces protease.
❑ (C) HIV produces reverse transcriptase.
❑ (D) HTLV infects CD4 T cells.
❑ (E) HTLV infects neurons.

135 Which pair of viruses has a similar antimicrobial target and could therefore be sensitive to the same FDA-approved antiviral drugs?

❑ (A) CMV and HPV
❑ (B) HAV and VZV
❑ (C) HBV and HIV
❑ (D) HSV and poliovirus
❑ (E) RSV and rubella virus

136 Approximately 10 days after returning from a trip to Mexico, a 25-year-old man develops flu-like symptoms. He begins suffering from arthralgia and a mild rash another 4 days later. The rash begins on his face, spreads to his body, and disappears in 4 days. The patient indicates that he did not receive all of the routine childhood vaccinations. The physician suspects that the infection was preventable and is caused by a virus. The most likely agent responsible for this disease is a virus that has which characteristic?

❑ (A) Has a broad range of hosts
❑ (B) Is a small DNA virus
❑ (C) Is resistant to detergents
❑ (D) Is spread by the fecal-oral route
❑ (E) Is spread by the respiratory route

137 A 20-year-old man visits the university health center because he has a rash on his face and neck. He says that he has been feeling "run down" and has had a cough and runny nose. Conjunctivitis, small vesicular lesions on the buccal mucosa, and fever are noted during the physical examination. Prevention of the patient's disease is normally accomplished by which action?

❑ (A) Passive immunization with immune globulin
❑ (B) Prophylactic treatment with amantadine
❑ (C) Vaccination with a live, attenuated vaccine
❑ (D) Vaccination with a subunit vaccine
❑ (E) Vaccination with an inactivated vaccine

138 Hodgkin's lymphoma develops in a kidney transplant patient who is taking immunosuppressive drugs. A biopsy specimen from the tumor expresses EBNA. When the dosage of immunosuppressive drugs is decreased, the lymphoma regresses. Tumor development is related to which property of EBV?

❑ (A) Atypical lymphocytes associated with infectious mononucleosis
❑ (B) Immortalization of B cells in tissue culture
❑ (C) Increased WBC count associated with infectious mononucleosis
❑ (D) Production of EBV during the development of oral hairy leukoplakia
❑ (E) Production of heterophil antibody during infectious mononucleosis

139 A 22-year-old man who works in the pediatric ward of a hospital suffers from malaise, sneezing, and a runny nose, but he does not have a fever. He subsequently develops a mild sore throat, headache, and stuffy nose. The symptoms resolve within 4 days. Which virus is most likely to be responsible for these symptoms?

❑ (A) Coronavirus
❑ (B) Hantavirus
❑ (C) Norwalk virus
❑ (D) Rubella virus
❑ (E) Vesicular stomatitis virus

140 A 42-year-old man with a history of heroin addiction complains of jaundice, dark urine, anorexia, abdominal pain, and malaise. The disease progresses rapidly to fulminant hepatitis and cirrhosis. Which virus is responsible for these findings?

❑ (A) Calicivirus
❑ (B) Deltavirus
❑ (C) Flavivirus
❑ (D) Hepadnavirus
❑ (E) Picornavirus

141 A farmer in China lives in close contact with his pigs and ducks. The farmer and a pig each appear to have the flu. A duck is coinfected with influenza A virus strains from the pig and the farmer, and a new virus results from this infection. This is an example of which genetic process?

☐ (A) Complementation

☐ (B) Reassortment

☐ (C) Recombination

☐ (D) Transcapsidation

☐ (E) Transposition

142 A 7-year-old boy has vesicular lesions in three areas: the hand, the foot, and the mouth. Which agent is responsible for this disease?

☐ (A) Large-sized, detergent-sensitive virus that encodes a DNA and an RNA polymerase

☐ (B) Medium-sized, detergent-resistant virus that replicates in the nucleus

☐ (C) Medium-sized, detergent-resistant virus with a genome that is infectious

☐ (D) Small-sized, detergent-resistant virus that replicates in the nucleus

☐ (E) Small-sized, detergent-resistant virus with a genome that is infectious

143 A 10-year-old boy experiences a sudden onset of sneezing, a runny nose, a mild headache, a cough, and fatigue but no fever. The symptoms last for approximately 1 week, and then the boy feels fine. Approximately 2 weeks later, he has a similar attack, so his parents take him to see the pediatrician. The parents are surprised by the pediatrician's diagnosis because they thought that protection from the disease should have resulted from the previous occurrence. Which condition is the best reason for the second occurrence?

☐ (A) Chédiak-Higashi syndrome

☐ (B) DiGeorge syndrome

☐ (C) IgA deficiency

☐ (D) Multiple viral serotypes

☐ (E) Recurrent viral disease

144 What is a target cell receptor for poliovirus?

☐ (A) C3d complement receptor on B lymphocytes

☐ (B) CD4 molecule and chemokine coreceptor on T lymphocytes

☐ (C) Immunoglobulin superfamily protein on epithelial cells

☐ (D) Acetylcholine receptor on neurons

☐ (E) Sialic acid receptor on epithelial cells

145 A 35-year-old man complains of extreme fatigue, has difficulty catching his breath, and has recently lost 9 lb without dieting. Examination shows a thrush infection in his mouth. A chest radiograph of the lung shows signs consistent with diffuse interstitial pneumonitis. Blood studies indicate a CD4 T cell count of $200/\mu l$. Detection of an enzyme with which activity would confirm the diagnosis?

☐ (A) Degradation of DNA

☐ (B) Degradation of RNA

☐ (C) Degradation of sialic acid

☐ (D) Generation of double-stranded DNA from RNA templates

☐ (E) Generation of double-stranded DNA from single-stranded DNA templates

146 A 65-year-old man who smokes one pack of cigarettes a day has an upper respiratory tract infection, headache, malaise, and generalized body ache. He is surprised to hear that his disease is caused by an influenza virus. He says that he had influenza just 5 years ago. Which explanation about the current disease should be provided to this patient?

☐ (A) Immunosuppression due to age allowed infection to develop.

☐ (B) Smoking allowed the virus to cause a recurrent infection.

☐ (C) The virus does not establish a long-lasting immune response, so there is no lifelong immunity.

☐ (D) The virus strain that caused influenza 5 years ago is not the same strain that caused the current disease.

☐ (E) The virus was able to infect a different site in the respiratory system this time and was able to escape immune detection.

147 A 1-month-old boy is brought to the emergency department suffering from severe diarrhea and dehydration. There are no leukocytes or blood in his stool. Which description identifies the etiologic agent?

☐ (A) Double-stranded, segmented RNA virus with a double capsid

☐ (B) Gram-negative rod that does not ferment lactose

☐ (C) Gram-positive anaerobe

☐ (D) Pear-shaped trophozoite with two nuclei and four pairs of flagella

☐ (E) Single-stranded, positive-sense RNA virus with a capsid

148 Premalignant cells are seen in a Pap smear from a 40-year-old woman, and a virus is found to be associated with the cells. This virus acts by which mechanism?

☐ (A) Causing cell lysis

☐ (B) Inhibiting the activity of p53 and RB

☐ (C) Producing a cDNA intermediate

☐ (D) Promoting the expression of viral glycoprotein on the cell surface

☐ (E) Stimulating the activity of p53

149 A 35-year-old man is brought to the emergency department in January suffering from a fever and headaches. His wife says that he has been acting strangely, has become very forgetful, and started to vomit that morning. While in the emergency department, the patient has a seizure. A CSF sample contains lymphocytes and a few red blood cells, but there are no polymorphonuclear leukocytes or organisms, and there is no increase in the man's glucose level. An MRI indicates the presence of a focal lesion affecting the left temporal lobe. Which drug would be the most appropriate therapy for this patient?

- ❐ (A) Acyclovir
- ❐ (B) Amantadine
- ❐ (C) Amphotericin B
- ❐ (D) Ceftriaxone
- ❐ (E) Rifampin

150 A 23-year-old man who is working as a camp counselor during the summer suddenly begins to experience headaches, nausea, and vomiting. He develops a stiff neck and fever and becomes lethargic. After 5 days, the symptoms resolve, without sequelae. Which infectious agent is the most likely cause of the disease?

- ❐ (A) California encephalitis virus
- ❐ (B) Coxsackievirus A
- ❐ (C) *Cryptococcus neoformans*
- ❐ (D) CMV
- ❐ (E) Group B *Streptococcus*

151 A 39-year-old man complains of fever, fatigue, nausea, vomiting, abdominal pain, and loss of appetite. He says that he became concerned because his urine is abnormally dark but does not recall when his symptoms started. Examination shows a yellow tinge to the sclerae of his eyes. Which serologic result is most consistent with the patient's symptoms? Answers A through E are presented horizontally in the table.

	HB$_s$Ag	HB$_e$Ag	Anti-HB$_e$	Anti-HB$_c$	Anti-HB$_s$
A.	+	+	+	+	+
B.	+	+	−	+	+
C.	+	+	−	+	−
D.	−	+	−	−	+
E.	−	−	−	−	+

HB$_s$Ag, hepatitis B surface antigen; HB$_e$Ag, hepatitis B e antigen; anti-HB$_e$, antibody to hepatitis B e antigen; anti-HB$_c$, antibody to hepatitis B core antigen; anti-HB$_s$, antibody to hepatitis B surface antigen; +, present; −, absent.

152 A 2-year-old boy has a sudden onset of fever of 38.9°C that lasts for 3 days, and then he develops a faint macular (sandpaper-like) rash that covers his body and lasts only 48 h. The agent causing the disease cannot be grown on blood agar and is sensitive to detergent inactivation. Which agent is the most likely cause of this boy's symptoms?

- ❐ (A) Coxsackievirus A
- ❐ (B) Human herpesvirus 6
- ❐ (C) Measles virus
- ❐ (D) Parvovirus B19
- ❐ (E) Rubella virus

153 A previously healthy 70-year-old woman complains of severe headaches, appears apathetic, and has a constant tremor of the right hand. As her condition deteriorates, she begins to show evidence of memory loss and confusion. She subsequently lapses into a coma but continues to experience spontaneous clonic twitching of the arms and legs; she eventually dies. An autopsy reveals vacuolation of neurons and the presence of amyloid-containing plaques and fibrils. No inflammation is observed. Which description is appropriate for the agent causing this disease?

- ❐ (A) Detergent-resistant agent controlled by antibody
- ❐ (B) Detergent-resistant agent that elicits no inflammation
- ❐ (C) Detergent-resistant, opportunistic agent
- ❐ (D) Detergent-sensitive agent controlled by cell-mediated immunity
- ❐ (E) Detergent-sensitive agent that is vaccine-preventable

154 A 35-year-old man experiences the rapid onset of a headache, myalgia, malaise, a dry cough, and a fever. A nasal wash is obtained, and a virus is isolated in a culture of primary monkey kidney cells. The virus causes absorption of erythrocytes to infected cells, and syncytia are seen in the infected cells. Which virus is most likely the cause of these symptoms?

- ❐ (A) Coronavirus
- ❐ (B) Influenza A virus
- ❐ (C) Influenza B virus
- ❐ (D) Influenza C virus
- ❐ (E) Parainfluenza virus type I

155 A 35-year-old woman who is positive for HIV infection goes to the emergency department because she has been suffering for 3 days from fever, headache, anorexia, fatigue, joint pain, nausea, and vomiting. She also has a hive-like rash (urticaria) on her chest. She has a hematocrit of 35%; white blood cell count of 6500/mm³, with 40% neutrophils, 3% bands, 47% lymphocytes, and 10% atypical lymphocytes; elevated levels of liver enzymes; and normal levels of bilirubin and alkaline phosphatase. Serologic tests yield the results shown in the table.

Laboratory test	Result
Antibodies to EBNA	+
Antibodies to HIV	−
Antibodies to CMV	+
Antibodies to HAV	+
Anti-HB$_s$	−
Anti-HB$_c$	−
HB$_s$Ag	+
HB$_e$Ag	+

CMV, cytomegalovirus; EBNA, Epstein-Barr nuclear antigen; HIV, human immunodeficiency virus; HAV, hepatitis A virus; anti-HB$_c$, antibody to hepatitis B core antigen; anti-HB$_s$, antibody to hepatitis B surface antigen HB$_s$Ag, hepatitis B surface antigen; HB$_c$Ag, hepatitis B core antigen; HB$_e$Ag, hepatitis B e antigen; +, positive result; −, negative result.

	Anti-HB$_c$	Anti-HB$_e$	Anti-HB$_s$	HB$_s$AG
A.	+	!	!	+
B.	!	!	+	!
C.	+	+	!	+
D.	!	!	!	+
E.	!	!	+	+

Anti-HB$_c$, antibody to hepatitis B core antigen; anti-HB$_e$, antibody to hepatitis B e antigen; anti-HB$_s$, antibody to hepatitis B surface antigen; HB$_s$Ag, hepatitis B surface antigen; +, present; −, absent.

Which risk factor is most likely associated with the manifestations of disease in this case?

- ☐ (A) Alcoholism
- ☐ (B) Ingestion of contaminated water
- ☐ (C) Multiple sexual partners
- ☐ (D) Smoking
- ☐ (E) Travel to underdeveloped countries

156 A 1-month-old breast-fed infant is exposed to HAV. The mother has been seropositive for this virus for several years. Which type of antibody is most likely to provide protection for the infant?

- ☐ (A) IgA
- ☐ (B) IgD
- ☐ (C) IgE
- ☐ (D) IgG
- ☐ (E) IgM

157 The table shows five serologic profiles of individuals screened for hepatitis B. An individual with which profile would be an appropriate candidate for donating blood? Answers A through E are listed horizontally in the table.

158 Approximately 6 months after receiving a corneal transplant, a 56-year-old woman begins to experience confusion, anxiety, memory loss, muscle spasms, and difficulty in walking steadily. Over a period of 8 weeks, her condition deteriorates, and she eventually loses all mental functions and dies in the hospital. Postmortem analysis of brain tissue shows vacuolation of neuronal cells but no abnormal presence of inflammatory or immune cells. Which additional finding would be consistent with these results?

- ☐ (A) Absence of antiviral antibody but presence of an abnormal protein in the brain
- ☐ (B) High titers of antibody to measles virus and isolation of a measles variant from the brain
- ☐ (C) History of recurrent cold sores and isolation of an enveloped DNA virus from the brain
- ☐ (D) Isolation of a small, naked capsid virus from the brain
- ☐ (E) Isolation of an enveloped and encapsidated RNA virus from the brain

159 A 9-year-old boy is carried into the emergency department suffering from bilateral paralysis. His parents report that he started experiencing flu-like symptoms approximately 2 weeks earlier. Recently, he had a high fever and began to complain of muscle pain and a stiff neck. The boy did not receive the normal course of childhood immunizations. What is the most likely route of infection with the causative agent?

- ☐ (A) Arthropod bite
- ☐ (B) Contact with lesions of an infected individual
- ☐ (C) Fecal-oral route
- ☐ (D) Parenteral route
- ☐ (E) Respiratory route

160 The blood in blood banks is screened for HIV. The initial screening of serum is based on which process?

- ☐ (A) Amplification of the viral genome and subsequent detection of the genome by gel techniques
- ☐ (B) Antibody-induced lysis of antigen-loaded erythrocytes in the presence of complement

(C) Binding of antibody to antigen that is bound to nitro-cellulose paper

(D) Binding of antibody to immobilized antigen

(E) Binding of antigen to immobilized antibody

161 A 32-year-old man who recently spent several weeks in Malaysia suffers from a high fever, a serious retro-orbital headache, and severe joint and back pain. The symptoms last for 4 days, and then a rash appears on his trunk and lower extremities for 2 days. His physician consults with the CDC and finds that an outbreak of dengue fever has been reported for the region visited by the patient. Which agent is transmitted by the same means as dengue virus?

(A) *Borrelia burgdorferi*

(B) Hantavirus

(C) *Plasmodium vivax*

(D) St. Louis encephalitis virus

(E) Yellow fever virus

162 A 15-month-old girl has been suffering from irritability, mild fever, diarrhea, and vomiting for 2 days. In the ELISA analysis of stool used to confirm the diagnosis, which immunosorbent and enzyme-labeled immunoreactant are used?

(A) Anti-IgG and enzyme-linked anti-immunoglobulin

(B) Anti-IgM and enzyme-linked anti-immunoglobulin

(C) Antirotavirus antibody and enzyme-linked anti-rotavirus antibody

(D) Rotavirus antigen and enzyme-linked anti-immunoglobulin

(E) Rotavirus antigen and enzyme-linked antirotavirus antibody

163 What is a target cell receptor for influenza A virus?

(A) C3d complement receptor on B lymphocytes

(B) CD4 molecule and chemokine coreceptor on T lymphocytes

(C) Immunoglobulin superfamily protein on epithelial cells

(D) Erythrocyte P antigen

(E) Sialic acid receptor on epithelial cells

164 A 5-year-old girl has a temperature of 40°C and mild flu-like symptoms for 6 days, and then the fever subsides. After 8 days without fever, she develops a rash that lasts several days, is prominent on her face (giving her a "slapped cheek" appearance), and is accompanied by achy joints. Which agent causes this condition?

(A) Gram-negative diplococcus

(B) Gram-positive coccus

(C) Virus with a double-stranded RNA genome

(D) Virus with a single-stranded, negative-sense DNA genome

(E) Virus with a single-stranded, negative-sense RNA genome

165 A 75-year-old man has been exposed to influenza A virus but has not developed symptoms. Which therapy would be most appropriate?

(A) Active immunization against influenza

(B) Passive immunization with anti-influenza A antibodies

(C) Treatment with ribavirin

(D) Treatment with rimantadine

(E) Treatment with vitamin supplements and orange juice

166 Which virus has a segmented genome?

(A) CMV

(B) HBV

(C) Influenza virus

(D) JC virus

(E) Parvovirus B19

167 Reports indicate that an outbreak of spongiform encephalopathies in Britain is associated with the ingestion of beef. In affected humans and cattle, no immune response to the agent of these encephalopathies has been observed. Which explanation accounts for this lack of immune response?

(A) The agent does not cause lytic infection.

(B) The agent does not express unique immunogenic epitopes.

(C) The agent infects T cells.

(D) The agent is immunosuppressive.

(E) The agent replicates in a privileged site.

168 The emergency department is filled with patients complaining of diarrhea, gastric distress, and vomiting. Their diarrhea started abruptly and has lasted for approximately 2 days. Electron microscopy of a stool sample shows a 27-nm virus with the characteristics shown in the photomicrograph (see figure). Which virus is most likely responsible for these symptoms?

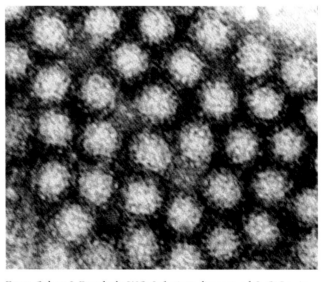

From Cohen J, Powderly WG: *Infectious diseases*, ed 2, St Louis, 2004, Mosby.

☐ (A) Adenovirus
☐ (B) Coronavirus
☐ (C) Echovirus 11
☐ (D) Norwalk virus
☐ (E) Rotavirus

169 A 45-year-old woman has been suffering from nausea, fever, inability to eat, and abdominal pains for the past several days. Her eyes have a yellowish color, and her urine is dark. Serologic tests yield results shown in the table.

Laboratory test	Result
IgG antibodies to HAV	+
IgG antibodies to HB$_c$Ag	−
IgG antibodies to HB$_s$Ag	−
IgM antibodies to HAV	−
IgM antibodies to HB$_c$Ag	+
HB$_s$Ag	+

HAV, hepatitis A virus; HB$_e$Ag, hepatitis B e antigen; HB$_s$Ag, hepatitis B surface antigen; HB$_c$Ag, hepatitis B core antigen; +, positive response; −, negative response.

The most likely cause of her symptoms has which property?

☐ (A) Encodes reverse transcriptase
☐ (B) Has an icosahedral capsid
☐ (C) Immortalizes B lymphocytes
☐ (D) Has a replication cycle with a double-stranded RNA intermediate
☐ (E) Is transmitted by mosquitoes

170 An 11-year-old girl who is attending summer camp in Ohio is brought to the emergency department because she has been suffering from a fever, vomiting, and a severe headache for 3 days. While in the emergency department, she is lethargic and confused and has a seizure. She recovers after 10 days of illness. The most likely cause of her symptoms would be confirmed by which finding?

☐ (A) Anticardiolipin (reagin) antibody in the blood
☐ (B) Cells with owl's eye inclusion bodies in the urine
☐ (C) Heterophil antibody in the cerebrospinal fluid
☐ (D) IgG antibody to HSV in the blood
☐ (E) IgM antibody to California encephalitis virus in the blood

171 Immunization against the measles virus will prevent measles and which disease?

☐ (A) CJD
☐ (B) Kawasaki disease

☐ (C) Kuru
☐ (D) Progressive multifocal leukoencephalopathy
☐ (E) SSPE

172 A 21-year-old college student visits the health clinic because of a maculopapular rash that started on his head and has spread to his trunk; the rash is accompanied by fever, cough, coryza, and conjunctivitis. Immune control of this infection requires a response involving which factor?

☐ (A) IgA
☐ (B) IgE
☐ (C) IgG
☐ (D) Neutrophils
☐ (E) T cells

173 The 5-year-old son of a migrant worker has a cough, conjunctivitis, coryza, and a diffuse maculopapular rash on his face and trunk. Lesions in his mouth have white centers that appear like grains of sand. How is this disease predominantly transmitted?

☐ (A) Blood
☐ (B) Mosquitoes
☐ (C) Respiratory droplets
☐ (D) Saliva
☐ (E) Sexual contact

174 A 50-year-old man undergoing a routine physical examination complains of fatigue, an inability to concentrate, and epigastric pain that has gotten worse during the past year. His medical records show that he received a blood transfusion during surgery in the late 1980s. His blood contains elevated transaminase levels. A PCR-based blood test for flavivirus sequences yields positive results. Which hepatitis virus is the most likely diagnosis?

☐ (A) HAV
☐ (B) HBV
☐ (C) HCV
☐ (D) HDV
☐ (E) HEV

175 A 65-year-old man recently exposed to influenza experiences a headache, myalgia, malaise, dry cough, and fever. His symptoms subside after 5 days. On day 7, he again becomes febrile and his cough worsens. Physical examination shows signs of pneumonia. Which drug treatment would be most appropriate for pneumonia?

☐ (A) Acyclovir
☐ (B) Amantadine
☐ (C) Levofloxacin
☐ (D) Ribavirin
☐ (E) Rimantadine

176 A 16-year-old boy has a sore throat, swollen cervical lymph nodes, fever, malaise, and hepatosplenomegaly. Laboratory findings include the presence of atypical lymphocytes and heterophil antibodies. Ampicillin is administered, and the patient develops an intense rash on his chest. Which agent is the most likely cause of the condition?

- ❐ (A) Adenovirus
- ❐ (B) CMV
- ❐ (C) EBV
- ❐ (D) HSV
- ❐ (E) *Streptococcus pyogenes*

177 A 5-month-old girl is brought to the emergency department in January because she has a fever and is wheezing, as well as having difficulty in breathing. Bronchiolitis is suspected. The structural characteristics of the virion infecting the patient are most similar to those of which virus?

- ❐ (A) Adenovirus
- ❐ (B) Poliovirus
- ❐ (C) Rabies virus
- ❐ (D) Rotavirus
- ❐ (E) Rubella virus

178 A 74-year-old man who underwent bypass surgery 8 years ago develops cirrhosis. He does not drink alcohol and does not participate in risky behavior. The physician suspects that his cirrhosis is caused by a virus. Which etiologic agent is the cause of his condition?

- ❐ (A) Enveloped, double-stranded DNA virus
- ❐ (B) Enveloped, single-stranded, circular RNA virus
- ❐ (C) Enveloped, single-stranded, positive-sense RNA virus
- ❐ (D) Enveloped, single-stranded, positive-sense RNA virus with a reverse transcriptase
- ❐ (E) Nonenveloped, single-stranded, positive-sense RNA virus

179 Which step in viral replication is inhibited by nucleoside analogues?

- ❐ (A) Penetration
- ❐ (B) Uncoating
- ❐ (C) Transcription
- ❐ (D) Replication
- ❐ (E) Viral assembly

1 (E) Its replication requires an RNA-dependent DNA polymerase. The patient's clinical and serologic findings are consistent with the diagnosis of hepatitis B. Hepatitis B e antigen (HB$_e$Ag) is the best indicator for the presence of hepatitis B virus (HBV) infection; hepatitis B surface antigen (HB$_s$Ag) is also an indicator. HBV has a circular DNA genome that replicates through an RNA intermediate using reverse transcriptase (RNA-dependent DNA polymerase). Picornaviruses, such as the hepatitis A virus (HAV), have a messenger RNA (mRNA) genome that encodes a polyprotein. Hepatitis D virus (HDV) requires HBV as a helper virus. Herpesviruses and adenoviruses have linear double-stranded DNA genomes, and retroviruses have RNA genomes that replicate through a DNA intermediate.
MM5 680

2 (A) It is assayed by reverse transcriptase polymerase chain reaction (RT-PCR) technology. The patient's history and symptoms suggest hantavirus pulmonary syndrome. This case is descriptive of the initial diagnosis of the Sin Nombre hantavirus outbreak, which led to the identification of this virus. Hantaviruses are bunyaviruses with RNA genomes, hence the use of RT-PCR. Primers with sequences found in many hantaviruses were used in RT-PCR techniques to amplify virus sequences from the patient and thereby provide the first description of the virus. Like other bunyaviruses, hantaviruses are enveloped, single-stranded, negative-sense, segmented RNA viruses. Hantavirus almost always causes serious disease. It is not spread by mosquitoes but is maintained in rodents. An increase in the rodent population increases contact with the vector. Amantadine is a treatment for influenza A.
MM5 651

3 (A) Blockade of nucleocapsid release into the cytoplasm. The symptoms of influenza A, but not influenza B, can be reduced or prevented if amantadine or rimantadine treatment is begun within the first few days of exposure. By blocking a channel formed by the M2 protein, both drugs inhibit the "uncoating" (release of nucleic acid from the nucleocapsid) of influenza A virus. The Food and Drug Administration has not approved any antiviral drugs that block viral glycoprotein synthesis or inhibit RNA-dependent RNA polymerase. Interferon (IFN) is an agent that inhibits viral protein synthesis, but no chemotherapy is directed at this target. Some drugs that are used in the treatment of human immunodeficiency virus (HIV) infection act by inhibiting RNA-dependent DNA polymerase, which is also known as reverse transcriptase. These drugs include zidovudine (azidothymidine, or AZT) and other nucleotide analogues.
MM5 510, 616

4 (A) C3d complement receptor on B lymphocytes. Binding of the viral attachment proteins (VAPs) to specific cell receptors determine which cells are infected by the virus. The receptors may be proteins, glycoproteins, or glycolipids. The VAPs for the Epstein-Barr virus (EBV) are glycoproteins gp350 and gp220. The glycoproteins attach to the C3d complement receptor on B

cells. Examples of other receptors for viruses include HIV that binds to the CD4 molecule and chemokine coreceptor on T lymphocytes, poliovirus that binds to the immunoglobulin superfamily protein on epithelial cells, rabies virus that binds to the acetylcholine receptor on neurons, and influenza A virus that binds to sialic acid receptors on epithelial cells.
MM5 553

5 (D) Interferon-gamma (IFN-γ). The patient's disease manifestations are consistent with the diagnosis of AIDS, a syndrome caused by infection with HIV. Pneumonia, thrush, and other opportunistic infections occur when the CD4+ T cell count falls to low levels. IFN-γ is produced primarily by CD4 Th1 cells and activates macrophages to promote clearance of fungal and viral infections. Despite CD4 depletion, complement components continue to be produced by the liver and other cells. Immunoglobulin G (IgG) continues to be produced, possibly uncontrolled. Interferon-alpha (IFN-α) continues to be produced by epithelial, fibroblast, and leukocyte cells in response to viral infections. Interleukin-1 (IL-1) continues to be produced by macrophages and monocytes, which are still functional.
MM5 665

6 (E) Nonenveloped, double-stranded DNA virus with spikes at its vertices. The patient's history and clinical manifestations are consistent with the diagnosis of pharyngoconjunctival fever. This disorder is also called "swimming pool conjunctivitis." It is caused by an adenovirus and is usually diagnosed only by clinical presentation. Although the description of the causative agent may suggest a toxin-producing bacterium, an adenovirus (a nonenveloped virus) is the most likely agent for two reasons. First, adenoviruses are the most frequent cause of conjunctivitis in swimmers. Second, adenoviruses commonly cause conjunctivitis that is accompanied by pharyngitis. An enveloped, double-stranded DNA virus, such as herpes simplex virus, can cause keratoconjunctivitis and is a common cause of blindness. A gram-negative diplococcus is *Neisseria gonorrhoeae*, a bacterium that causes eye infections in infants. A gram-negative, oxidase-positive rod is *Pseudomonas aeruginosa*, a bacterium that can cause corneal ulcers and endophthalmitis. A gram-positive diplococcus is *Streptococcus pneumoniae*, a bacterium that is usually associated with upper respiratory tract infections and not ocular infections.
MM5 533

7 (A) Blood transfusion. Some areas of Japan have a high incidence of acute T cell lymphocytic leukemia, a disease that can be caused by the human T lymphotropic virus (HTLV). Like HIV, HTLV is a retrovirus that is transmitted in blood products and via sexual contact. Unlike HIV, HTLV is a C-type retrovirus and is not lytic. There is a long latency period between infection and the onset of leukemia. Although endogenous retroviruses are transmitted through the germ line, their association with human cancers has not been clearly defined. HTLV is not transmitted via contact with saliva or via the fecal-oral or respiratory route. EBV is transmitted in saliva and is associated with infectious mononucleosis ("kissing disease"), Burkitt's lymphoma, nasopharyngeal carcinoma, and some Hodgkin's lymphomas. The fecal-oral route is a common route of infection with enteric viruses (such as adenoviruses and HAV), none of which are tumorigenic in humans. The respiratory route is the most common route of virus transmission. HTLV is a retrovirus, and retroviruses integrate into host chromatin. Endogenous retroviruses, but not HTLV, are transmitted through the germ line by vertical genetic transmission.

MM5 671

8 (B) Activation of interleukin-2 (IL-2) receptor expression. HTLV-I is a retrovirus that slowly induces leukemia. HTLV leukemia is more common in parts of Japan than in the rest of the world. The Tax protein of HTLV is a transactivator that promotes mRNA production for IL-2 and IL-2 receptor genes. This stimulates cell growth. After many years of growth, genetic errors occur and lead to leukemia. Activation of IFN-γ by HTLV-I may occur, but this cytokine would stimulate protection and not leukemogenesis. Expressions of a virus-encoded growth hormone receptor, of a virus-encoded guanosine triphosphate binding protein, and of a virus-encoded tyrosine kinase are characteristic of oncogenes produced by retroviruses that are rapid inducers of cancer. For example, the *erb*B and *erb*A oncogenes are receptors to the epidermal growth factor and thyroid hormone, respectively. The *Ha-ras* and *Ki-ras* oncogenes are guanosine triphosphate-binding proteins. The *abl, fes,* and *src* oncogenes are tyrosine kinases.

MM5 671

9 (D) Nonenveloped, double-stranded DNA virus with penton fibers at its vertices. In 1941, an adenovirus was responsible for 10,000 cases of keratoconjunctivitis among shipyard workers in Pearl Harbor. This virus is airborne and is easily transmitted. Eye irritation due to foreign materials, such as paint chips, facilitates the infection. Adenovirus is a nonenveloped DNA virus with fibers attached to its icosadeltahedral capsid. The fiber proteins at the pentons are the VAPs. Arenaviruses, bunyaviruses, filoviruses, orthomyxoviruses, paramyxoviruses, and rhabdoviruses have enveloped, single-stranded, negative-sense RNA. Enveloped, single-stranded, positive-sense RNA viruses include coronaviruses, flaviviruses, retroviruses, and togaviruses. Papovaviruses have nonenveloped, double-stranded, circular DNA. Nonenveloped, single-stranded, positive-sense RNA viruses are astroviruses, caliciviruses, and picornaviruses.

MM5 534

10 (C) Endogenous reactivation of an earlier infection. Varicella-zoster virus (VZV) is the agent of chickenpox (also called varicella) and shingles (also called herpes zoster). An individual may acquire chickenpox via inhalation of aerosolized droplets of VZV or via contact with a lesion. After an individual has chickenpox, VZV becomes latent. The VZV virions reside in the nerve ganglia and reactivate when the conditions are favorable. The

distribution of lesions is restricted to a dermatome as in this case. Contaminated food or water can transmit some nonenveloped viruses, but VZV has an envelope and cannot be transmitted by the fecal-oral route. Needle sticks may transmit viruses that cause chronic viremia, such as HIV and HBV, but they do not transmit VZV. Some viruses, such as HIV, HBV, cytomegalovirus, herpes simplex viruses, and Papillomaviruses, are sexually transmitted; however, VZV cannot be transmitted in this manner.

MM5 550

11 (D) IFN-α. Treatment with this agent inhibits a step in virus replication, such as protein synthesis, that is common to most viruses. The compound probably induces IFN-α. Influenza and other single-stranded, negative-sense RNA viruses are sensitive to the interferon because they produce a double-stranded RNA intermediate during replication of the genome. The double-stranded RNA induces the interferon and also activates the antiviral state in an interferon-treated cell. The double-stranded RNA activates protein kinase R (PKR), an inhibitor of protein synthesis, and a ribonuclease to degrade mRNA. Acyclovir is a nucleotide analogue with a truncated sugar. It is activated by the thymidine kinase of herpes simplex virus (HSV) or VZV and then inhibits the viral DNA polymerase. It is specific for the HSV and VZV herpesviruses. Amantadine is not effective against influenza B virus. It inhibits the uncoating of influenza A virus. Because viral mRNA is present, the degradation of the coating must have occurred. AZT inhibits the reverse transcriptase of HIV. Ribavirin, a guanosine analogue that is approved for the treatment of respiratory syncytial virus infection, inhibits replication and promotes hypermutation of viruses. It is effective against RNA viruses.

MM5 144

12 (D) Norwalk virus. Norwalk virus, a member of the family Noroviridae, is an extremely small virus with an icosahedral capsid and a single-stranded, positive-sense RNA genome. The Norwalk virus causes outbreaks that affect a large number of exposed individuals. Adenoviruses are large, double-stranded DNA viruses with an icosahedral capsid that has fibers. Some adenoviruses cause diarrhea (e.g., adenoviruses 41 and 42). Coronaviruses are medium, single-stranded, positive-sense RNA viruses with an envelope and a halo-like appearance. Coronaviruses are resistant to the conditions of the gut and are suspected of causing diarrhea. Rotaviruses, which are reoviruses, are large, double-stranded RNA viruses with a double capsid. They are a major cause of diarrhea in infants and can also cause similar symptoms in adults. Coxsackieviruses are small, single-stranded, positive-sense RNA viruses with an icosahedral capsid. Coxsackieviruses are picornaviruses and do not usually cause diarrhea.

MM5 594

13 (E) Yellow fever virus. Sensitivity to detergents indicates the presence of an envelope. A genome is infectious if the DNA or RNA can be injected into a cell and is sufficient to infect the cell. The only genomes that are infectious are DNA viral genomes and positive-sense RNA viral genomes. Yellow fever virus and other flaviviruses have an envelope and a single-stranded, positive-sense RNA genome. Papillomaviruses, adenoviruses, HAV, and hepatitis E virus (HEV) do not have envelopes and are therefore not sensitive to detergents. Papillomaviruses and other papovaviruses have a double-stranded, circular DNA genome. Adenoviruses have a linear double-stranded DNA genome. The HAV and other picornaviruses have a single-stranded, positive-sense RNA genome. The HEV also has a positive-sense RNA genome. Therefore all of the viruses listed in the answers to this question have infectious genomes.

MM5 51, 637

14 (B) Breast-feeding the infant. A secretory antibody in the mother's milk can protect the infant from infection with rotavirus. Rotavirus infection occurs by the fecal-oral route. Although utensils may be the source of infection, the virus is more likely to be passed from hand to mouth. It is almost impossible to keep infants' hands clean. The vaccine against rotavirus is a genetic mixture of RNA segments from rotaviruses of different species and is a live vaccine. Amantadine is used to prevent or treat infection with influenza A virus, not rotavirus.

MM5 111, 631

15 (D) Norwalk virus. Norwalk virus is a member of the Noroviridae family and is composed of single-stranded RNA surrounded by an icosahedral capsid. No envelope is present, which can account for the environmental stability of this virus. Other RNA viruses listed in the answers to this question are influenza virus (member of the Orthomyxoviridae family), Lassa fever virus (Arenaviridae), and respiratory syncytial virus (Paramyxoviridae). Each of these has an envelope. Herpes simplex virus is an enveloped DNA virus.

MM5 51, 594

16 (D) Immunofluorescence of tear-infected tissue culture fibroblasts. Although the findings of atypical lymphocytes in the serum sample, epithelial cells in the urine sample, and viral DNA in the blood sample would suggest the presence of a CMV infection, they are not taken from the affected site (the eye) and are therefore not relevant to the diagnosis of CMV retinitis. The presence of atypical lymphocytes also would not confirm the diagnosis of CMV retinitis. Atypical lymphocytes are seen during infectious mononucleosis (which is caused by EBV) and even during the initial phase of HIV disease. CMV is an opportunistic pathogen. In patients with AIDS, the immunosuppression allows the reactivation of CMV in many tissue sites, and systemic infection spreads the virus throughout the body. Tissue culture isolation is the gold standard for analysis. The only relevant samples are those taken from the affected site (in this case, tears from the infected eye); thus immunofluorescence of tear-infected tissue culture fibroblasts would help diagnose this patient's CMV retinitis.

MM5 514, 561

17 (B) H1N2. The mobilities of the RNA for the hemagglutinin (HA) match the 1991 isolate, and those for the neuraminidase (NA) match the 1989 isolate. The influenza virus has a segmented RNA genome that can reassort its segments when it is coinfected. This reassortment generates diversity, especially if viruses from human and animal coinfect a common host. H1N1 is the designation for the 1991 isolate, and H3N2 is the designation for the 1989 isolate. The coinfection described in the question differs from each of these. The data indicate that reassortment (not gross change in genetic composition) occurred.

MM5 613, 615

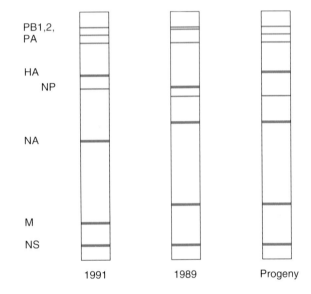

18 (D) nef. The patient's disease manifestations are consistent with the diagnosis of AIDS, a syndrome caused by infection with HIV. HIV mutants lacking nef do not cause AIDS, but the mutants replicate and have been considered for vaccine development. Viral replication requires gag, gp120, integrase, and protease. The group-specific antigen (gag) includes the capsid proteins required for the virion structure. The VAP gp120 is required to initiate infection. Integrase is required to insert the viral cDNA into the chromosome to allow replication. Protease is necessary for maturation of the virion.

MM5 660

19 (C) Icosahedral capsid. The patient's age and symptoms as well as the results of the Gram stain and other laboratory findings suggest the diagnosis of meningitis caused by echovirus 11. This virus is associated with outbreaks of meningitis in children and is transmitted via the fecal-oral route and possibly via aerosols. Like other picornaviruses, echoviruses have a virion capsid that is impervious to the conditions of the gastrointestinal tract and to drying. Echoviruses and other picornaviruses do not have an envelope. Envelopes are membranes that are labile. Enveloped viruses that may cause meningitis include mumps virus, herpes simplex virus, varicella-zoster virus, HIV, lymphocytic choriomeningitis virus, and some togaviruses and flaviviruses. Echoviruses do not have hemagglutinin. Hemagglutinins are the attachment proteins for orthomyxoviruses and paramyxoviruses. Echoviruses also do not have NA. NA removes the binding structure (sialic acid) from the virus receptor and is present in orthomyxoviruses and some paramyxoviruses. Echoviruses and other picornaviruses are capsid viruses that have a valley into which the cellular virus receptor inserts. In contrast, adenoviruses and reoviruses are capsid viruses with structures sticking out of the capsid. Enveloped viruses have glycoproteins, but picornaviruses do not.

MM5 579

20 (C) Presence of retroviral DNA may be due to an endogenous virus. The stem of the question does not define the retroviral sequences that were amplified by PCR. Because PCR is such a highly sensitive technique, endogenous retroviruses can be amplified when it is used. Although HTLV-I is endemic in southern Japan, the presence of retroviral DNA is not proof that HTLV-I is involved in the disease. Environmental factors have not been identified for induction of HTLV-I leukemia. HTLV-I does not express an oncogene. HIV and HTLV-I infect the same cell type. However, HIV kills CD4 T cells, whereas HTLV-I stimulates the growth of these cells. HTLV-I has a lag period of up to 30 years before the leukemia occurs.

MM5 673

21 (E) Ribavirin. Although ribavirin is mainly used for the treatment of infants with respiratory syncytial virus infections, it is also effective against hepatitis C virus (HCV) and against Lassa virus, an arenavirus that causes Lassa fever as is suspected in the patient. Ribavirin is a guanosine analogue that inhibits virus replication and other guanosine-related activities. Acyclovir is used to treat HSV and VZV infections. Amantadine is used to treat influenza A (but not influenza B or C). Azidothymidine, which is also called zidovudine, is used to treat HIV infection. Foscarnet is used to treat HSV, VZV, and cytomegalovirus (CMV) infections.

MM5 504

22 (A) Assembly. Virus assembly is one of the last steps in viral replication and is a likely target of antiviral drugs. The order of the steps in viral replication is as follows: binding to host cells, penetration of host cells, uncoating, protein and DNA synthesis, assembly of new virions, and escape from host cells. The ability of the new drug to inhibit viral replication when it is added as late as 5 h after exposure indicates that the steps preceding assembly are not affected.

MM5 61

23 (D) The vaccine is usually administered with an adjuvant. Inactivated vaccines use a large antigenic exposure to stimulate an immune response without the risk of an active infection. Because the inactivated vaccine material will not persist in the host as long as a live vaccine, however, inactivated vaccines are usually administered with an adjuvant such as alum, which boosts the immunogenicity of the vaccine. The adjuvant can also influence the type of the immune response induced by the vaccine. Booster doses are commonly administered with the vaccine. Most inactivated vaccines do not induce a local IgA response, immunity is primarily humoral, and immunity is not usually lifelong as with many live vaccines.

MM5 160-162

24 (D) Polio vaccine. The oral polio vaccine (OPV) is a live, attenuated vaccine and is also called the Sabin vaccine. The inactivated polio vaccine (IPV) is a killed virus vaccine and is also called the Salk vaccine. The Centers for Disease Control and Prevention (CDC) now recommends that children in the United States receive the IPV rather than the OPV. The hepatitis B vaccine is a subunit vaccine consisting of HB_sAg prepared in yeast by recombinant DNA technology. The annual influenza vaccine is a mixture of killed viruses representing the predicted virus threats for the year. The Lyme disease vaccine, LYMErix, was a killed vaccine that prevents transmission of the bacteria from the tick. Only a live, attenuated varicella vaccine is effective.

MM5 163, 587

25 (E) Thymidine kinase. The lesions are characteristic of herpes gladiatorum and oral herpes, diseases caused by HSV. The disease is spread when one person's vesicular lesion (usually orofacial) comes into contact with another person's skin and the infectious agents are rubbed into an abrasion of the skin. Thymidine kinase is a scavenging enzyme that is encoded by HSV and is the target for some drugs that are effective in the treatment of HSV infections. HSV does not encode the enzymes in the incorrect answers to this question. Integrase is made by retroviruses. The 5N-methyl capping enzyme is a cellular enzyme found in the nucleus and also encoded by reoviruses. NA is made by influenza viruses. RNA-dependent RNA polymerase is encoded by RNA viruses but not by retroviruses or DNA viruses.

MM5 547

26 (D) In situ DNA hybridization analysis of cells from the cervical smear. Human papillomavirus (HPV) types 16 and 18 cause wart-like lesions characterized by koilocytotic cells. These HPV types are also associated with cervical carcinoma. The viral DNA is present and can be detected in the cells, but virus is not produced and immune responses are minimal. Immune responses to HPV are minimal. Hemadsorption, or binding of erythrocytes to the cell surface, is useful for viruses with a hemagglutinin but not for HPV. HPV generally does not replicate in infected cells and does not produce readily detectable antigen in those cells. The virus is not produced in detectable amounts, and no tissue culture growth system is available for clinical laboratory use.

MM5 178, 527

27 (A) Cowdry type A inclusion bodies. Cowdry type A inclusion bodies, syncytia, and margination of chromatin are characteristic of HSV infection. HSV can cause encephalitis throughout the year, unlike arboviral encephalitis viruses. Downey cells, hemagglutinin, Negri bodies, and owl's eye inclusion bodies are not associated with HSV infections. Downey cells are abnormal lymphocytes associated with EBV infections. Hemagglutinin is associated with influenza, parainfluenza, and other viruses. Negri bodies are seen in rabies virus infected cells. Owl's eye inclusion bodies are seen in cytomegalovirus-infected cells.

MM5 548

28 (D) Parvovirus B19. The genetic material in a virus can be either DNA or RNA and can present in the double-strand or single-strand arrangement. Poliovirus is a member of the Picornaviridae family of RNA viruses. All of the other viruses listed in the answers to this question are DNA viruses. Most DNA viruses contain double-stranded DNA. The exceptions are the Parvoviridae that include parvovirus B19 and adeno-associated virus (AAV).

MM5 50-52, 574

29 (A) Circular double-stranded DNA. The history and findings in this case are consistent with the diagnosis of progressive multifocal leukoencephalopathy (PML), a disease that affects immunosuppressed patients and is caused by a ubiquitous polyomavirus called JC virus. Polyomaviruses have a circular double-stranded DNA genome and encode T antigen as an early protein. Viruses with linear double-stranded DNA include herpesviruses, adenoviruses, and poxviruses. HSV and VZV can cause encephalitis. Rhabdoviruses and paramyxoviruses are examples of viruses with linear single-stranded negative RNA genomes that cause neuronal disease. Rabies, a rhabdovirus, and measles and its variant, subacute sclerosing panencephalitis (SSPE) virus, cause neuronal disease. Picornavirus (polio), togavirus (equine encephalitis), and flavivirus (St. Louis encephalitis) are examples of positive-stranded RNA viruses that cause neuronal disease. Hepatitis B (a hepadnavirus) is the only human virus with partially double-stranded DNA.

MM5 529

30 (E) VZV. A live, attenuated vaccine for VZV, the Oka strain, is administered to children at the same time as the measles, mumps, and rubella (MMR) vaccine. A formalin-inactivated HAV vaccine has been developed and is highly effective, with a strong antibody response after a single dose is administered. HBV vaccines are subunit vaccines. Vaccination is recommended for infants, children, and people in high-risk groups. A series of three injections are highly protective. The influenza virus vaccine is prepared using formalin-inactivated virus. The rabies vaccine is a killed-virus vaccine prepared through the chemical inactivation of rabies-infected tissue culture human diploid cells. This vaccine is administered as postexposure prophylaxis in a series of five immunizations during the course of 1 month.

MM5 164, 553

31 (B) Disease is sexually transmitted. HTLV-I is a retrovirus that can cause adult T cell leukemia or lymphoma (ATLL) and tropical spastic paraparesis. The virus is transmitted sexually, congenitally, or via contact with contaminated blood products or breast milk. ATLL and HTLV are endemic in many parts of Japan. There is no vaccine against HTLV. HTLV-1 infection does not rapidly promote lymphomagenesis. The latent period can be 30 or more years. Oncogene-encoding retroviruses rapidly cause tumors, but HTLV-I does not encode an oncogene. HIV infection, not HTLV infection, is susceptible to treatment with azidothymidine (zidovudine). An RNA-dependent RNA polymerase is present in cells infected with RNA viruses other than retroviruses. Retroviruses encode an RNA-dependent DNA polymerase.

MM5 672

32 (D) Restriction fragment length polymorphism (RFLP) techniques. There are two types of HSV, called HSV-I and HSV-II. Samples from a common source would be identical in terms of their strain and their HSV type. RFLP identifies DNA sequence differences of strains from different individuals and is the only technique that can identify specific virus strains harbored by individuals. Although examination of tissue cultures may reveal differences in the cytopathologic effects of virus strains (with some strains producing more syncytia, for example, or causing a greater extent of cell damage), this method is too imprecise to identify and compare the strains of a virus. Immunofluorescence and in situ DNA hybridization can distinguish the types of HSV (HSV-I versus HSV-II) but cannot distinguish the different strains of HSV. The Western blot assay of the antibody will not indicate the strain of infecting virus. Serologic tests for HSV are generally not useful.

MM5 178, 548

33 (E) Virus infection targets erythrocyte precursor cells. The patient has a parvovirus B19 infection. Parvovirus B19 is an extremely small, simple virus that requires a rapidly growing cell to replicate. Infection of erythrocyte precursor cells causes a decrease in the already reduced number of erythrocytes found in patients who have a potential for anemia. The sickle cell trait does not affect an individual's susceptibility to parvovirus B19 infection. The erythrocyte does not have a nucleus and cannot be infected or produce a virus. Malaria has nothing to do with parvovirus B19 infection. The sickle cell trait reduces an individual's risk for serious falciparum malaria. An IFN may be responsible for some of the flu-like symptoms but is not responsible for anemia.

MM5 573

34 (B) Modifies the host cell membrane during replication. Members of the family Herpesviridae and DNA viruses with the genome are surrounded by an icosahedral capsid and covered with an envelope. DNA replication and assembly into the capsids occurs in the nucleus of infected cells. The envelope is acquired from the host nuclear or Golgi membrane as the viruses exit the nucleus. The viruses exit the cell by exocytosis or by lysis of the cell. Enveloped viruses are more labile than nonenveloped viruses. Because they are susceptible to drying and detergents, they are not easily spread by fomites or by hand contact.

MM5 51, 514

35 **(B) The viral genome contains many nonessential genes.** The vaccinia vector contains and causes expression of inserted genes that replace nonessential genes. These infected cells will then process and present antigens (including the incorporated antigen) as if the host had a normal vaccinia virus infection. This initiates a natural immune response, with the host responding as if the vector were a live virus vaccine. Routine vaccination for smallpox is no longer performed. Spread to other hosts is not relevant to this vaccine. A broad range of hosts would indicate the ability to infect humans and animals. This would facilitate vaccine production but not vaccine action. A noncytolytic virus may be better for presenting antigen than a cytolytic virus.

MM5 567

36 **(B) Uncoating.** Antiviral agents can disrupt a variety of steps in viral attachment and penetration to the host cell; can disrupt uncoating, transcription, protein synthesis, and nucleic acid replication; and can affect assembly and release of viral particles. After the uptake of many viruses, the acidic environment of the endocytic vesicle is used to initiate uncoating, which is the release of nucleic acid from the nucleocapsid. Specifically, the acidic pH promotes conformational changes in the attachment proteins that promote fusion or membrane disruption. Amantadine, a weak organic base, can neutralize the pH of these compartments and inhibit uncoating. Also, amantadine has specific activity against influenza A virus by inhibiting the ion channel activity of influenza A virus M2 protein, thus preventing viral uncoating and release of viral RNA into the cytoplasm. This antiviral activity does not interfere with attachment, transcription, replication, or viral assembly.

MM5 56

37 **(A) Influenza vaccine.** A child who has leukemia and is undergoing treatment is assumed to be immunosuppressed. The only safe vaccine is therefore an inactivated vaccine. The influenza vaccine is an inactivated vaccine that is prepared in eggs and consists of protein from influenza virus strains representing the predicted epidemic or pandemic strains of the next year. Live vaccines, such as for measles, mumps, and varicella, and the oral polio vaccine (OPV), may initiate disease in the weakened host. The inactivated polio vaccine is a safe alternative to the OPV.

MM5 161, 616

38 **(A) Rubella virus causes asymptomatic infection.** To eliminate a disease, it is important to eliminate the source of transmission. For smallpox, everyone who was infected with variola virus showed obvious symptoms and therefore could be quarantined to prevent spread of the virus. Not everyone who is infected with rubella virus is symptomatic. Asymptomatic unvaccinated individuals can spread rubella. Both rubella virus and variola virus cause viremia, so antibody is important to limit the spread of these viruses in the body. Variola virus and rubella virus each have only one serotype. Therefore only one vaccine strain is required, and immunity prevents subsequent infections. The host range of both rubella virus and variola virus is limited to humans. This means that there are no animal reservoirs that can reintroduce these viruses into the population. Live vaccines are used to prevent both smallpox and rubella. The smallpox vaccine consists of live vaccinia virus that shares antigenicity with variola virus. The rubella vaccine consists of live, attenuated rubella virus.

MM5 646

39 **(D) Establish latent infections.** The herpesviruses are able to establish latent infections in their hosts. HSV and VZV establish latency in neuron cells, EBV establishes latency in B cells, and cytomegalovirus establishes latency in monocytes and lymphocytes.

MM5 545

40 **(D) Persistence in erythrocytes that establishes prolonged viremia.** The Colorado tick fever virus infects erythroid precursors and persists in a protected manner in erythrocytes. When the tick takes a blood meal from a mammal, it is likely to acquire the virus. Like other reoviruses, the Colorado tick fever virus is a double-stranded RNA virus that has a double capsid. Its capsid protein is the VAP. Its genome is segmented, but reassortment is not relevant to transmission. Persistence of the virus in erythrocytes is the property most relevant to transmission. Replication of virions in the salivary gland of ticks allows the virus to pass from ticks to mammals, not from mammals to ticks.

MM5 633

41 **(A) Cowdry type A inclusion bodies.** The history and findings in this case are consistent with the diagnosis of herpetic whitlow, a skin infection that is caused by HSV and is an occupational hazard for dental and medical care workers. Cowdry type A inclusion bodies are a characteristic of HSV-infected cells. Downey cells are abnormal lymphocytes associated with EBV infections. Koilocytotic cells are seen in association with HPV infections. Although HPV strains infect the cervix, they are unlikely to infect a gynecologist's finger, and they would not cause vesicular lesions. Negri bodies are seen in rabies virus B-infected cells. Owl's eye inclusion bodies are found in cytomegalovirus-infected cells.

MM5 548

42 **(A) Circular double-stranded DNA.** The patient's clinical manifestations are consistent with the diagnosis of scalded skin syndrome, a toxin-mediated disease caused by *Staphylococcus aureus.* In addition to causing scalded skin syndrome, staphylococcal toxins cause staphylococcal food poisoning and toxic shock syndrome. Like other bacteria, *S. aureus* has circular double-stranded DNA. Adenoviruses have linear double-stranded DNA with protein attached to the 5N ends. Fungi and parasites are eukaryotes that have multiple linear diploid DNA strands (chromatin). Bunyaviruses, orthomyxoviruses, paramyxoviruses, and rhabdoviruses are examples of viruses that have negative-sense single-stranded RNA. Caliciviruses, coronaviruses, flaviviruses, picornaviruses, and togaviruses are examples of viruses that have positive-sense single-stranded RNA.

MM5 50

43 **(B) Influenza virus.** The influenza virus vaccine is prepared using formalin-inactivated virus. Killed whole-virus vaccines are prepared from virus grown in embryonated eggs and then chemically inactivated. Detergent-treated virion preparations and extracts of viral hemagglutinin and NA are also available. HBV vaccines are subunit vaccines. The rubella vaccine is a live, attenuated virus (e.g., cold-adapted RA27/3 strains). Vaccination for smallpox includes a live vaccinia virus. A live, attenuated vaccine is used for VZV, the Oka strain.

MM5 160, 616

44 **(D) VZV establishes viremia.** Circulating antibody is most effective at blocking viremia. VZV but not HSV is disseminated in the body by viremia. Both HSV and VZV produce syncytia, are neurotropic, and encode thymidine kinase. Unlike HSV, VZV is transmitted by the respiratory route. The immune globulin, however, has no effect on respiratory transmission.

MM5 550

45 **(A) Activation of unrelated antibody production.** The patient's clinical and laboratory findings are consistent with the diagnosis of infectious mononucleosis due to EBV. The monospot test detects heterophil antibodies, which are characteristic of an EBV infection and react with sheep, horse, and bovine erythrocytes. This virus is not associated with the activities of binding of erythrocytes to infected cell surfaces, continued release of surface antigen, and integration of cDNA into host chromatin. Influenza virus and some paramyxoviruses make hemagglutinins that are expressed on the surface of infected cells and will bind erythrocytes. HBV causes continued release of HB$_s$Ag until the viral infection is controlled. Retroviruses make a cDNA intermediate that can be integrated into the chromosome. EBV is associated with heterophil antibodies. CMV, another agent of mononucleosis, is not associated with heterophil antibodies; it is associated with owl's eye inclusion bodies in infected cells.

MM5 555

46 **(A) DNA-dependent DNA polymerase.** CMV is a member of the family Herpesviridae and the subfamily Betaherpesviri-

nae. Unlike members of the subfamily Alphaherpesvirinae, CMV does not encode thymidine kinase. Ganciclovir is phosphorylated by a viral enzyme, and then it inhibits the viral DNA polymerase. NA is a new drug target for the influenza virus. It is not the target for ganciclovir. Ribonucleotide reductase is a potential drug target for herpesviruses, but it is not the target for ganciclovir. RNA-dependent DNA polymerase is reverse transcriptase (RT). It is encoded by retroviruses, such as HIV, and is a major target for anti-HIV drugs. It is not the target for ganciclovir. Thymidine kinase is encoded by HSV and VZV, which are members of the subfamily Alphaherpesvirinae. Thymidine kinase is not encoded by CMV, which is a member of the subfamily Betaherpesvirinae. Thymidine kinase activates acyclovir and penciclovir, which then inhibit the viral DNA polymerase. Valacyclovir and famciclovir are prodrugs of acyclovir and penciclovir, respectively.

MM5 506, 561

47 **(B) Rabies.** Passive immunity in the form of immune globulin is used to prevent disease after a known exposure to a specific pathogen (e.g., rabies), to ameliorate the symptoms of an ongoing disease, to protect immunosuppressed patients, and to block the action of bacterial toxins. Human immune serum globulin preparations are available for HBV, VZV, rabies, and tetanus. Diphtheria is treated by the early administration of diphtheria antitoxin that neutralizes the bacterial exotoxin. Streptococcal necrotizing fasciitis is treated with antibiotics and aggressive surgery. Toxic shock syndrome and typhoid fever are treated with antibiotics.

MM5 159, 623

48 **(B) Ebola virus.** Like other filoviruses, Ebola virus has a filamentous shape and is an enveloped, single-stranded, negative-sense RNA virus. Ebola virus causes such deadly outbreaks that hosts are killed before they can spread the disease. All of the viruses listed in the answers to these questions are RNA viruses that cause hemorrhagic fever. Only a filovirus, such as Ebola virus, has the filamentous shape shown in the figure. Dengue virus is a flavivirus. Lassa virus is an arenavirus. Hantavirus and Rift Valley fever virus are bunyaviruses.

MM5 623

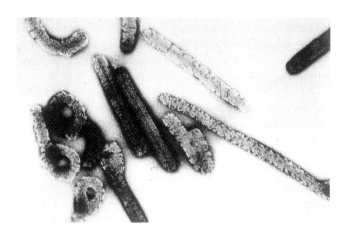

49 **(D) Profile D.** The presence of antibody to VCA and MA, components of the virion, are developed at the same time during the course of disease. IgM to VCA may also be present, but antibody to Epstein-Barr nuclear antigen (EBNA) arises during convalescence.

MM5 556-558

50 **(D) Treatment with rimantadine.** An individual who is 80 years old and living in a nursing home is likely to be at high risk for serious disease if infected with influenza. The patient should immediately begin taking rimantadine or another anti-influenza drug. Like amantadine, rimantadine inhibits the uncoating of the influenza A (but not B) virus. These drugs are efficacious in the prevention of influenza A if given within the first 24 h of exposure. Because of the nature of the disease, the drugs are not effective if treatment is delayed. As soon as practicable, he should also be immunized with influenza vaccine. After the influenza vaccine is given, it takes 2 weeks for an adequate antibody response to form. Although the vaccine will have no impact on the patient's current infection, it will prevent subsequent infections with the particular influenza strains that are covered in the vaccine. Acyclovir is a drug used to treat HSV and has no activity on influenza. There is no specific immune globulin for influenza.

MM5 510, 616

51 **(A) Viral genome is produced in the cytoplasm; virus is encapsulated in the cytoplasm.** This correct answer describes picornaviruses; coxsackieviruses are encapsulated RNA viruses that replicate in the cytoplasm and are members of the family Picornaviridae. Enveloped viruses have a single-stranded, negative-sense RNA genome that is produced in the cytoplasm; the virus is enveloped at the plasma membrane. Adenoviruses have a viral genome that is produced in the nucleus, and the virus is encapsulated in the nucleus. The herpesvirus genome is produced in the nucleus, and the virus is enveloped at the nuclear membrane. Last, the retrovirus nucleus produces the viral genome, and the virus is enveloped at the plasma membrane.

MM5 59

52 **(E) Virus whose replication is dependent on the epithelial cell differentiation stage.** The growth is a common wart. It is caused by HPV and is transmitted by contact. Replication of the virus is tightly controlled by the transcriptional apparatus of the skin or mucoepithelial cell. Fungi that exhibit septate hyphae, are not thermally dimorphic, and metabolize keratin are dermatophytes, which commonly cause tinea pedis (athlete's foot) and other superficial mycoses. Koilocytosis is not associated with dermatophyte infections. A large, enveloped, linear double-stranded DNA virus describes a herpesvirus. Herpesviruses cause vesicular lesions. HPV does not grow in tissue culture.

MM5 523

53 **(B) Coxsackievirus A.** This patient has aseptic meningitis. Enteroviruses are the most common cause of viral meningitis during the summer months, with flaviviruses such as St. Louis encephalitis virus and West Nile virus also common during epidemic periods. The blisters in the patient's throat and mouth are consistent with a preceding coxsackievirus A infection. Specific diagnosis of coxsackievirus A infections is most commonly made by molecular methods such as PCR amplification of viral nucleic acids. If bacteria, such as *S. pneumoniae*, were responsible for this patient's infection, the progression of disease would have been more rapid, and the CSF profile would have been different (i.e., predominance of polymorphonuclear leukocytes, low glucose, and elevated protein). *C. neoformans* can cause a similar clinical picture; however, without treatment, the yeast would have been seen on Gram stain and would have grown on both the bacterial and fungal media. HSV can produce vesicular lesions and aseptic meningitis as seen in this patient. However, this diagnosis is less likely because the viral cultures were negative. In addition, aseptic meningitis is more commonly associated with genital vesicular lesions. *N. fowleri* can cause a primary meningoencephalitis; however, this disease is rapidly fatal, and the amoeba would be observed in the CSF upon careful examination.

MM5 585

54 **(C) Chickens are the incubators for new strains of influenza virus.** Influenza A virus has a broad range of hosts, including pigs, ducks, chickens, and humans. When an animal is coinfected with several different virus strains, the segments of the virus genome can undergo reassortment (mix and match) to produce a new strain of influenza virus, and the new strain may subsequently infect humans. In this way, chickens can serve as incubators for new strains. Although chicken feathers may harbor the virus that causes Marek's disease, they do not harbor influenza virus. Influenza viruses do not elicit viremia, so influenza would not be transmitted by mosquitoes. Influenza viruses do not usually spread systemically, so an outbreak due to contamination of chicken meat is unlikely. Furthermore, influenza is not acquired by the fecal-oral route. Infection with a particular strain of influenza virus provides immunity only against that strain of virus. The authorities eliminated all the chickens in the region of Hong Kong because they were worried about a new strain of virus.

MM5 613

55 **(B) Echovirus 11.** The negative results of a Gram stain and the presence of a predominantly mononuclear cell infiltrate, a slightly elevated protein concentration, and a normal glucose concentration indicate that the patient is suffering from aseptic meningitis. RT-PCR converts RNA into DNA. All RNA viruses, including echovirus 11 and other picornaviruses, encode polymerases. Echovirus 11 is a common cause of meningitis. *C. neoformans* is an encapsulated yeast that causes chronic fungal meningitis. *E. coli* causes acute bacterial meningitis in neonates but usually does not cause this disease in children. *S. pneumoniae* is a common cause of bacterial meningitis. RT-PCR converts RNA into DNA. HSV is not an RNA virus and does not usually cause meningitis in children.

MM5 585

56   (E) Sudden onset of symptoms. Hepatitis A differs from hepatitis B, C, or D in that it has an abrupt onset of symptoms and is more often accompanied by rigor. HAV is transmitted via the fecal-oral route, not through sexual contact. Although 3-year-olds are susceptible to hepatitis A infection, they may not show symptoms of this infection and are likely to be the means of virus transmission. The symptoms described for this patient represent the prodrome of hepatitis but are not specific for infection with hepatitis A. The presence of jaundice suggests hepatitis or biliary tract obstruction. Jaundice appears after the prodrome of hepatitis. Its appearance after 5 days does not offer clues regarding the causative agent. The symptoms of fever, fatigue, nausea, stomach pain, and loss of appetite are also characteristic of other hepatitis viruses.

MM5 677

57   (D) Smallpox virus. Smallpox, the most important member of the genus *Orthopoxvirus*, is among the largest and most complex viruses. The central core of double-stranded DNA and protein is surrounded by a core membrane and then an outer membrane and envelope. Hepatitis C and West Nile viruses are members of the family Flaviviridae, which are enveloped single-stranded RNA viruses. Respiratory syncytial virus, a member of the family Paramyxoviridae viruses, is also an enveloped, single-stranded RNA virus. Papillomavirus is a nonenveloped, double-stranded DNA virus.

MM5 565

58   (D) Smallpox virus. The patient's clinical manifestations are consistent with the diagnosis of molluscum contagiosum, a disease caused by a poxvirus. Smallpox virus is in the same family of viruses. Coxsackievirus A is a picornavirus that causes vesicular lesions. HPV type 11 is a papovavirus that causes wart-like lesions. Mumps, like measles, is a paramyxovirus; measles is an exanthematous disease, whereas mumps is characterized by swollen glands. VZV, like HSV, is a herpesvirus that causes vesicular lesions.

MM5 565

59   (C) HSV. HSV is an increasingly important cause of pharyngitis, especially in sexually active individuals between the ages of 18 and 35 years. HSV induces the cellular changes noted in the patient described. Adenoviruses are agents of pharyngitis and pharyngoconjunctival fever. They will cause cell death and nuclear inclusion bodies but will not produce syncytia. EBV causes infectious mononucleosis, a disease in which pharyngitis is a major manifestation. The virus, however, is not isolated in the laboratory and does not produce the cytopathologic effects described. Influenza viruses cause pharyngitis in association with other respiratory tract symptoms. The viruses can cause

hemagglutination or hemadsorption but would not produce the cytopathologic effects described. The classic manifestations of measles do not include pharyngitis. The measles virus will cause syncytia but, like the influenza viruses, will not result in the other cytopathologic effects.

MM5 544

60   (D) Genome that is infectious. California encephalitis virus is a bunyavirus with a negative-sense RNA genome. St. Louis encephalitis virus is a flavivirus with a positive-sense RNA genome; this type of genome is sufficient to initiate infection upon microinjection into a cell. Both viruses have RNA genomes and a broad range hosts, including humans, animals, and mosquitoes. The vectors are *Culex* (forest) mosquitoes for California encephalitis virus and *Aedes* (city) mosquitoes for St. Louis encephalitis virus.

MM5 637, 651

61   (B) Protein. The findings in this patient are characteristic of Creutzfeldt-Jakob disease (CJD). A modified host protein that is infectious causes the disease. This agent is called a prion. No genome has been detected for prions. Glycoproteins are found in the envelope of viruses. Most enveloped viruses are made of proteins, glycoproteins, and lipids. Enveloped viruses do not only contain glycoproteins and lipids or only proteins and lipids.

MM5 691

62   (D) Acetylcholine receptor on neurons. Binding of VAPs to specific cell receptors determine which cells are infected by the virus. The receptors may be proteins, glycoproteins, or glycolipids. Rabies virus binds to the acetylcholine receptor on neurons. Examples of other receptors for viruses include the following: EBV binds to the C3d complement receptor on B lymphocytes, HIV binds to the CD4 molecule and chemokine coreceptor on T lymphocytes, poliovirus binds to the immunoglobulin superfamily protein on epithelial cells, and influenza A virus binds to sialic acid receptors on epithelial cells.

MM5 55

63   (D) HPV type 16. HPV type 16 or type 18 is found in association with most cervical cancers. Adenovirus type 2 is a virus that commonly infects the respiratory tract. Some adenoviruses have been found to cause tumors in hamsters but not in humans. *C. trachomatis* and parvovirus B19 are not associated with dysplasia and cancer. *C. trachomatis* causes eye infections, urethritis, and lymphogranuloma venereum. Parvovirus B19 causes fifth disease, an exanthematous disease. HSV type 2 causes genital infections, but it has only a weak association with cancer. The virus usually kills the infected cells.

MM5 526

64   (E) The infant will be healthy. Vaccination against rubella provides lifelong immunity; hence the woman will not spread the virus to her fetus. Cataract, deafness, and mental retardation are symptoms of congenital rubella. Only the infants of unvaccinated women who are exposed to rubella virus during pregnancy are at risk for congenital rubella. Mental retardation, microcephaly, and blindness are symptoms of congenital cytomegalovirus infection. Vesicular lesions and life-threatening encephalitis are symptoms of neonatal HSV infection.

MM5 645

65 **(C) ELISA for p24 antigen.** The protein called p24 is a component of the HIV virion and is therefore an early marker of HIV infection. The antigen is shed with the virus into the blood and indicates virus replication. A capture ELISA would be used to detect the protein. RT-PCR or a similar procedure could also be used to amplify and detect the viral genome in the blood. Cell culture isolation of HIV is difficult and is not done. An ELISA for antibodies to gp120, a latex agglutination test for antibodies to gp41, and a Western blot test are all used to detect antibodies. An antibody response to HIV would not be present early in the infection.

MM5 669

66 **(B) Coronavirus.** Coronaviruses are helical, enveloped, positive-sense RNA viruses that are usually associated with the common cold but may also cause diarrhea. Of the options listed, only coronaviruses have envelopes. Coronavirus is an exception to the rule that enveloped viruses are labile to acid and bile in the gastrointestinal tract. Adenovirus, Norwalk virus, reovirus, and rotavirus can cause diarrhea but do not have envelopes. Adenoviruses are icosahedral, nonenveloped DNA viruses. The Norwalk virus is an example of a norovirus, which is a small, icosahedral, nonenveloped, positive-sense virus. Rotaviruses are in the reovirus family and have double-stranded RNA and a double capsid.

MM5 591, 698

67 **(C) Translation.** IFN-α triggers a cascade of biochemical events that block viral replication at the level of transcription and protein synthesis. Specifically, the degradation of viral and cellular mRNA is enhanced, and mRNA binding to the ribosome is blocked, preventing protein synthesis and subsequent viral replication. IFN does not affect attachment of viruses to the host cell or uncoating and only indirectly affects nucleic acid replication and viral assembly.

MM5 144

68 **(E) Thymidine kinase.** Thymidine kinase activates acyclovir but not foscarnet. Both drugs act on the virus-encoded DNA-dependent DNA polymerase. DNA-dependent RNA polymerase is encoded by host cells and poxviruses. RNA-dependent DNA polymerase is encoded by retroviruses. These enzymes are not encoded by herpesviruses. Protease is encoded by many viruses, including herpesviruses, but only HIV protease is a target for pharmacologic agents approved by the Food and Drug Administration (FDA).

MM5 508, 549

69 **(A) CMV.** The most frequent causes of congenital infection are the so-called TORCH agents (*Toxoplasma*, other infections, rubella virus, cytomegalovirus, and herpes simplex virus). In this group, CMV is the only agent associated with owl's eye inclusion bodies. CMV is the most common viral cause of congenital malformation, and it is likely that in this case the mother suffered a primary asymptomatic CMV infection as a result of her blood transfusion. Infants infected with HSV may have vesicular lesions but would not have calcifications. Infants infected with rubella virus usually suffer from cataracts and deafness. Congenital malformations are not associated with streptococcal disease.

MM5 560

70 **(B) Formalin-treated, rabies virus-infected cells.** The current vaccine consists of inactivated rabies virus grown in human diploid fibroblasts. Although several injections are required, this vaccine requires fewer injections than the previous vaccine and is associated with fewer adverse effects. A live, attenuated rabies vaccine is administered to pets but not to humans. The original (Pasteur) vaccine contained formalin-treated, rabies virus-infected rabbit spinal cord, but it is no longer used. Egg-grown rabies vaccines are also no longer used. Subunit vaccines (e.g., glycoprotein G) have not been developed. A vaccinia virus that expresses G protein is being used to immunize forest animals, such as raccoons. The vaccine is administered by impregnating the food with the vaccine and dropping the food into endemic regions.

MM5 623

71 **(B) Influenza virus.** Although great care is taken in predicting the most likely influenza strains of the coming year and then incorporating those strains into a multivalent vaccine, the predictions may be wrong. As a result, a person can acquire influenza despite receiving an influenza vaccine. California encephalitis is transmitted by a forest mosquito, so it is unlikely to cause a nosocomial infection. Rubella vaccine is administered as part of the MMR vaccine during childhood and elicits lifelong immunity. Chickenpox is caused by VZV. An individual who had chickenpox during childhood is not at risk of having chickenpox again. A varicella vaccine is available to prevent this disease, and the CDC now recommends its routine use in children. Variola virus is the cause of smallpox. This is the only disease that has been eradicated worldwide via the use of a vaccine.

MM5 164, 616

72 **(E) The T cells react with an antigen other than hemagglutinin.** CD8 cytolytic T cells recognize antigens that are processed by the cell and presented as peptides on the major histocompatibility complex (MHC) class I molecules. The man was exposed to the H3N2 virus because he had antibody to the H3N2 virus but not to the H1N1 virus. His T cell response would also be directed at the H3N2 virus. The response to the H1N1 virus indicates a different target than the hemagglutinin (HA) or neuraminidase (NA). The internal NS protein produces a major T cell antigen, and this protein does not necessarily differ among viruses whose HA or NA differs. HA and NA are the major structures recognized by antibody. Although HSV encodes a complement receptor that reduces complement activity, influenza virus does not. Because the infected cells do not show significant lysis in the absence of T cells or antibody and complement, it is unlikely that one virus is more cytolytic than the other. Moreover, there was no antibody reaction to the H1N1 virus, so it is unlikely that the man has a history of infection with this virus. The man has been infected with H3N2 virus some time during his life, but the data do not support recent infection.

MM5 612

73 (C) Parainfluenza virus. Viruses are classified by their genetic material (single-stranded or double-stranded DNA or RNA), capsid structure (icosahedral or helical), and the presence or absence of an outer envelope. Parainfluenza virus, Norwalk virus, and rotavirus are RNA viruses; adenovirus and VZV are DNA viruses. Rotavirus is a double-stranded RNA virus. Parainfluenza virus has an envelop, and Norwalk virus does not have one.

MM5 48-50

74 (C) Inhibition of DNA polymerase. This patient has fever blisters, which are usually caused by HSV. The drugs of choice for treating herpes labialis are acyclovir, valacyclovir, penciclovir, or famciclovir. These nucleotide analogues are activated by the viral thymidine kinase, but they act by inhibiting the viral DNA polymerase. Antiviral drugs do not act via the blockade of peptidoglycan cross-linkage, inhibition of 70S ribosome, and inhibition of topoisomerase; however, some antibacterial drugs do. For example, vancomycin and beta-lactam antibiotics (including penicillins and cephalosporins) act by inhibiting peptidoglycan cross-linkage and thereby inhibit bacterial cell wall synthesis. Fluoroquinolones act by inhibiting topoisomerase. The 70S ribosome is a useful target for many antibacterial drugs, including clindamycin, chloramphenicol, erythromycin, tetracyclines, and aminoglycosides. Amantadine, a drug used in the prevention and treatment of influenza A, is an example of an agent that acts by blocking the uncoating and entry of a specific virus (e.g., influenza A virus).

MM5 508, 549

75 (E) Sheep erythrocytes. The patient's clinical and laboratory findings are consistent with the diagnosis of infectious mononucleosis, a disease caused by EBV. The heterophil antibody is directed against glycolipids on sheep, horse, or bovine erythrocytes. Heterophil antibody does not recognize cardiolipin. Cardiolipin is recognized in the VDRL test for syphilis. Antibodies to the EBV capsid antigen are generated during acute disease and are confirmation of the diagnosis. Antibodies to EBNA are generated after resolution of the disease. Antibodies to DNA are detected in patients with some autoimmune diseases (e.g., systemic lupus erythematosus, or SLE).

MM5 557

76 (B) Destruction of ciliated columnar epithelial cells. Ciliated epithelial and mucus-secreting cells in the respiratory tract normally block the movement of bacteria into the lungs. The influenza virus destroys these cells and thereby allows bacteria to establish a lung infection. Influenza may cause a change in the pharyngeal microflora. Moreover, patients known to have a positive tuberculin reaction may experience a loss of skin reactivity during influenza. Neither of these changes, however, would predispose the patient to bacterial lung infections. There is no loss of alveolar macrophages in patients with influenza. Alveolar macrophages are very much involved in the defense against influenza. Influenza does not cause severe immunosuppression.

MM5 612

77 (A) Dengue virus. Infections with dengue virus, a member of the flavivirus family, can range from asymptomatic to a life-threatening hemorrhagic fever. Most infections are characterized by a 4- to 7-day incubation period followed by an acute onset of fever, headache, retro-orbital pain, myalgias, and rash. Disease is typically self-limiting after a 6- or 7-day course, although progression to dengue hemorrhagic fever and dengue shock syndrome can occur. Infections with HAV, *L. interrogans*, *P. falciparium*, and *S. typhi* can all produce febrile illnesses in travelers to developing countries. Hepatitis A can initially present as a mild flu-like illness with fever, headache, myalgias, and malaise. Symptoms will progress to development of dark urine (i.e., bilirubinuria), followed by pale stools and yellow discoloration of the skin and mucous membranes. Development of a rash is not characteristic. Symptomatic *L. interrogans* infections are typically characterized by high fevers, myalgias, and headaches. Conjunctival suffusion may be present. A rash is not commonly seen. *P. falciparum* would present as a febrile illness with nausea, vomiting, and diarrhea. This disease is unlikely with the history of compliant malaria prophylaxis. *S. typhi* infections are characterized by fever, headache, myalgias, and malaise. Although a rash may develop, it is not a prominent feature of the infection.

MM5 644

78 (D) Influenza virus. Orthomyxoviridae (e.g., influenza virus), Arenaviridae (e.g., Lassa fever virus), and Reoviridae (e.g., rotavirus) are families of RNA viruses that have segmented genomes (multiple, discrete segments of genetic material within the viral capsid or shell). Reassortment of the genomes between two different strains of virus can create a novel strain. This reassortment does not occur with the other viruses listed in the answers to this question, because they do not have segmented genomes.

MM5 63

79 (C) VEE virus infection causes only limited viremia in humans. Venezuelan equine encephalitis (VEE) virus and yellow fever virus are both transmitted by mosquitoes. To be transmitted from one person to another, the virus must be present in the blood in sufficiently high concentration when the mosquito takes a blood meal. VEE does not establish extensive viremia in humans, whereas yellow fever does. Yellow fever virus is transmitted by *Aedes* mosquitoes, whereas VEE virus is transmitted by either *Culex* or *Aedes* mosquitoes. The habitat of the mosquito determines the area (urban or sylvan) in which the virus will be acquired. Yellow fever virus is a flavivirus and encodes one glycoprotein. VEE virus is a togavirus and encodes three glycoproteins that form a complex. Production of mild disease does not inhibit or facilitate transmission of the virus; however, the host may live long enough to transmit the virus. The ability of the virus to replicate in the mosquito promotes transmission but is not relevant to why humans are a dead-end host.

MM5 643

80 **(E) There are too many agents that cause this disease.** The common cold can be caused by picornaviruses (including over 100 serotypes of rhinovirus), coronaviruses, orthomyxoviruses (including influenza viruses), and paramyxoviruses. A vaccine would be unable to initiate a protective response against all of these agents. A cytolytic T cell response would not likely be important. Secretory IgA and possibly IgG would be important. As the name implies, the common cold is common. Although it is not life threatening, it is considered a significant condition because its incidence is so high and because it has such a large impact on the activities and productivity of the population. Herpesviruses, retroviruses, and hepadnaviruses have the potential to establish chronic or transforming infections, especially if some but not all of the viral activities are inactivated. The viruses that are responsible for the common cold, however, do not have this potential.

MM5 698-699

81 **(E) Viral assembly.** HIV protease is essential for production of a functional virion. This enzyme cleaves the precursor polyproteins encoded by the *gag* and *pol* genes. Protease inhibitors competitively bind to the active site of the enzyme, thus preventing its activities on the polyproteins. The inhibitor does not affect penetration, uncoating, transcription, or nucleic acid replication. Viral assembly is indirectly affected.

MM5 61, 663

82 **(C) In situ DNA hybridization.** Infection with HPV 18 can cause cervical dysplasia and cancer. In situ DNA hybridization is the method of choice because it will detect and identify the HPV genome whether or not viral proteins are made. Papillomaviruses do not grow in tissue culture. They do not replicate to any great extent, so antigens are generally not detectable by ELISA, immunofluorescence testing, or Western blot assays.

MM5 178, 527

83 **(E) Replication in a privileged site.** Rabies virus infects the area around the bite and then proceeds quickly to the neuron. It travels through the central nervous system to the salivary glands and the brain with minimal replication and remains in the neuron. This is a privileged site that is inaccessible to immune cells. No immune response is made until the virus resurfaces in and near the brain and the symptoms are observed. The rabies virus does not have the properties listed in the incorrect answers. HIV and influenza virus are viruses that undergo antigenic shift (change via mutation). HIV and measles virus are examples of viruses that infect T cells and reduce their ability to attack infected cells. *Neisseria gonorrhoeae* produces an IgA protease. HSV and *Staphylococcus aureus* are examples of infectious agents that produce proteins that act as Fc receptors.

MM5 620

84 **(C) RNA-dependent DNA polymerase.** HBV replicates through an RNA intermediate and uses the virus-encoded reverse transcriptase to synthesize the DNA genome. DNA-dependent DNA polymerases are encoded by adenoviruses, herpesviruses, and poxviruses but not by hepatitis B. DNA-dependent RNA polymerases are encoded by poxviruses and host cells. RNA-dependent RNA polymerases are encoded by RNA viruses other than retroviruses. Thymidine kinase is encoded by HSV and VZV.

MM5 679

85 **(C) Chronic hemolytic anemia.** The patient's clinical manifestations are consistent with the diagnosis of erythema infectiosum, a disease caused by parvovirus B19. The virus infects and destroys erythroid precursors that are undergoing rapid multiplication. This places individuals with chronic hemolytic anemia at risk for an aplastic crisis. Patients with Chédiak-Higashi syndrome and patients with chronic granulomatous disease have a defect in granulocyte function, and this places them at risk for certain bacterial infections. Patients with cystic fibrosis have poor pulmonary and secretory function, and they are prone to recurrent bacterial infections of the respiratory tract. The patient in this question's scenario has a viral disease. Patients with diabetes are at risk for bacterial and fungal diseases due to a reduction in blood flow.

MM5 575

86 **(C) Monospot test to screen for EBV infection.** The patient's clinical manifestations suggest the diagnosis of infectious mononucleosis, a disease that is caused by EBV and is confirmed by the monospot test. Patients infected with CMV, HIV, or *Treponema* may have many mononucleosis-like symptoms but would not have exudative pharyngitis. Exudative pharyngitis is associated with EBV infection and with *S. pyogenes* infection. If the patient had streptococcal pharyngitis, the disease would be expected to resolve in 5 days or less. In this case, the diagnosis of EBV infection is more likely not only because of the longer duration of disease but also because of the presence of hepatosplenomegaly.

MM5 557

87 **(C) Enveloped, single-stranded, negative-sense RNA virus.** The virus shown in the figure is rabies virus, a rhabdovirus. Like other rhabdoviruses, it is an enveloped, single-stranded, negative-sense RNA virus. Herpesviruses and poxviruses have an enveloped, double-stranded DNA structure. No single-stranded DNA viruses have an envelope. Parvoviruses are single-stranded DNA viruses that have a capsid. Coronaviruses, flaviviruses, and togaviruses have an enveloped, single-stranded, positive-sense RNA structure. Adenoviruses and papovaviruses have an enveloped, double-stranded DNA structure.

MM5 619

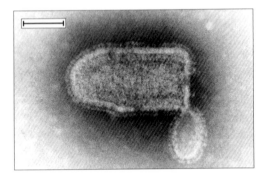

From Hart CA, Shears P: *Color atlas of medical microbiology* ed 2, St Louis, 2004, Mosby.

88 **(A) The antibody to HIV has not risen to detectable levels.** Serologic testing is the standard method for evaluating HIV infection. The ELISA for HIV and the Western blot analysis are serologic tests that measure a patient's antibody titer; they do not detect virions or viral antigen. Recent infection would not be detectable because antibody would not be produced for at least 3 weeks up to 6 weeks. The Western blot is a confirmatory test that is given after the ELISA is given. HIV is not isolated in tissue culture. HIV starts replicating as soon as the infection is initiated. The virus may be detected at an early stage by using an RT-PCR to assay for viral RNA or by testing for p24 antigen (not the antibody but the actual viral protein). The levels of p24 rise with virus replication.

MM5 669

89 **(C) JC virus.** SV40 and JC virus are both polyomaviruses. JC virus causes progressive multifocal leukoencephalopathy, a disease that is virtually restricted to immunosuppressed individuals. Echovirus 11 is a picornavirus that causes meningitis and is not related to SV40. HSV is a neurotropic agent that causes a variety of diseases, including encephalitis, but it is not related to SV40. The risk of severe HSV disease is higher in immunosuppressed individuals than in immunocompetent individuals. Both measles virus (a paramyxovirus) and Western equine encephalitis (WEE) virus (a togavirus) can cause encephalitis but are not related to SV40.

MM5 530

90 **(C) RNA viruses must encode an RNA polymerase.** Because cells do not have a means of replicating RNA, RNA viruses must encode RNA-dependent RNA polymerases. Encoded polymerases must be available soon after infection, or the unstable viral RNA will degrade and infection will be aborted. Except for influenza viruses, transcription and replication of negative-stranded RNA viruses (e.g., rhabdoviruses, orthomyxoviruses, paramyxoviruses, filoviruses, and bunyaviruses) occur in the cell cytoplasm and not in the nucleus. All positive-stranded RNA viruses (e.g., picornaviruses, noroviruses, coronaviruses, flaviviruses, togaviruses) replicate in the cytoplasm. Retroviruses can produce latent infections, but these infections are not observed with other RNA viruses. Although the larger DNA viruses encode a DNA polymerase, the smaller viruses are dependent on the host cell enzymes. Viral DNA is stable in contrast to viral RNA.

MM5 59

91 **(B) Giant cell pneumonia.** The older sibling's clinical manifestations are consistent with the diagnosis of measles. In immunosuppressed individuals, such as those being treated for leukemia, measles virus tends to cause a serious condition at the first site of infection (i.e., in the lungs). Therefore the 3-year-old is at risk for giant cell pneumonia. Exanthema subitum is caused by human herpesvirus 6. Hemorrhagic pulmonary syndrome is caused by a hantavirus. Orchitis may be caused by the mumps virus, an echovirus, or coxsackievirus B. Progressive multifocal leukoencephalopathy is caused by a papovavirus called JC virus.

MM5 602

92 **(A) Binding of C3d receptors on B lymphocytes.** The patient's clinical and laboratory findings are consistent with the diagnosis of infectious mononucleosis, a disease caused by EBV. This herpesvirus binds exclusively to CR21, the C3d receptor, and infects B lymphocytes. EBV causes their immortalization if the process is unchecked by T cells. EBV infection is also associated with Burkitt lymphoma, nasopharyngeal carcinoma, and Hodgkin's disease. CD8 T cells may be infected by other members of the herpesvirus family, such as human herpesviruses 5 (cytomegalovirus, or CMV), 6 (roseola), and 7. The CD4 T cell, rather than the CD8 T cell, is the usual target for virus infections. Induction of immunosuppression due to killing of CD4 T cells is a property of HIV, which binds to the CD4 molecule on T cells and macrophages. The patient's laboratory findings are characteristic of an infection with EBV. EBV is not susceptible to acyclovir. HSV types I and II (human herpesviruses I and II) encode a thymidine kinase that can activate acyclovir via phosphorylation and thereby cause the drug to inhibit the viral polymerase. Tumor promotion in keratinocytes is a property of some human papillomaviruses, such as papillomavirus types XI, XVI, and XVIII, which infect epithelial cells, cause a wart-like disease, and are associated with human cancers.

MM5 553

93 **(B) Blocking IL-1 and TNF-mediated inflammation.** Poxviruses are able to inhibit inflammation by blocking the activity of IL-1 and tumor necrosis factor. This property is shared with adenoviruses.
MM5 144, 149, 567

94 **(B) Inhibition of viremic spread by antibodies.** The infant's clinical manifestations are consistent with the diagnosis of congenital rubella. The key to the diagnosis is the presence of cataract. Congenital CMV infection has many of the same manifestations but is not associated with cataracts. If the mother had been immune to rubella virus (had been seropositive for the virus) before she became pregnant, she would have generated antibody upon re-exposure to the virus, and this antibody would have prevented the viremic transfer of rubella virus to the fetus. IFN may limit local replication of rubella virus but would not prevent viremic spread of the virus to the fetus. Cytotoxic T cells and natural killer cells may cause local killing of cells infected with rubella virus, but they also would not prevent viremic spread of the virus to the fetus. Macrophages are not helpful in preventing the spread of rubella virus to the fetus.
MM5 646, 559

95 **(B) HSV.** The patient's clinical manifestations are consistent with the diagnosis of herpes zoster (shingles), a disease caused by VZV. HSV and VZV are both members of the family Herpesviridae and the subfamily Alphaherpesvirinae, so they share many features. In addition to causing herpes zoster, VZV causes varicella (chickenpox). HSV usually causes oral and genital lesions but can also cause eye infections, encephalitis, and disseminated disease. HSV and VZV are not similar to the other viruses listed in the answers to this question. Coxsackievirus A is a picornavirus that causes hand-foot-and-mouth disease. Measles virus is a paramyxovirus that causes an exanthematous disease characterized by cough, conjunctivitis, coryza, and Koplik spots. Parvovirus B19 is the parvovirus that is responsible for erythema infectiosum (fifth disease), a pediatric disease that begins with flu-like symptoms, remits, and then erupts into a rash. Rubella virus is a togavirus that causes German measles and congenital rubella syndrome.
MM5 552

96 **(C) In situ hybridization.** In situ hybridization can detect viral DNA in the cells that harbor the HPV 16 genome. Hemadsorption and microscopic examination for owl's eye inclusion bodies are not useful in the diagnosis of HPV infections. Hemadsorption is useful for finding evidence of influenza virus-infected cells, which express the viral hemagglutinin on their cell surface. Owl's eye inclusion bodies are found in CMV-infected cells. Like all papovaviruses, HPVs are DNA viruses that have a naked capsid and therefore do not have glycoproteins. RT-PCR is used for detecting the genome of an RNA virus or viral mRNA in solution.
MM5 178, 527

97 **(D) Stavudine.** Like zidovudine (azidothymidine), stavudine (4-deoxythymidine) is a thymidine analogue that acts by inhibiting reverse transcriptase. Nelfinavir and ritonavir are protease inhibitors. Nevirapine is a non-nucleoside reverse transcriptase inhibitor. Zidovudine and nevirapine have different binding sites on reverse transcriptase. Zovirax is a trade name for acyclovir, a drug used in the treatment of herpesvirus infections.
MM5 506, 667

98 **(C) The infection site was close to the brain.** The closer the site of infection is to the brain, the smaller is the amount of time required for the rabies virus to travel from the site of infection to the brain. All rabies virus infections, regardless of the strain or amount of virus transmitted, are assumed to be fatal unless treated. The dose of virus from dog bites may influence the course of disease but to a much lesser extent than the site of infection. The virus does not elicit an immune response until the last stages of disease, so it is lethal in both immunocompetent and immunocompromised individuals. The age of the patient is not significant to the progression of the disease. Rabies vaccine is not given routinely to children or adults. It is given only to individuals who are at increased risk for rabies (such as veterinarians and other animal handlers) and to individuals who may have been infected.
MM5 620

99 **(C) RNA-dependent DNA polymerase.** Opportunistic infections, such as pneumonia and thrush, are a hallmark of AIDS. In patients with AIDS, pneumonia is often caused by *Pneumocystis carinii.* Thrush is caused by *Candida albicans.* RNA-dependent DNA polymerase is another name for reverse transcriptase, an enzyme that is present in HIV virions and infected cells. HIV, the cause of AIDS, is a single-stranded, positive-sense RNA virus and a member of the family Retroviridae. The enzymes listed in the other answers to this question are not encoded by retroviruses. DNA-dependent DNA polymerases are encoded by large DNA viruses, such as adenoviruses, herpesviruses, and poxviruses. DNA-dependent RNA polymerases are used in the transcription of mRNA; they are encoded by host cells (which transcribe mRNA) and by poxviruses (which replicate in the cytoplasm). RNA-dependent RNA polymerases are encoded by RNA viruses other than retroviruses. Thymidine kinase is encoded by specific herpesviruses.
MM5 659, 663

100 **(B) Parainfluenza virus.** The patient's symptoms are consistent with the diagnosis of laryngotracheobronchitis (croup). This disease can be caused by a variety of agents, including parainfluenza viruses, respiratory syncytial virus, influenza viruses, and *Haemophilus influenzae.* The patient's age, response to humidified air, and laboratory data (syncytia formation) implicate one of the paramyxoviruses, probably parainfluenza virus type II. The paramyxoviruses are enveloped viruses with a nonsegmented, single-stranded, negative-sense RNA genome.

Influenza viruses, parvoviruses, reoviruses, and rhinoviruses do not promote syncytia formation in cell culture.
MM5 603

101 **(C) Genetic change after infection.** The most significant way in which HIV escapes immune control is by its ability to undergo mutation, altering its antigenicity and escaping antibody clearance.
MM5 63, 661

102 **(D) No serious, definable disease symptoms.** The neonate has congenital CMV infection, and the photomicrograph shows a CMV-infected cell with a basophilic nuclear inclusion body. CMV is ubiquitous, and 30% to 50% of adults harbor the virus. CMV infection, however, usually causes no serious, definable disease symptoms in the majority of these adults. Infection presents a problem only for previously uninfected pregnant women and immunocompromised individuals. A pregnant woman who is infected with CMV for the first time during her pregnancy (primary infection) can transmit the infection to her fetus. An immunocompromised patient may develop serious disease manifestations. A person with AIDS is susceptible to opportunistic diseases. A person infected with the rubella virus can be affected by a mild arthritic condition with a fine lacy rash, and a person who has EBV can develop mononucleosis with production of antibody to sheep red blood cells, whereas CMV can cause mononucleosis without heterophil antibody. Last, a person with adenovirus is prone to getting pharyngoconjunctivitis.
MM5 560

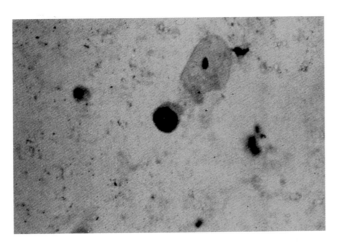

103 **(C) Deafness.** A maculopapular rash can be caused by parvovirus B19, measles, or rubella virus. Rubella is indicated by the presence of virus-specific IgM and IgG in an unvaccinated individual. Deafness is associated with rubella virus infection in any trimester. The earlier the infection, the more severe is the outcome and the higher is the infant's risk for mental retardation, cardiac problems, and cataracts. Cerebral calcification is associated with congenital CMV infection. Chorioretinitis is the most common congenital defect associated with *Toxoplasma*

infection. Hydrops fetalis is associated with parvovirus B19 infection. Keratoconjunctivitis is a manifestation of HSV infection in adults.
MM5 647

104 **(B) Poxviruses have a large genome and encode many accessory genes.** Because the genome of each poxvirus is large and many of the genes are expendable, one of these expendable genes (i.e., accessory genes) can be replaced with the gene of a pathogen. The foreign gene will be expressed by the poxvirus and can elicit immune responses relevant to infection, including T cell responses. Poxviruses assemble and replicate in the cytoplasm, but this does not facilitate antigen presentation or immunization. Use of a live vaccinia vaccine made it possible to eliminate smallpox in 1980, but this does not mean that use of the vaccinia virus or other poxviruses in vaccines will eliminate other infectious diseases. Visible symptoms might show that a virus replicated, but replication is not necessary. Canarypox does not replicate in humans, and replication may interfere with booster shots.
MM5 567

105 **(A) Echovirus meningitis.** Rhinoviruses and echoviruses are picornaviruses and have similar capsid structures. A canyon within the viral capsid is the binding site for pleconaril and for the viral receptor. The interaction of the drug and receptor has been confirmed by x-ray crystallography of the drug/virus complex. HSV is a herpesvirus. HSV encephalitis can be treated with famciclovir, valacyclovir, or acyclovir. Influenza A virus pneumonia is not treatable, but it can be prevented by prophylactic use of amantadine, rimantadine, zanamivir, or oseltamivir. Measles virus encephalitis is not treatable with antiviral drugs. Respiratory syncytial virus (RSV) is a paramyxovirus. RSV pneumonia in infants can be treated with ribavirin.
MM5 585

106 **(C) Enveloped, positive-sense, single-stranded RNA virus that makes a polyprotein.** Like other flaviviruses, yellow fever virus is an enveloped, positive-sense, single-stranded RNA virus that makes a polyprotein. Examples of viruses with the characteristics described in the incorrect answers to this question are as follows: Bunyaviruses viruses are enveloped, negative-sense, single-stranded RNA viruses without a matrix protein; influenza viruses are enveloped, negative-sense, single-stranded, segmented RNA viruses; togaviruses are enveloped, positive-sense, single-stranded RNA viruses that make early and late proteins from RNA of different sizes; and reoviruses are nonenveloped, double-stranded, segmented RNA viruses with a double capsid.
MM5 644

107 **(C) HIV.** The combination of thrush and pneumonia frequently occurs in patients who are infected with HIV and have AIDS. Thrush can only be caused by an infection with *Candida*

albicans. Pneumonia could be caused by an adenovirus, *C. immitis,* or *S. pneumoniae;* however, in this case, it is more likely caused by *P. carinii.* HTLV causes leukemia and spastic paraparesis.
MM5 667

108 (B) Nonsegmented, single-stranded, negative-sense RNA. The patient's symptoms are consistent with the diagnosis of laryngotracheobronchitis (croup). This disease can be caused by a variety of agents, including parainfluenza viruses, respiratory syncytial virus, influenza viruses, and *Haemophilus influenzae.* The patient's age, response to humidified air, and laboratory data (syncytia formation) implicate one of the paramyxoviruses, probably parainfluenza virus type II or respiratory syncytial virus. The paramyxoviruses are enveloped viruses with a nonsegmented, single-stranded, negative-sense RNA genome. Reoviruses have double-stranded RNA and double capsids, but they usually cause gastroenteritis. Orthomyxoviruses (influenza) have segmented, single-stranded, negative-sense RNA genomes, but they usually do not cause croup and do not promote syncytia formation in cell culture. The only single-stranded DNA viruses are parvoviruses. Parvovirus B19 causes erythema infectiosum (fifth disease). Parvoviruses do not promote syncytia formation. Picornaviruses are single-stranded, positive-sense RNA viruses. They can cause respiratory tract symptoms similar to those of the common cold, but they usually do not cause croup and do not promote syncytia formation in cell culture.
MM5 603

109 (E) Sialic acid. An anti-idiotype antibody (anti-id) is directed against the portion of the antibody that recognizes the original antigen and, in many ways, will resemble the original antigen (like making a mold of a hand and then casting a replica of the hand in plaster). Sialic acid is the receptor for influenza virus. Because the original antibody prevents the binding of HA (or hemagglutinin) to sialic acid, the anti-id may resemble the binding portion of HA and also bind to sialic acid. Binding to complement is a normal property of IgG. By definition, the anti-id will bind to the anti-HA because anti-HA was the immunogen to which the anti-id was made. The primary antibody recognizes HA, but the anti-idiotype antibody does not. An anti-HA antibody could neutralize infection. The M1 protein lines the inside of the viral envelope and cannot be seen by antibody. The M2 protein is an ion channel important for virion coating and is the target for amantadine. Antibody to NA (or neuraminidase) does not block infection.
MM5 609

110 (E) The patient is not infected with HBV. Having antibodies to HB$_s$Ag without having antibodies to hepatitis B core antigen (HB$_c$Ag) indicates that the anti-HB$_s$ is due to vaccination and not to infection with HBV. A patient with acute HBV infection would have antibodies to HB$_c$Ag but not anti-HB$_s$ or HB$_e$Ag.

The latter two antibodies are not detectable until HB$_s$Ag and HB$_e$Ag are no longer synthesized and are absent from the blood (after the disease is resolved). A patient with chronic HBV infection would have HB$_s$Ag and anti-HB$_c$, but not anti-HB$_s$. HBV is less likely to cause fulminant disease unless the patient is coinfected with hepatitis D. During the prodrome of HBV infection, the patient may have HB$_s$Ag, HB$_e$Ag, and either no antibodies or IgM anti-HB$_c$ antibodies.
MM5 685

111 (B) IFN-β production, NK cell activation, CD4 T cell activation, and IgG production. These steps are in the proper order. VZV is spread via the respiratory route. The infection of lung cells initiates the production of IFN-β or IFN-α; this is the earliest host response to the virus. The interferon activates natural killer (NK) cells. After cells die and antigen is delivered to the lymph nodes by dendritic cells and macrophages, IgM is produced and CD4 T cells become activated. Then helper cells activate CD8 T cells and promote the switch in B cells from IgM to IgG production. (Note that IFN-γ is primarily a CD4 T cell product.)
MM5 143-150

112 (C) Two inhibitors of RT and one inhibitor of protease. The patient's disease manifestations are consistent with the diagnosis of AIDS, a syndrome caused by infection with HIV. Most of the anti-HIV cocktails have two RT inhibitors (one or both of which may be nucleoside analogues) and at least one protease inhibitor. The FDA has not approved integrase inhibitors. HIV does not encode TK, DNA polymerase, or an *src* gene. TK is important for activating such drugs as acyclovir and famciclovir to inhibit DNA polymerase in the treatment of HSV infections. The *src* gene is an oncogene found in Rous sarcoma virus.
MM5 667

113 (D) A vaccine administered on the same schedule as the mumps vaccine. The figure shows cataracts in an infant with congenital rubella. The rubella vaccine is a component of the MMR vaccine. This vaccine is given no sooner than 15 months after birth. Varicella vaccine would have the same schedule. The rubella vaccine is a live vaccine. The *Haemophilus influenzae* type B (Hib) vaccine consists of a capsular polysaccharide attached to a carrier protein. Influenza vaccines and the inactivated polio vaccine are formalin-treated. The hepatitis B vaccine is a subunit vaccine. The inactivated polio vaccine (IPV) is administered at 2, 4, 6, and 15 months and again at 6 years of age. The oral polio vaccine (OPV, or live polio vaccine) can be administered at 2, 4, and 15 months of age and again at 6 years of age. Current guidelines make the OPV an optional immunization but only after a regimen of IPV.
MM5 165, 648

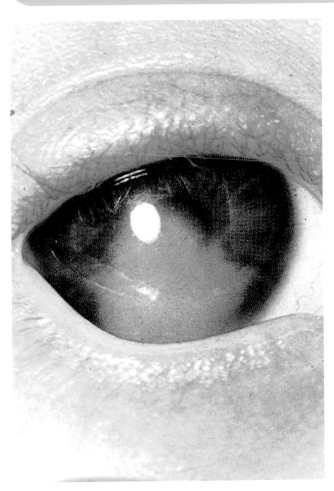

From Emond et al: *Colour atlas of infectious diseases*, St Louis, 2004, Mosby.

114 **(C) Hemagglutination inhibition (HAI) test.** The symptoms described are characteristic of influenza, a disease caused by a hemagglutinating virus. The HAI test uses specific antibodies in an attempt to block the binding of hemagglutinating viruses to erythrocytes. The HAI test can be used not only to identify the hemagglutinating virus but also to establish a serologic history. The complement fixation test is a serologic test that is used to detect specific antibody. The test is difficult to perform but is used for some nonhemagglutinating viruses and for histoplasmosis and coccidioidomycosis. The hemadsorption test detects any virus that encodes a hemagglutinin (HA). In this test, infected cells will bind erythrocytes to their cell surface. Unlike the HAI test, the hemadsorption test does not identify the virus or viruses that are detected. The Ouchterlony test uses gel diffusion and precipitin techniques to detect antigen from fungi, such as *Histoplasma* and *Blastomyces*. This test is more difficult to perform than HAI. The cytopathologic effects exhibited when an infectious agent is grown in tissue culture would give an indication of the agent's identity, but it would not conclusively identify the agent.
MM5 520, 615

115 **(C) During the fever.** The patient's symptoms are consistent with the diagnosis of roseola infantum (which is caused by human herpesvirus type 6) or the diagnosis of erythema infectiosum (which is also called fifth disease and is caused by parvovirus B19). Both infections are highly contagious. In either infection, the virus is being produced and spread when the fever is present. The infection has been controlled by the time there is a break in the fever. The rash is due to a nonspecific immune response and not due to the virus itself. Chickenpox (which is caused by VZV) is an example of an infection whose primary period of contagion precedes the fever.
MM5 562, 576

116 **(E) RSV.** Aerosolized ribavirin is administered to infants with RSV infections. There is no antiviral drug for the treatment of infections caused by California encephalitis virus or Ebola virus. CMV infections can be treated with foscarnet or ganciclovir. Amantadine or rimantadine can be used to treat influenza A. The newer NA inhibitors, such as oseltamivir and zanamivir, are effective against both influenza A and influenza B viruses.
MM5 606

117 **(E) Rhinovirus.** The patient's symptoms are characteristic of the common cold. Colds are usually caused by rhinoviruses and other picornaviruses. However, they may also be caused by coronaviruses and paramyxoviruses. EBV is a herpesvirus that causes infectious mononucleosis, a disease with a long incubation and symptomatic period. Although infection with an influenza virus causes many of the same symptoms as rhinovirus infection, the disease is usually more severe and is accompanied by fever. Norwalk virus is a calicivirus that causes outbreaks of diarrheal disease. Parvovirus B19 is the virus responsible for erythema infectiosum (fifth disease), a pediatric disease that begins with flu-like symptoms, remits, and then erupts into a rash.
MM5 588

118 **(A) Adenovirus.** The symptoms are consistent with the diagnosis of an adenovirus infection. This infection may present with pharyngitis in children under 2 years old but more commonly presents with pharyngitis and conjunctivitis (pharyngoconjunctival fever). HSV causes keratoconjunctivitis without a concurrent sore throat. Measles virus causes cough, conjunctivitis, Koplik spots (vesicle-like lesions in the mouth), and coryza (runny nose), followed by a rash. Rhinoviruses cause the common cold, which may be accompanied by a sore throat but not conjunctivitis. *S. pyogenes* causes a sore throat without conjunctivitis.
MM5 537

119 **(E) Tetanus toxoid skin test.** AIDS results when the CD4 T cell count drops below the level required for maintaining delayed-type hypersensitivity (DTH) and helper functions. The tetanus toxoid skin test is a DTH test for an antigen against which almost all adults have been immunized. The heterophil antibody test is useful in the diagnosis of infectious mononucleosis, a disease caused by EBV. The test measures the induction of unusual antibody formation directed toward the Paul-Bunnell antigen on sheep erythrocytes. The test results would not provide useful information about the progression toward AIDS. The titer of IgG antibody to measles virus would be expected to remain normal because most adults have been vaccinated against measles as children, and the B cells should continue to make a basal level of antibody. IgM antibody to HIV is seen during the initial HIV infection, when there is minimal immunodeficiency, so it does not provide useful information about the progression toward AIDS. Virus-specific IgM is useful for the diagnosis of acute diseases. Serum levels of IL-1 are elevated during bacterial and other infections and during inflammatory responses. Elevated levels are not related to HIV disease.

MM5 663

120 **(E) Ability to withstand acids and detergents and be transmitted via the fecal-oral route.** Hepatitis A and E viruses are the viral hepatitis agents that cause an abrupt onset of symptoms. Both viruses are encapsidated and are transmitted by the fecal-oral route. Hepatitis E is an uncommon illness. The hepatitis B, C, and D viruses are transmitted in blood products. HSVs and EBVs are examples of agents transmitted in saliva. The arboviruses must maintain sufficient viremia to allow acquisition by mosquitoes taking a blood meal. Influenza, measles, mumps, rubella, and varicella-zoster viruses are examples of agents that replicate in the lung and spread by aerosols.

MM5 51, 675

121 **(E) Nonenveloped virus with a single-stranded DNA genome.** The patient's clinical manifestations are consistent with the diagnosis of erythema infectiosum (fifth disease). This childhood exanthem is caused by parvovirus B19, which is a nonenveloped virus with a single-stranded DNA genome. The rash appears first on the face, typically spares the mouth, and causes the cheeks to become bright red ("slapped cheek" syndrome). The rash then spreads to the extremities and trunk before it fades away. In most patients, there are no complications. The occurrence of a parvovirus B19 infection in an individual with hemolytic anemia, however, can lead to an aplastic crisis because the virus infects and weakens erythroid precursors.

MM5 575

122 **(A) The causative agent cannot produce DNA polymerase during the initial infection of neurons.** The patient's clinical findings are consistent with the diagnosis of herpes labialis, a disease caused by HSV. This DNA virus initiates herpes labialis and then infects the ennervating neuron, establishing a latent-recurrent infection. Latency results because the neuron allows synthesis of only the latency-associated transcript (LAT) RNA but no proteins. Activation of the neuron promotes progression into the replicative cycle and viral protein synthesis. HSV activates T cell control mechanisms. It does not have variable major proteins, and it does not produce integrase or RNA

polymerase. *Borrelia* species that cause relapsing fever have variable major proteins (VMPs) on their outer membranes. Retroviruses encode integrases. RNA viruses and poxviruses encode RNA polymerase.

MM5 546

123 **(A) Expresses an F (fusion) protein.** Paramyxoviruses have an F glycoprotein that promotes syncytia formation and entry into the target cell. This family of viruses includes parainfluenza viruses (PIVs) and RSV. PIVs are the main causes of croup. Other causes include influenza viruses (which are orthomyxoviruses) and RSV. Rhinoviruses grow optimally at 33°C and are resistant to detergent. They cause respiratory tract disease but do not cause croup. Paramyxoviruses have a negative-sense RNA genome that is not infectious. A DNA or positive-sense RNA genome would be infectious. There is no vaccine against PIVs or other paramyxoviruses. Killed vaccines would make matters worse for paramyxoviruses by initiating an incorrect immune response. RSV, PIVs, and other paramyxoviruses are not susceptible to acyclovir although RSV is susceptible to ribavirin. Acyclovir is used in the treatment of HSV and VZV infections.

MM5 597

124 **(A) CD4 count <200/μl.** The patient's manifestations suggest an oral *Candida* infection and *Pneumocystis* pneumonia. The combination of two opportunistic diseases, night sweats, fever, and weight loss is indicative of a late-stage infection with HIV. AIDS is defined by a CD4 count that drops below 200/μl. A CD4 count of 400/μl is not low enough to allow for opportunistic infections. A CD4 count above 500/μl is normal. The CD8 counts of 400/μl and 500/μl are not abnormal.

MM5 663

125 **(E) Varicella-zoster immune globulin.** Varicella-zoster immune globulin (VZIG) is used to prevent infection in exposed susceptible individuals who are immunosuppressed and are therefore at risk of serious VZV infection. VZV is the only herpesvirus that responds well to antibody protection. The antibody prevents the spread of VZV from the lungs to other tissues. Amantadine is used for the prevention and treatment of influenza A. Beta-lactam antibiotics are used for the treatment of various bacterial infections, and pentamidine is used for the treatment of *Pneumocystis carinii* infections. Although the live VZV vaccine is safe for patients with Hodgkin's disease and leukemia, development of protective immunity by immunization with a varicella vaccine would take too long to be effective.

MM5 159, 553

126 **(A) Absence of HB$_e$Ag antigen.** The HB$_e$Ag and HB$_s$Ag are indicators that HBV is being produced. When HBV is produced, these antigens are released into the blood. Anti-HB$_e$ and anti-HB$_s$ titers cannot be detected because they are bound to the antigens in the blood. Decreased jaundice would indicate resolution of an acute disease with liver swelling. Chronic disease, however, is often less severe, and jaundice is not always present.

If it is present, the virus infection may persist despite its reduction. The presence of anti-HB$_s$ indicates resolution of the infection but at a later time. A decrease in anti-HB$_s$ would be a normal consequence of time. An increase in the anti-HB$_c$ titer occurs at the start of acute infection. IgM anti-HB$_c$ is a good indicator of recent infection, whereas IgG anti-HB$_c$ indicates previous exposure. An increase in the serum alanine aminotransferase level indicates liver damage, not success at therapy. This is an indicator of hepatitis.

MM5 685

127 **(B) The patient was not recently infected with a strain containing H3 but was infected with it earlier in life.** The HAI test identifies the presence of antibody that blocks the interaction of viral HA with red blood cells. Seroconversion upon progression from acute disease to convalescence requires that there be a fourfold increase in antibody titer. The figure shows only a twofold increase, so the patient was not recently infected. However, the titer is high enough to indicate infection earlier in life. The assay evaluates only the HA; no information can be obtained regarding the NA.

MM5 520

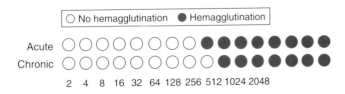

128 **(D) Erythrocyte P antigen.** Binding of the VAPs to specific cell receptors determines which cells are infected by the virus. The receptors may be proteins, glycoproteins, or glycolipids. Parvovirus B19 binds to erythrocyte P antigen on erythroid precursors. Examples of other receptors for viruses include the following: EBV binds to the C3d complement receptor on B cells, HIV binds to the CD4 molecule and chemokine coreceptor on T lymphocytes, poliovirus binds to the immunoglobulin superfamily protein receptor on epithelial cells, and influenza A virus binds to sialic acid receptors on epithelial cells.

MM5 55, 573

129 **(B) Development of an antibody response that blocks viremia.** Polio vaccines have virtually eliminated disease caused by wild-type polioviruses. Vaccination elicits an antibody response that blocks viremia and thereby prevents the spread of the virus from the primary sites of infection (the oral pharynx and Peyer patches in the intestinal mucosa) to the anterior horn cells of the spinal cord. Although HSV travels from the skin to the nerve, poliovirus does not. Antibody targeting of the infected cell is not protective because the virus will kill the cell anyway. Antibody blocking of viral spread through the nervous system would be too late and too inefficient to prevent disease. CD8 T cell immunity may not be initiated by the killed polio vaccine. In any case, this type of immunity is not necessary because the

poliovirus kills the cells that it enters. Only the extracellular virions must be stopped.

MM5 146, 587

130 **(B) Viremia in a horse is not sufficient to promote transmission.** WEE virus is an arbovirus transmitted by *Culex* mosquitoes, and the natural reservoirs are birds. Humans and horses are dead-end hosts because the viremia is insufficient to allow other mosquitoes to acquire the virus from them. There is no approved or standard vaccination against the WEE virus. WEE virus can infect humans and can cause symptoms ranging from mild flu-like disease to encephalitis. It is not transmitted sexually nor in marsh water.

MM5 643

131 **(A) Hepatitis A.** All of the symptoms are characteristic of hepatitis, but the abrupt onset indicates HAV or HEV. HAV and HEV are spread by the fecal-oral route. HEV is uncommon in the United States. The presence of antibodies to only HB$_s$Ag indicates either vaccination against hepatitis B. Hepatitis B, C, and D, which are spread in blood and by sexual contact, are insidious in onset. HDV requires coinfection with HBV. HEV, which is spread by the fecal-oral route, is uncommon in the United States but causes symptoms similar to HAV. HEV has more serious consequences for pregnant women, with a mortality rate as high as 25% for the women.

MM5 678

132 **(E) Rotavirus.** For this patient, the history, clinical manifestations, and description of the virus all point to rotavirus. This virus is a frequent cause of diarrhea in children and is transmitted by the fecal-oral route. Like other members of the family Reoviridae, rotavirus is a nonenveloped, double icosahedral, double-stranded RNA virus (double/double). This virus is a major cause of infant mortality worldwide, causing over 1 million deaths per year. Of the answers listed, only rotavirus is a virus with a double-stranded RNA genome and a double capsid. Some types of adenoviruses cause diarrhea, but all members of the family Adenoviridae are icosahedral, nonenveloped, double-stranded DNA viruses, so they do not fit the description provided. Coronaviruses can cause diarrhea, but all members of the family Coronaviridae are helical, enveloped, single-stranded, positive-sense RNA viruses. Coxsackievirus A, a member of the genus *Enterovirus* and the family Picornaviridae, is not associated with diarrhea. Furthermore, the picornaviruses are icosahedral, nonenveloped, single-stranded, positive-sense RNA viruses. Norwalk virus, a member of the family Noroviridae, causes a short bout of diarrhea, usually accompanied by vomiting that lasts 1 to 2 days. All noroviruses are icosahedral, nonenveloped, single-stranded, positive-sense RNA viruses.

MM5 631

133 **(D) Change in viral glycoprotein.** The results indicate a change in the host range (the cell types and species a virus can infect). Infection is initiated when the viral glycoprotein recognizes the host cell receptor. Passage of the virus in chicken cells allows viral mutants to become dominant under these unnatural conditions. A change in the replicative machinery may also have occurred because mosquito cells grow at a different temperature than do tissue culture cells. It is unlikely that a change in the horse would occur to make it become resistant to infection. A change in the mosquito or its cells is also unlikely to occur. The WEE virus is a togavirus and is enveloped. The viral capsid is inside the envelope and will not affect the virus/cell interaction. The lipid composition of the enveloped virus has little influence on the infection.

MM5 644

134 (A) HIV causes a lytic infection of T cells. Both HTLV and HIV are retroviruses. However, HTLV is an oncovirus, whereas HIV is a lentivirus. HTLV causes a slow, transforming infection, whereas HIV causes a lytic infection of the CD4 T cells. As a result, the nature of the diseases is extremely different. As retroviruses, both HTLV and HIV produce protease and reverse transcriptase. Protease facilitates breakdown and final assembly of the polyprotein components of the capsid. Both HTLV and HIV infect CD4 T cells and neurons. Neuronal infection by HTLV causes spastic paraparesis. HIV causes dementia in patients with AIDS.

MM5 659

135 (C) HBV and HIV. HBV and HIV encode reverse transcriptases that share sensitivity to lamivudine, an FDA-approved drug that is also called 3-thiacytosine (3TC). CMV, VZV, and HSV are herpesviruses. Foscarnet is an anti-CMV drug that targets the herpesvirus-encoded polymerase. Acyclovir, famciclovir, and valacyclovir are anti-VZV and anti-HSV drugs that are activated by viral thymidine kinase and inhibit the herpesvirus-encoded polymerase. Papillomaviruses do not encode a polymerase. Poliovirus and HAV do not encode a thymidine kinase or a polymerase. Ribavirin is approved for the treatment of severe RSV infection and hepatitis C (with IFN-γ). The drug inhibits RSV and several other viruses but not rubella virus. No antiviral drug has been approved for the treatment of rubella.

MM5 505, 667, 685

136 (E) Is spread by the respiratory route. The patient's history and clinical manifestations are consistent with the diagnosis of rubella, a disease that can be prevented by use of the MMR vaccine. Rubella virus is transmitted by the respiratory route and only infects humans. Like other togaviruses, rubella virus is an enveloped, single-stranded, positive-sense RNA virus. Detergent removes the viral envelope and inactivates the virus.

MM5 645

137 (C) Vaccination with a live, attenuated vaccine. The patient's clinical manifestations are consistent with the diagnosis of measles. This disease is normally prevented by routine childhood immunization with the MMR vaccine. The MMR vaccine contains live, attenuated viruses. An inactivated measles vaccine was once used; however, it was withdrawn from use because it was found to promote more serious disease (atypical measles) in some individuals who had been vaccinated with it and were subsequently exposed to natural infection. Although immune globulin will ameliorate the symptoms of measles, it is not the standard means for preventing the disease. Measles cannot be prevented with amantadine or a subunit vaccine. Amantadine is used to prevent influenza A. A subunit vaccine is used to prevent hepatitis B.

MM5 163, 603

138 (B) Immortalization of B cells in tissue culture. Hodgkin's lymphoma is a B cell neoplasm. In the absence of T cells, EBV activates and promotes the outgrowth of B cells. Immunosuppression can reduce the number of T cells and thereby allow the outgrowth of latently infected B cells or newly infected B cells. In infectious mononucleosis, the lymphocytosis is due to proliferation of T cells responding to EBV infection. Atypical lymphocytes are T cells. Patients infected with this virus may develop oral hairy leukoplakia (a white patch on the tongue or buccal mucosa). Virus production by a DNA virus results in cell death, however, so continued growth of lymphocytes (lymphoma) will not occur. Heterophil antibody is produced by EBV-infected B cells. It is not responsible for tumor development.

MM5 557

139 (A) Coronavirus. The patient's clinical manifestations are consistent with the diagnosis of a common cold, which is usually caused by a rhinovirus or a coronavirus. Hantavirus is a bunyavirus that is spread by rodents and causes a severe hemorrhagic respiratory disease. Norwalk virus is a norovirus that causes a diarrheal disease. Rubella virus is a togavirus that causes German measles. Although togaviruses can cause flu-like symptoms, they do not cause colds. Like rabies virus, vesicular stomatitis virus (VSV) is a rhabdovirus. VSV does not usually cause disease in humans.

MM5 591

140 (B) Deltavirus. The patient has HDV infection. HDV is an RNA virus that is referred to as the deltavirus or delta agent. HDV requires HBV for replication. HDV will replicate faster if the HBV infection is already established (chronic disease) and if the patient is superinfected, rather than coinfected, with HDV. Similarly, symptoms will progress faster in patients who are superinfected rather than coinfected. HAV is a picornavirus; HBV is a hepadnavirus; HCV is a flavivirus; and HEV is a calicivirus. HAV and HEV are transmitted via the fecal-oral route and rarely cause fulminant disease or cirrhosis. HBV, HCV, and HDV are transmitted sexually or via contact with blood or other body fluids. HBV is also transmitted transplacentally. HBV rarely causes fulminant disease or cirrhosis. HCV causes cirrhosis but with slow, insidious onset.

MM5 688

141 **(B) Reassortment.** Reassortment is the mixing of gene segments within a single infected cell to produce a new virus with components of each of the parental viruses. Complementation occurs when one virus (or a cell expressing viral proteins) provides an enzyme or protein required by another virus (i.e., a defective mutant), thereby allowing replication of the virus. Recombination is the process in which coinfection and exchange of genes occurs within a single strand to create two hybrid viruses. Transcapsidation (camouflage) occurs when the genome of one virus is wrapped in the shell or envelope of a different virus. Transposition occurs when genes are rearranged by recombination or other means.

MM5 63

142 **(E) Small-sized, detergent-resistant virus with a genome that is infectious.** The patient's clinical manifestations are consistent with the diagnosis of hand-foot-and-mouth disease. This disease is caused by coxsackievirus A (probably A16), which like other picornaviruses is a small, naked-capsid virus whose genome consists of a single positive-sense strand of RNA. This genome is the same as mRNA, and when it is inserted into a cell, it is capable of causing infection. Coxsackieviruses are enteroviruses and are resistant to detergents. Poxvirus is a large-sized, detergent-sensitive virus that encodes a DNA and an RNA polymerase. Although poxviruses are DNA viruses, they replicate in the cytoplasm and must make their own RNA. An adenovirus is a medium-sized, detergent-resistant virus that replicates in the nucleus; this virus is a naked-capsid DNA virus whose penton base and fibers are cytotoxic. A medium-sized, detergent-resistant virus with a genome that is infectious could be a coronavirus or an encapsidated DNA virus, such as an adenovirus. A small-sized, detergent-resistant virus that replicates in the nucleus could be a papovavirus or a parvovirus. Coronaviruses and hepadnaviruses are the only enveloped viruses that are resistant to detergents.

MM5 51, 579

143 **(D) Multiple viral serotypes.** The patient has the symptoms of a common cold, which in 85% of cases is caused by one of more than 100 different serotypes of rhinovirus. Coronaviruses are also a frequent cause of the common cold. Rhinovirus is a picornavirus that causes only upper respiratory tract infections because it cannot replicate in the higher temperatures of the lung. Although some viruses (such as herpesviruses) can cause recurrent viral disease, rhinovirus and other picornaviruses cannot. Therefore the second occurrence was caused by a different serotype of rhinovirus or other cold-causing virus. Chédiak-Higashi syndrome results in neutrophil dysfunction, which would have little effect on this viral infection. DiGeorge syndrome is characterized by T cell deficiency, and T cells are not essential for control of a rhinovirus infection. IFN is probably the main host protection. IgA might contribute to protection, but there are too many rhinovirus serotypes to be immune to all of them.

MM5 588, 697

144 **(C) Immunoglobulin superfamily protein on epithelial cells.** Binding of VAPs to specific cell receptors determine which cells are infected by the virus. The receptors may be proteins, glycoproteins, or glycolipids. Poliovirus binds to the immunoglobulin superfamily protein receptor on epithelial cells. Examples of other receptors for viruses include the following: EBV binds to the C3d complement receptor on B cells, HIV binds to the CD4 molecule and chemokine coreceptor on T lymphocytes, rabies virus binds to the acetylcholine receptor on neurons, and influenza A virus binds to sialic acid receptors on epithelial cells.

MM5 55

145 **(D) Generation of double-stranded DNA from RNA templates.** Weight loss, opportunistic infections (thrush caused by *Candida albicans* and pneumonia caused by *Pneumocystis carinii*), and a low CD4 T cell count suggest the diagnosis of HIV infection and AIDS. HIV is a retrovirus that is released into blood and produces reverse transcriptase. DNA and RNA are degraded by deoxyribonuclease and ribonuclease, respectively. These enzymes are produced by the host and several viruses, so they would not confirm the diagnosis of a specific type of viral infection. NA from orthomyxoviruses or paramyxoviruses degrades sialic acid. Most DNA polymerases will make double-stranded DNA from single-stranded DNA, both viral and cellular, so this would not confirm the diagnosis of a specific type of viral infection.

MM5 659

146 **(D) The virus strain that caused influenza 5 years ago is not the same strain that caused the current disease.** Influenza viruses undergo shift and drift. Every year, different strains of influenza A and B virus predominate. Periodically, a totally new virus evolves and causes a pandemic. As a result, it is difficult to be immune to all of the influenza viruses. Immunosuppression would increase an individual's susceptibility to influenza. Although smoking compromises the ciliated epithelium and would increase the risk of infection with influenza viruses, all individuals are at risk of infection with strains of influenza virus that have not infected them previously. After a person is infected with a strain of influenza virus, he or she will have long-lasting immunity against that particular strain. Influenza does not infect an immune-privileged site.

MM5 613

147 **(A) Double-stranded, segmented RNA virus with a double capsid.** Severe nonbloody diarrhea in an infant is usually caused by rotavirus. This virus has a double-stranded, segmented RNA genome and a double capsid. A gram-negative rod that does not ferment lactose describes *Shigella*, a bacterium that causes bloody diarrhea. The patient has nonbloody diarrhea. A gram-positive anaerobe could indicate *Clostridium difficile*. In patients taking high doses of antibiotics, *C. difficile* sometimes causes pseudomembranous colitis, which is characterized by profuse watery or mucoid diarrhea but is accompanied by pseudomembrane formation. A pear-shaped trophozoite with two nuclei and four pairs of flagella describes the trophozoites of *Giardia lamblia*, a protozoan parasite that causes smelly, crampy, watery diarrhea in people who drink contaminated water. A single-stranded, positive-sense RNA virus with a capsid describes Norwalk virus, a norovirus that is implicated in community outbreaks of diarrhea. The diarrhea caused by Norwalk virus is usually of short duration and is commonly accompanied by vomiting.

MM5 631

148   (B) Inhibiting the activity of p53 and RB. HPV types 16 and 18 are found in association with most cervical cancers. These viruses inhibit the cell growth-suppressing activities of p53 and RB. As a result, cell growth remains unchecked. A lytic virus will kill the target cell, and this is inconsistent with tumorigenicity. Production of a cDNA intermediate and promotion of viral glycoprotein expression on the cell surface are characteristics of retroviruses. Unlike retroviruses, papillomaviruses are DNA viruses and therefore do not produce cDNA intermediates. Papillomaviruses have a naked capsid and do not encode glycoproteins on the cell surface. Cell growth suppressors p53 and RB normally prevent tumor production, cell growth, and HPV replication.

MM5 526

149   (A) Acyclovir. The patient's manifestations are consistent with the diagnosis of encephalitis caused by HSV. Lymphocytes but no polymorphonuclear leukocytes in the CSF suggests a viral etiology. One of the key clues that the agent is HSV is the time of year (it is not mosquito season), and another clue is that the disease is limited to one temporal lobe. Acyclovir is a nucleotide analogue that is activated by HSV thymidine kinase and inhibits HSV polymerase. Amantadine is an anti-influenza A drug. Amphotericin B is an antifungal agent. Ceftriaxone is a third-generation cephalosporin that is used to treat bacterial meningitis. Rifampin is an antibacterial agent that is used to prevent meningococcal meningitis.

MM5 548, 549

150   (A) California encephalitis virus. The patient's clinical manifestations are consistent with the diagnosis of meningoencephalitis. The prodrome and short course of the disease, the time of year, and the likelihood of exposure to forest-dwelling mosquitoes (*Culex* species) all implicate California encephalitis virus as the cause of the disease. Coxsackievirus A may be responsible for similar symptoms, but the epidemiologic data do not support this choice. The fungus *C. neoformans* would cause a more serious and longer-lasting disease than that described in the patient. CMV is not a common cause of meningitis, and it rarely causes symptoms in immunocompetent individuals. Group B *Streptococcus* causes meningitis in infants rather than in adults, and the disease does not resolve quickly.

MM5 644

151   (C) Profile C. The patient has experienced a gradual, insidious onset of hepatitis, likely to be caused by HBV. HB$_s$Ag

and HB$_e$Ag are present during symptoms. HB$_e$Ag is present while the virus is being shed. Anti-HB$_c$ may be seen before other antibodies. Anti-HB$_s$ and anti-HB$_e$ cannot be detected or are not present when their antigens are also detected in the blood. Anti-HB$_s$ and HB$_s$Ag are not detectable at the same time. The presence of HB$_e$Ag signifies the presence of virus (either during the early phase of infection or during chronic infection), whereas anti-HB$_s$ denotes resolution of disease. An individual who has anti-HB$_s$ but lacks other markers of infection has been immunized with the HBV vaccine.

MM5 684, 685

152   (B) Human herpesvirus 6. The patient's clinical manifestations are consistent with the diagnosis of roseola infantum, or exanthema subitum. This disease, caused by human herpesvirus 6 (HHV-6), is one of the five exanthematous diseases of early childhood. Detergent sensitivity indicates an enveloped virus, such as a herpesvirus. Coxsackievirus A can cause herpangina, with vesicles in the mouth, and can cause hand-foot-and-mouth disease, with vesicles in these locations. However, the virus is a picornavirus and is resistant to detergent. Like HHV-6, measles virus and rubella virus are enveloped viruses that cause exanthematous diseases. Measles and rubella, however, infect a person for a longer duration than roseola, and fever and rash occur together. Rubella is also accompanied by lymphadenopathy. Parvovirus B19 causes fifth disease, a childhood exanthem with symptoms similar to those seen in the patient. However, parvoviruses are encapsidated and resistant to detergents.

MM5 562

153   (B) Detergent-resistant agent that elicits no inflammation. The patient's clinical and autopsy findings are consistent with the diagnosis of CJD. This disease is caused by a prion. The prion is resistant to detergents, DNase, and most of the other agents that normally inactivate classic viruses. Prions are mutated versions of host proteins and do not elicit inflammation. A detergent-resistant agent controlled by antibody describes a naked-capsid (detergent-resistant) virus, such as a picornavirus. Poliovirus is a picornavirus that is neurotropic and causes paralysis. Antibody is sufficient to control viremic spread of poliovirus and disease production. A detergent-resistant, opportunistic agent describes a naked-capsid (detergent-resistant) virus. The JC papovavirus is an opportunistic capsid virus that causes neurologic disease. JC virus causes progressive multifocal leukoencephalopathy, which is a slow viral disease, but JC elicits and is controlled by the immune response. A detergent-sensitive agent controlled by cell-mediated immunity describes an enveloped virus. Most enveloped viruses are controlled by cell-mediated immunity, and those that produce neurologic disease include HSV and measles viruses, togaviruses, and flavi-encephalitis viruses. Cell-mediated immunity controls and contributes to the pathogenesis by these viruses. A detergent-sensitive agent that is vaccine preventable also describes an enveloped virus. The vaccine-preventable enveloped virus infections that can cause neurologic symptoms are measles virus (and the subacute sclerosing panencephalitis, or SSPE, measles variant) and VZV. Cell-mediated immunity controls and contributes to the pathogenesis by these viruses.

MM5 591

154   (E) Parainfluenza virus type I. Of the options listed, only parainfluenza virus type I causes syncytia formation. The patient's clinical manifestations are similar to the symptoms of a common cold, which can be caused by a coronavirus, or to the symptoms of influenza, which is most frequently caused by influenza A or B virus but is rarely caused by influenza C virus. Coronavirus can be ruled out because it is not isolated and cannot form syncytia. Influenza viruses and parainfluenza viruses all cause hemadsorption, but influenza viruses can be ruled out because they do not form syncytia.

MM5 603

155   (C) Multiple sexual partners. The patient has the symptoms of mild hepatitis. An ongoing infection with HBV is indicated by the presence of HB_sAg and HB_eAg in the absence of anti-HB_s. Risk factors for HBV infection include multiple sexual partners and contact with contaminated blood products (via needle sharing and other means). Antibodies to HAV, EBV, and CMV indicate prior exposure. Although alcoholism can cause serious liver disease, the serologic results for this patient suggest that HBV is the cause. Contaminated water may be a source of infection by HAV but not HBV. Travel to regions with poor sanitation may put one at risk for HAV infection, HEV infection, and other diseases but not necessarily for HBV infection. If HAV were the cause of the patient's hepatitis, then the onset of symptoms would be sudden and not subtle, just as for a person infected with HBV. Antibody to HAV indicates prior exposure. Smoking is not a direct risk factor for liver disease.

MM5 684, 685

156   (D) IgG. The infant should be protected by maternal anti-HAV IgG. Maternal IgG, which crosses the placenta and is also present in breast milk, has a half-life of 120 days in the infant. Antibody in the infant's blood would block progression of HAV to the liver. IgA can be a secretory or a serum antibody. It might be secreted in breast milk, but its production is transient and would require that the mother be exposed shortly before the infant is exposed. IgD is an early antibody present on B-cell surfaces. IgE is produced in relatively low levels and binds tightly to mast cells to initiate allergic reactions. IgM is an early antibody that would not be provided by the seropositive mother because the maternal IgM molecules are too big to cross the placenta. IgG is the only immunoglobulin that is transferred across the placenta.

MM5 111, 677

157   (B) Profile B. Profile B resembles the profile of an individual who was vaccinated against hepatitis B. Vaccinated individuals develop anti-HB_s but not the other types of antibodies. The presence of HB_sAg, seen in all of the other profiles, is an early marker of current acute or chronic infection. A person who was infected with HBV in the past would have antibodies to other viral antigens (as in profiles A and C). The combination of findings shown in profile E is not possible because the presence of HB_sAg would preclude the detection of unbound antibody (anti-HB_s).

MM5 684, 685

158   (A) Absence of antiviral antibody but presence of an abnormal protein in the brain. Presenile dementia, myoclonic jerks, the absence of an immune reaction (encephalopathy), and the presence of spongiform vacuolation are findings that suggest CJD. The patient may have acquired the disease from a contaminated cornea, and this route of infection would decrease the incubation period. The agent of the disease is a modified form of prion protein (PrP) that promotes the generation of scrapie-like PrP. The findings of high titers of antibody to measles virus and isolation of a measles variant from the brain suggest the diagnosis of SSPE, a slow viral disease caused by a mutant strain of measles virus. This disease, however, is not associated with the vacuolation of neuronal cells. A history of cold sores suggests encephalitis caused by HSV. Like VZV and CMV, HSV is an enveloped DNA virus. However, herpesvirus-induced encephalitis would elicit an immune response and would not cause vacuolation of neuronal cells. Isolation of a small, naked capsid virus from the brain suggests an infection with JC virus, a papovavirus that causes progressive multifocal leukoencephalopathy. This disease, however, is not associated with the vacuolation of neuronal cells. A virus with an enveloped capsid containing an RNA genome might describe an arboviral encephalitis virus or even HIV or HTLV, but these viruses are not associated with the vacuolation of neuronal cells.

MM5 691

159   (C) Fecal-oral route. The patient's history and clinical findings are consistent with the diagnosis of poliomyelitis. This disease is caused by poliovirus, a picornavirus that is produced by epithelial cells in the gastrointestinal tract and is transmitted via the fecal-oral route. Although some picornaviruses can be transmitted by the respiratory route, poliovirus is not transmitted in this manner. Viruses must generate a significant and long-lasting viremia to be transmitted via arthropod bites (as is the case with flaviviruses responsible for yellow fever and dengue viruses) or via parenteral means (as is the case with HBV and HIV). Viruses that cause dermatologic and sexually transmitted diseases may be transmitted by contact with lesions. Although many picornaviruses are transmitted by the respiratory route, poliovirus is a picornavirus that is not transmitted in this manner.

MM5 582

160   (D) Binding of antibody to immobilized antigen. An ELISA procedure is used to initially screen blood for HIV. In this ELISA, HIV antigen is affixed to a plastic plate. Donor blood is added to the well and bound antibody is then detected by a second antibody that has an attached enzyme. The enzyme converts a chromophore to color. Amplification of the viral genome and subsequent detection of the genome by gel techniques describe a PCR procedure that is useful for following the course of HIV infection but is not useful for screening. Antibody-induced lysis of antigen-loaded erythrocytes in the presence of complement describes an older test that is not commonly used today. Binding of antibody to antigen that is bound to nitrocellulose paper describes the Western blot analysis that is used for confirmation of HIV infection but not for screening. Binding of antigen to immobilized antibody describes an ELISA procedure designed to detect antigen (e.g., rotovirus); the current screening test for HIV is an ELISA procedure designed to detect antibody, rather than antigen.

MM5 185

161 (E) Yellow fever virus. Yellow fever virus and dengue virus are transmitted by *Aedes* mosquitoes. These viruses have a jungle and urban pattern of transmission because humans can act both as host and reservoir. *B. burgdorferi*, the agent of Lyme disease, is transmitted by *Ixodes* ticks. Hantavirus, an agent of respiratory disease, is transmitted via contact with rat droppings. *P. vivax*, an agent of malaria, is transmitted by *Anopheles* mosquitoes. St. Louis encephalitis virus is transmitted by *Culex* mosquitoes.

MM5 642

162 (C) Antirotavirus antibody and enzyme-linked antirotavirus antibody. A stool sample would contain large amounts of rotavirus, which can be detected by a capture ELISA. In the capture assay, the antigen is concentrated and held in the plastic well for detection by the enzyme-linked virus-specific antibody. Use of anti-IgG or anti-IgM with enzyme-linked anti-immunoglobulin describe serologic tests for IgG and IgM, respectively. These tests would not confirm the diagnosis, because they are not virus-specific. A serologic test to detect the presence of antibody to rotavirus uses rotavirus antigen and enzyme-linked anti-immunoglobulin. The antibody will not be present in a stool sample. A serologic test with rotavirus antigen and enzyme-linked antirotavirus antibody would not work. Antibody to rotavirus present in a serum sample would bind to the antigen affixed to the plastic well, as would the enzyme-linked antibody. All wells would give a positive signal.

MM5 633

163 (E) Sialic acid receptor on epithelial cells. Binding of the VAPs to specific cell receptors determine which cells are infected by the virus. The receptors may be proteins, glycoproteins, or glycolipids. Influenza A virus binds to sialic acid receptors on epithelial cells. Examples of other receptors for viruses include the following: EBV binds to the C3d complement receptor on B cells, HIV binds to the CD4 molecule and chemokine coreceptor on T lymphocytes, poliovirus binds to the immunoglobulin superfamily protein receptor on epithelial cells, and parvovirus B19 binds to erythrocyte P antigen on erythroid precursors.

MM5 55

164 (D) Virus with a single-stranded, negative-sense DNA genome. The patient has erythema infectiosum, also called fifth disease, which is one of the five childhood exanthems. The disease is caused by parvovirus B19, a single-stranded, negative-sense DNA virus. *N. meningitidis* is a bacterium that is a gram-negative diplococcus and can cause petechiae. *S. pyogenes* is a gram-positive coccus and can cause scarlet fever. Rotavirus is a virus with a double-stranded RNA genome but causes diarrhea. Rhabdoviruses, paramyxoviruses, orthomyxoviruses, and several other viruses have a single-stranded, negative-sense RNA genome.

MM5 573

165 (D) Treatment with rimantadine. Rimantadine and amantadine are active against influenza A virus but not influenza B virus. If treatment is initiated early, it can block viral replication and thereby prevent influenza. However, if treatment is initiated after 3 days of symptoms, the virus has already replicated and elicited a response, so treatment is not effective. Active immunization does not take effect for approximately 2 to 3 weeks. This would be too long to help a person who has already been exposed to an influenza virus. There are several reasons that passive immunization is not effective against influenza viruses. One is that influenza viruses cause a respiratory disease rather than causing viremia. Passive immunization would only prevent viremia. Another is that there are many influenza virus strains, so it would be difficult to provide the appropriate antibodies for passive immunization. Ribavirin is indicated for the treatment of respiratory syncytial virus in infants. It is difficult to administer and is not appropriate for the treatment of influenza in adults. Liquids and vitamin C are helpful in the management of influenza symptoms, but they cannot prevent the disease. Only active immunization or early administration of rimantadine or amantadine can prevent influenza.

MM5 510, 616

166 (C) Influenza virus. Viruses with segmented genomes have an enhanced capability to exchange genetic information and rapidly evolve into new strains through mutation and reassortment of the gene segments among different human and animal strains of virus. This genetic instability is responsible for epidemics and pandemics of influenza virus infections. Arenaviridae (e.g., Lassa fever virus, Junin virus, Machupo virus, lymphocytic choriomeningitis virus) and Reoviridae (e.g., rotavirus, Colorado tick fever virus) also have segmented genomes. The other viruses listed in the answers to this question do not have a segmented genome.

MM5 63

167 (B) The agent does not express unique immunogenic epitopes. The spongiform encephalopathies include scrapie, CJD, and Gerstmann-Sträussler-Scheinker syndrome. Their agent, the prion, appears to be a mutant form of a cellular protein that binds to and induces a change in the conformation of the native protein, causing shedding and aggregation of the protein. The expression of the PrP is increased, and the cycle continues. The prion resembles the host protein and does not express unique immunogenic epitopes. It does not cause lytic infection; however, lytic infection is not a criterion for inducing an immune response. Unlike CMV, HIV, and various other infectious agents, prions do not infect T cells and are not immunogenic or immunosuppressive. Immunoprivileged sites include the eye and the central nervous system. Prions are found in these and other sites (e.g., blood, organs).

MM5 691

168 (D) **Norwalk virus.** The case describes a typical community outbreak of disease caused by Norwalk virus, a norovirus. Norwalk virus is a nonenveloped, single-stranded, positive-sense RNA virus. Under the electron microscope, it often appears as a star-like or pockmarked icosahedron. Adenoviruses and coronaviruses can cause diarrhea. Adenoviruses, however, are DNA viruses that are larger than 27 nm and have an icosadeltahedral capsid with fibers. Coronaviruses are single-stranded, positive-sense RNA viruses that are larger than 27 nm and have an envelope. Echovirus 11 is a picornavirus and is therefore small. However, it does not cause diarrhea. Rotavirus is a nonenveloped, double-stranded RNA virus. It may cause symptoms similar to those described, but it is larger than 27 nm, and it is usually benign in adults. Rotavirus is the major cause of infantile diarrhea.

MM5 594

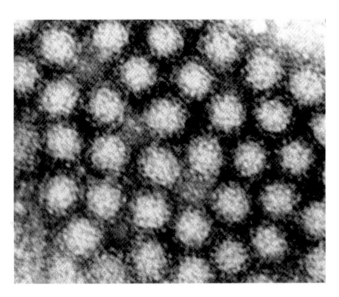

From Cohen J, Powderly WG: *Infectious diseases*, ed 2, St Louis, 2004, Mosby.

169 (A) **Encodes reverse transcriptase.** The presence of IgG antibodies to HAV in the absence of IgM antibodies to HAV indicates prior but probably not recent infection with HAV. The presence of HB_sAg and IgM antibodies to HB_cAg indicates recent infection with HBV. HBV is a DNA virus in the family Hepad-

naviridae. During replication, a longer than genome-length RNA is transcribed as a replicative intermediate, and the viral polymerase (reverse transcriptase) converts it into a DNA copy and then into double-stranded DNA within the virion. HAV has an icosahedral capsid, but the patient's serologic results suggest a recent infection with HBV rather than HAV. HBV does not immortalize B lymphocytes and is not transmitted by mosquitoes. EBV can cause hepatitis and also immortalizes B lymphocytes. Most RNA viruses, which would include HAV, HCV, and HEV, have a replication cycle with a double-stranded RNA intermediate. Yellow fever virus, which causes jaundice and hepatitis, is transmitted by mosquitoes.

MM5 676

170 (E) **IgM antibody to California encephalitis virus in the blood.** The patient's symptoms indicate encephalitis. Mosquitoes near a camp may be carriers, and California encephalitis virus is found in Ohio. IgM antibody indicates recent infection. Antibody to the phospholipid cardiolipin (reagin) occurs with syphilis. Although some patients with tertiary syphilis have neurologic manifestations, neurosyphilis is a chronic disease and would not be likely in an 11-year-old patient. Owl's eye inclusion bodies are characteristic of CMV infection. CMV and CMV-infected cells, however, are often shed in the urine of asymptomatic individuals, as well as of symptomatic individuals. CMV is unlikely to cause encephalitis, even in immunocompromised patients. Heterophil antibody is associated with the early stages of infectious mononucleosis caused by EBV. EBV infection is not usually associated with neurologic symptoms. HSV can cause encephalitis, with a serious outcome. However, the camp setting, season, and positive outcome suggest an arboviral encephalitis.

MM5 651

171 (E) **SSPE.** SSPE, or subacute sclerosing panencephalitis, results from infection with a defective measles virus that remains in neurons and elicits damaging inflammatory responses. The defective virus evolves during a primary infection, and the SSPE occurs later in life. CJD and kuru are spongiform encephalopathies caused by prions. Kawasaki disease, a disease whose cause is unknown, is also called mucocutaneous lymph node syndrome. JC virus, a polyomavirus that is ubiquitous, causes progressive multifocal leukoencephalopathy, a disease seen most frequently in immunosuppressed individuals.

MM5 602

172 (E) **T cells.** The patient's manifestations are consistent with the diagnosis of measles. The combination of Koplik spots plus cough, coryza, and conjunctivitis (the "three Cs"), one diagnostic for measles, T cells are essential for the control of a measles virus infection. T cell-deficient individuals have severe complications, such as giant cell pneumonia. IgG is important and will prevent the spread of measles virus via the blood, but it will not prevent local viral replication. IgA will prevent recurrent infection of the lung. IgE is not important for viral infections, but it is important for control of helminth infections. Neutrophils are mainly important for bacterial infections.

MM5 602

173   (C) Respiratory droplets. The patient has the classic symptoms of measles: the three Cs, the rash, and Koplik spots. The measles virus is a respiratory tract virus. Measles is not spread by blood or blood products, mosquitoes, or sexual contact. Although contact with contaminated saliva might transmit measles, this is not the predominant means of transmission.

MM5 600

174   (C) HCV. Transaminase levels are increased in patients with chronic liver infections. The HCV is the most common of the non-hepatitis A and non-hepatitis B viruses and is the most likely member of this group to cause chronic hepatitis. In the past, before donated blood was screened for HCV, the agent was readily transmitted via blood transfusion. HCV is a flavivirus that cannot be isolated or grown. HAV is a norovirus. HBV is a hepadnavirus, HDV is the deltavirus, and HEV is a nornovirus. HAV and HEV do not cause chronic infection. HDV requires coinfection or previous infection with HBV.

MM5 685

175   (C) Levofloxacin. The patient's symptoms and clinical course are consistent with the diagnosis of pneumonia caused by a bacterial superinfection. Cilia in the respiratory tract are an important protective mechanism against bacterial infection. In this case, the patient's initial bout of influenza caused the loss of cilia. Influenza viruses can themselves cause pneumonia; however, the patient's symptoms subsided before they reappeared or worsened, so a superinfection is more likely. Pneumonia after influenza is usually caused by a bacterium such as *Staphylococcus aureus, Streptococcus pneumoniae,* or *Haemophilus influenzae.* Treatment would include an appropriate antibacterial agent, such as levofloxacin or ceftriaxone. An antiviral agent would not be indicated. Acyclovir is used for the treatment of HSV and VZV infections. Amantadine and rimantadine are used for the prevention and treatment of influenza but are effective only if they are given shortly after exposure to an influenza virus. Ribavirin is approved for the treatment of respiratory syncytial virus infections.

MM5 614

176   (C) EBV. The patient's clinical and laboratory findings are consistent with the diagnosis of heterophil-positive infectious mononucleosis, a disease caused by EBV or Epstein-Barr virus. Adenovirus is a common cause of pharyngitis, with or without conjunctivitis. Adenovirus infection would not cause

hepatosplenomegaly or produce the laboratory findings described in this patient. CMV can cause mononucleosis with many of the clinical manifestations described in the patient. CMV infection, however, would not cause heterophil antibodies or an ampicillin-induced rash. HSV pharyngitis is becoming more prevalent but would not cause hepatosplenomegaly or atypical lymphocytes. *S. pyogenes* can cause most of the clinical findings described, including a rash. Infection with *S. pyogenes* would not cause the laboratory findings described and would not be associated with an ampicillin-induced rash.

MM5 556

177   (C) Rabies virus. Respiratory syncytial virus (RSV) is the most common cause of bronchiolitis in infants younger than 6 months of age and is especially prevalent in winter and spring. RSV is a paramyxovirus, and rabies virus is a rhabdovirus. Paramyxoviruses and rhabdoviruses are enveloped, single-stranded, negative-sense RNA viruses. Adenoviruses are double-stranded DNA viruses that have a naked capsid with fibers at the vertices. Like all picornaviruses, poliovirus is a nonenveloped, single-stranded, positive-sense RNA virus. Like all reoviruses, rotavirus is a nonenveloped, double-stranded RNA virus that has a double capsid. Like all togaviruses, rubella virus is an enveloped, single-stranded, positive-sense RNA virus.

MM5 620

178   (C) Enveloped, single-stranded, positive-sense RNA virus. The most likely etiologic agent is HCV, an enveloped, single-stranded, positive-sense RNA virus. The patient probably acquired HCV via a blood transfusion during his bypass surgery. Unlike screening procedures at the time of the surgery, the current screening procedures will limit HCV transmission via the blood supply. Risky behaviors, such as promiscuity and drug abuse, are usually associated with the acquisition of HBV infection, although HCV can also be spread by these means. HBV is more likely to cause hepatitis rather than the more severe symptoms of cirrhosis. HBV is an enveloped, double-stranded DNA virus; HDV is an enveloped, single-stranded, circular RNA virus; a retrovirus is an enveloped, single-stranded, positive-sense RNA virus with a reverse transcriptase; and HAV is a nonenveloped, single-stranded, positive-sense RNA virus.

MM5 685

179   (D) Replication. Many antiviral agents are nucleoside analogues, which are nucleosides with modifications of the base, sugar, or both. Nucleoside analogues selectively inhibit viral polymerases, leading to premature stoppage of DNA synthesis. Other steps in viral replication are not disrupted.

MM5 56, 505

Mycology Questions

1 Which antimicrobial agent would be used to treat infections with *Pneumocystis?*

- ❑ (A) Amphotericin B
- ❑ (B) Albendazole
- ❑ (C) Chloroquine
- ❑ (D) Metronidazole
- ❑ (E) Pentamidine

2 Which component is present in fungi?

- ❑ (A) Ergosterol
- ❑ (B) Lipid A
- ❑ (C) Peptidoglycan
- ❑ (D) Teichoic acid
- ❑ (E) 70S ribosome

3 An 8-year-old boy is taken to his pediatrician because his mother noticed a raised, scaly area on the back of his head. The physician notes that the area is approximately 5 cm in diameter with an inflamed, raised border. When he examines the boy's scalp with a Wood's lamp, he does not notice fluorescence. He collects scrapings of the area. No organisms are seen on microscopic examination, but a mold grows on Sabouraud dextrose agar (SDA). Numerous microconidia but no macroconidia are seen on microscopic examination (see figure). Which organism is most likely responsible for this patient's infection?

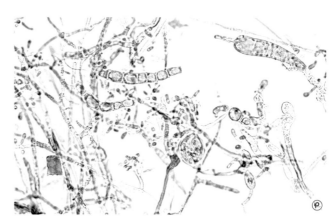

From Marler LM, Siders JA, et al: *Mycology* CD-ROM, Indiana Pathology Images, 2004.

- ❑ (A) *Epidermophyton*
- ❑ (B) *Malassezia*
- ❑ (C) *Microsporum*
- ❑ (D) *Trichophyton*
- ❑ (E) *Trichosporan*

4 A 55-year-old man receives a renal transplant. Approximately 1 month later, he returns to his physician with a productive cough of 1-week duration and a severe headache that developed over the previous 24 h. A patchy infiltrate is seen on the chest radiography. Sputum is induced and submitted for bacterial, mycobacterial, and fungal cultures. Cerebrospinal fluid (CSF) is also collected for stains and culture. Analysis of the CSF shows the presence of cells (predominantly mononuclear cells), increased protein, and decreased glucose levels. After 2 days of incubation, yeasts grow in the bacterial and fungal cultures. Subsequent tests identify the organism as *Cryptococcus neoformans*. Which test is most sensitive for early detection of infections with this organism?

- ☐ (A) Gram stain of CSF
- ☐ (B) India ink stain of CSF
- ☐ (C) Enzyme-linked immunosorbent assay (ELISA) test for *Cryptococcus* antigen in CSF
- ☐ (D) ELISA test for *Cryptococcus* antigen in urine
- ☐ (E) ELISA test for *Cryptococcus* antibody in blood

5 Which microscopic staining method should be used to detect *C. neoformans?*

- ☐ (A) Calcofluor white stain
- ☐ (B) Gram stain
- ☐ (C) Kinyoun stain
- ☐ (D) Trichrome stain
- ☐ (E) Wright-Giemsa stain

6 Approximately 10 days after bone marrow transplantation, a 36-year-old woman develops fevers with no localizing symptoms. Therapy with meropenem and vancomycin is initiated, but the fevers persist. A chest radiograph is performed and shows new bilateral fluffy infiltrates. Bronchoscopy with a biopsy is performed. The organism is observed in histopathology (see figure below). After 2 days of incubation, a mold grows; branching, septated, hyaline hyphae with fruiting structures are observed (see figure on the right). Which organism is responsible for this patient's infection?

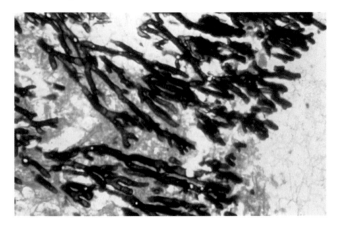

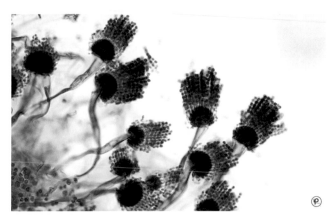

From Marler LM, Siders JA, et al: *Mycology* CD-ROM, Indiana Pathology Images, 2004.

- ☐ (A) *Aspergillus flavus*
- ☐ (B) *Aspergillus fumigatus*
- ☐ (C) *Aspergillus nidulans*
- ☐ (D) *Aspergillus niger*
- ☐ (E) *Aspergillus versicolor*

7 A 56-year-old woman who has been in her usual state of good health notices stiffness in her right knee after kneeling in her garden. This condition worsens during the next 6 months to the point where she finds her right knee to be persistently stiff, painful, and slightly swollen. She visits her physician, who feels the symptoms are consistent with a mild case of arthritis, and he prescribes symptomatic relief. Although this treatment initially helps, she soon finds that her knee becomes more swollen, erythematous, and warm. At another office visit, her physician aspirates the knee and orders a Gram stain and culture of the fluid. When the laboratory reports these tests as negative, her physician prescribes a course of steroids. These provided symptomatic relief, but at the conclusion of the treatment, the swelling, erythema, and pain return. Another 3 months have passed, and the physician decides to admit her to the hospital. Additional fluid is collected for stains and culture. Although the stains are negative, a darkly pigmented mold with delicate hyphae grows after 5 days of incubation at room temperature. Yeasts are also seen in the culture incubated at 37°C. Which organism is most likely responsible for this woman's infection?

- ☐ (A) *Blastomyces dermatitidis*
- ☐ (B) *Coccidioides immitis*
- ☐ (C) *Cryptococcus neoformans*
- ☐ (D) *Histoplasma capsulatum*
- ☐ (E) *Sporothrix schenckii*

8 Which disinfectant has activity against fungi and viruses?

- ☐ (A) Alcohol
- ☐ (B) Chlorine
- ☐ (C) Iodophor
- ☐ (D) Phenolic
- ☐ (E) Quaternary ammonium compound

9 A 59-year-old woman presents to the emergency department with a 3-day history of eye swelling, a frontal headache, and low-grade fevers. The woman is slowly responsive to questions on physical examination. Laboratory tests show the patient has an elevated white blood cell (WBC) count with a predominance of neutrophils and a blood glucose level of 475 mg/dl. A CT scan of the sinuses shows opacities in the ethmoid sinuses. A specimen from a sinus aspiration is collected for bacterial and fungal stains and cultures. An organism is observed in the stained aspirate (see figure), and a mold grows in 1 day from both the bacterial and fungal cultures. Which organism is most likely responsible for this infection?

- ☐ (A) *Aspergillus*
- ☐ (B) *Bipolaris*
- ☐ (C) *Curvularia*
- ☐ (D) *Histoplasma*
- ☐ (E) *Rhizopus*

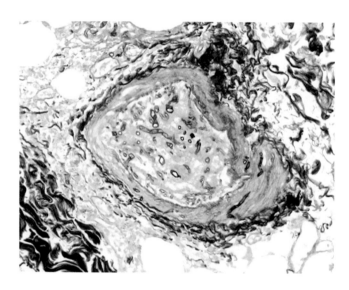

10 Which agent is used to treat lymphocutaneous infections with *Sporothrix schenckii?*

- ☐ (A) Amphotericin B
- ☐ (B) Caspofungin
- ☐ (C) Miconazole
- ☐ (D) Potassium iodide
- ☐ (E) Selenium sulfide

11 A 5-year-old girl living in St. Louis, Missouri, stumbles and injures her arm while playing. Radiographic studies reveal a closed fracture of the humerus involving the diaphysis of the bone. The arm is placed in a cast, but the girl starts to experience fevers, chills, and night sweats. This is attributed to a viral infection, and the girl is treated symptomatically. After 6 weeks, the cast was removed, and the arm is noted to be swollen, erythematous, and tender. Two small ulcers are also noted. She is admitted to the hospital, and radiographic studies of the arm demonstrate a large, destructive lesion involving the distal

humerus. When the original radiographs are reexamined, the initial fracture is noted to be in an area of bony demineralization. Biopsies of the skin ulcers and bone are collected and sent for pathologic examination and microbiological studies. After 10 days of incubation, growth is noted on the bacterial and fungal media. On cultures incubated at 37°C, colonies of cells 3 to 4 μm in diameter are observed. On cultures incubated at room temperature, filamentous growth with large (8 to 14 μm in diameter) and small (2 to 4 μm in diameter) cells is observed. The large cells have a rough surface. Which organism is most likely responsible for this infection?

- ☐ (A) *Blastomyces dermatitidis*
- ☐ (B) *Coccidioides immitis*
- ☐ (C) *Histoplasma capsulatum*
- ☐ (D) *Sporothrix schenckii*
- ☐ (E) *Staphylococcus aureus*

12 Which agent is used to treat disseminated infections with *Candida glabrata?*

- ☐ (A) Amphotericin B
- ☐ (B) Caspofungin
- ☐ (C) Miconazole
- ☐ (D) Potassium iodide
- ☐ (E) Selenium sulfide

13 A 45-year-old woman visits her physician because she has several sores on her arm that have developed during the preceding 2 weeks. The physician notes that the sores are ulcerative nodular lesions that followed the lymphatic system up her arm. Her axillary lymph nodes are also enlarged. The surface of one of the lesions is cleaned, and a specimen is aspirated from deep in the ulcer. The specimen is submitted for stains and cultures for bacteria, mycobacteria, and fungi. A few oval, fusiform yeast cells are observed on microscopy; after 1 week of incubation at room temperature, a small white mold grows in the fungal culture. Microscopic examination of the mold shows delicate structures (see figure). During the next week, the mold darkens to a brown-black color. Which organism is responsible for this woman's infection?

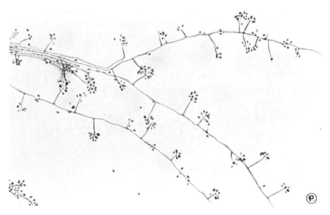

From Marler LM, Siders JA, et al: *Mycology* CD-ROM, Indiana Pathology Images, 2004.

☐ (A) *Candida*
☐ (B) *Blastomyces*
☐ (C) *Histoplasma*
☐ (D) *Microsporum*
☐ (E) *Sporothrix*

14 A 28-year-old man makes an appointment with his physician because toes on both of his feet are painful, and they are itching him. The physician notes that the areas between his toes are inflamed and scaling with some small vesicles present. His physician cultures the involved areas, and after 14 days, a mold is noted in the culture. The surface of the mold is white, but the bottom of the colony is deep red when the culture is examined from the bottom of the plate. Abundant single microconidia and rare macroconidia are seen on microscopic examination of the mold. Which organism is responsible for this patient's infection?

☐ (A) *Epidermophyton floccosum*
☐ (B) *Microsporum canis*
☐ (C) *Trichophyton mentagrophytes*
☐ (D) *Trichophyton rubrum*
☐ (E) *Trichophyton tonsurans*

15 Which organism can colonize the skin of humans?

☐ (A) *Bacteroides*
☐ (B) *Escherichia*
☐ (C) *Lactobacillus*
☐ (D) *Malassezia*
☐ (E) *Streptococcus*

16 Which agent is used to treat infections with *Trichophyton mentagrophyte*?

☐ (A) Amphotericin B
☐ (B) Caspofungin
☐ (C) Miconazole
☐ (D) Potassium iodide
☐ (E) Selenium sulfide

17 After returning from a trip to Arizona, a 30-year-old man experiences a respiratory illness with symptoms including a cough and fever. Approximately 1 week later, he develops red, tender nodules on his shin. His physician collects sputum specimens for stains and cultures. After 1 week of incubation, the fungal culture incubated at room temperature grows a white filamentous mold. Microscopic examination of the mold is conducted (see figure). Which organism is responsible for this man's infection?

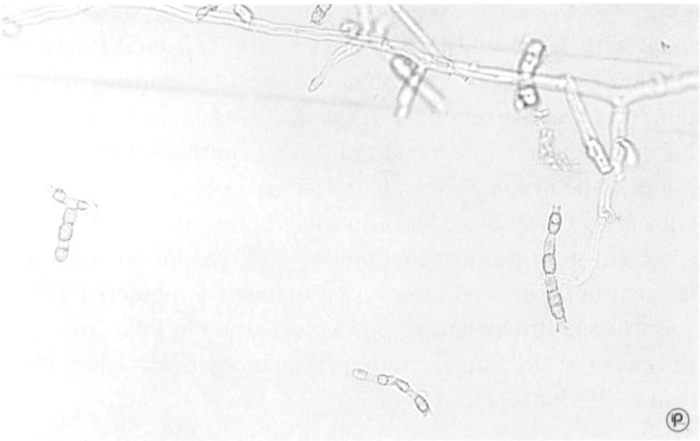

From Marler LM, Siders JA, et al: *Mycology* CD-ROM, Indiana Pathology Images, 2004.

☐ (A) *Aspergillus fumigatus*
☐ (B) *Blastomyces dermatitidis*
☐ (C) *Coccidioides immitis*
☐ (D) *Histoplasma capsulatum*
☐ (E) *Sporothrix schenckii*

18 Which component is responsible for fungi staining with acridine orange stain?

☐ (A) Chitin
☐ (B) DNA
☐ (C) Ergosterol
☐ (D) Glucan
☐ (E) Peptidoglycan

19 A 51-year-old bone marrow transplant patient became febrile 1 week after transplantation. The skin overlying an intravenous catheter is inflamed. Blood cultures are collected, and antibiotic therapy with ceftazidime and vancomycin is initiated. The catheter is removed and also cultured. After 2 days of incubation, the laboratory reports two blood cultures and the catheter as positive with yeast. Preliminary tests are performed and yield the following results: germ tube, positive; urease, negative; phenyl oxidase, negative; glucose utilization, positive. Which organism is responsible for this patient's infection?

☐ (A) *Candida albicans*
☐ (B) *Candida glabrata*
☐ (C) *Candida parapsilosis*
☐ (D) *Candida tropicalis*
☐ (E) *Cryptococcus neoformans*

20 A 64-year-old man is admitted to the hospital for the evaluation of a productive cough with blood-tinged sputum. During the preceding 3 months, he has had low-grade fevers and night sweats. He also complains of a persistent cough during this period and a 15-lb weight loss. A chest radiograph is performed, and densities are seen in the right upper lobe. A skin test for tuberculosis is negative. Sputum is collected for stains and cultures. The Gram stain and bacterial culture are negative, but a mold grows at room temperature after 2 weeks of incubation (see figure). Which organism is responsible for this man's infection?

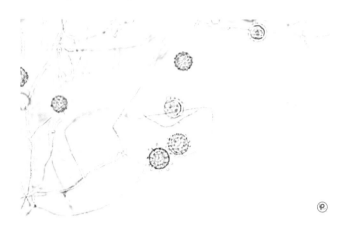

From Marler LM, Siders JA, et al: *Mycology* CD-ROM, Indiana Pathology Images, 2004.

- [ ] (A) *Blastomyces dermatitidis*
- [ ] (B) *Candida albicans*
- [ ] (C) *Coccidioides immitis*
- [ ] (D) *Cryptococcus neoformans*
- [ ] (E) *Histoplasma capsulatum*

21 Which agent is used to treat infections with *Histoplasma capsulatum?*

- [ ] (A) Amphotericin B
- [ ] (B) Caspofungin
- [ ] (C) Miconazole
- [ ] (D) Potassium iodide
- [ ] (E) Selenium sulfide

22 A 32-year-old woman, previously in good health, visits her family physician with a complaint of a low-grade fever, myalgias, and a nonproductive cough of 3 weeks duration. A chest radiograph shows infiltrate in the right middle lobe. The physician suspects the woman has an infection with *Mycoplasma pneumoniae* and prescribes an erythromycin. During the next 2 weeks, her symptoms persist, and she notices what she thinks is a small pimple that develops on her forearm. She returns to her physician who notes that her chest radiograph has worsened, she has developed a productive cough, and the lesion on her arm is 3 to 5 cm in diameter with an ulcer forming in the center. The physician collects sputum and exudates from the ulcer for stains and culture. The Gram stains and bacterial cultures are negative. No organisms are seen in the sputum specimen, but a wet mount of the exudates demonstrates organisms (see figure). After 14 days of incubation at room temperature, a mold grows in the cultures of sputum and exudates. Which fungus is responsible for this woman's infection?

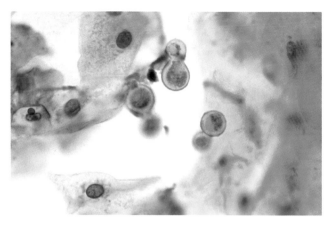

- [ ] (A) *Blastomyces dermatitidis*
- [ ] (B) *Candida albicans*
- [ ] (C) *Coccidioides immitis*
- [ ] (D) *Cryptococcus neoformans*
- [ ] (E) *Histoplasma capsulatum*

23 A 43-year-old woman with a history of alcoholic cirrhosis is brought to the emergency department of a local hospital. She is found to be febrile, disoriented, and hypotensive. Upon physical examination, she complains of abdominal pain. She is admitted to the hospital and is started on broad-spectrum antibacterial antibiotics. During the next 3 days, her fevers continue, and the abdominal pain intensifies. Paracentesis is performed, and the fluid is sent to the microbiology lab for stains and cultures. Gram stain reveals abundant polymorphonuclear leukocytes and poorly staining gram-positive cells, 3 to 5 μm in diameter. The organisms grows in 1 day on nonselective bacterial and fungal media. The organism is identified by suspending cells in serum and incubating the suspension for 2 h at 37°C. Hyphal outgrowths from the cells are observed. Which organism is responsible for this woman's infection?

- [ ] (A) *Candida albicans*
- [ ] (B) *Candida glabrata*
- [ ] (C) *Candida tropicalis*
- [ ] (D) *Cryptococcus neoformans*
- [ ] (E) *Enterococcus faecalis*

24 A 24-year-old man with AIDS develops a painful, thick, white exudate on the surface of his tongue and posterior pharynx. Gram stain reveals a gram-positive organism 2 to 3 times as large as *Staphylococcus aureus*. Which organism is most likely responsible for this man's infection?

- [ ] (A) *Blastomyces dermatitidis*
- [ ] (B) *Candida albicans*
- [ ] (C) *Cryptococcus neoformans*
- [ ] (D) *Histoplasma capsulatum*
- [ ] (E) *Paracoccidioides brasiliensis*

25 A 48-year-old man living in the western part of Texas is admitted to the community hospital with complaints of a productive cough with fever, chills, weight loss, and anorexia that have developed during the last 10 days. A chest radiograph demonstrates a right lower lobe infiltrate. Sputum is collected for stains and cultures. Microscopic examination of the specimen is negative for bacteria, mycobacteria, and yeasts, but organisms are present (see figure). A mold grows on the bacterial and fungal media after incubation for 5 days. Which organism is responsible for this man's infection?

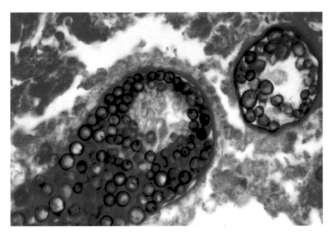

From Chandler FW, Watts JC: *Pathologic diagnosis of fungal infections*, Chicago, 1987, ASCP Press.

- ❏ (A) *Blastomyces dermatitidis*
- ❏ (B) *Candida albicans*
- ❏ (C) *Coccidioides immitis*
- ❏ (D) *Cryptococcus neoformans*
- ❏ (E) *Histoplasma capsulatum*

26 Which structural component is responsible for fungi staining with the periodic acid-Schiff stain (PAS)?

- ❏ (A) Chitin
- ❏ (B) DNA
- ❏ (C) Ergosterol
- ❏ (D) Glucan
- ❏ (E) Peptidoglycan

27 A 19-year-old homosexual man is admitted for evaluation of a 2-week history of a nonproductive cough, fever, and shortness of breath. A chest radiograph is performed and demonstrates bilateral pulmonary infiltrates with both interstitial and alveolar markings. The man is HIV positive and has a CD4+ count that is less than 200 cells/mm³. An induced sputum is collected, but all laboratory tests are negative. A bronchial alveolar lavage and biopsy are then performed. Histopathology reports indicate that 4 to 5 μm organisms are observed in the Gomori methenamine silver-stained (GMS) section of the biopsy (see figure). Which organism is responsible for this man's infection?

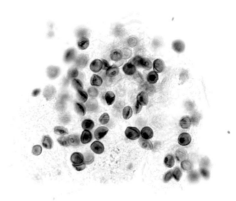

- ❏ (A) *Aspergillus fumigatus*
- ❏ (B) *Candida albicans*
- ❏ (C) *Cryptococcus neoformans*
- ❏ (D) *Histoplasma capsulatum*
- ❏ (E) *Pneumocystis (carinii) jiroveci*

28 Which agent is used to treat cutaneous infections with *Malassezia furfur?*

- ❏ (A) Amphotericin B
- ❏ (B) Caspofungin
- ❏ (C) Ketonazole
- ❏ (D) Potassium iodide
- ❏ (E) Selenium sulfide

29 A 26-year-old man with AIDS develops interstitial pneumonitis. His CD4 T cell count is below 200/mm³, and his serum levels of lactamase dehydrogenase are markedly elevated. A chest radiograph shows infiltrates that have a diffuse, fluffy appearance and that spread outward from the hilar areas. Which test would have the greatest accuracy in diagnosing this infection?

- ❏ (A) Acid-fast stain
- ❏ (B) Culture
- ❏ (C) Fluorescent antibody test
- ❏ (D) Gram stain
- ❏ (E) Trichrome stain

30 Which structural component is responsible for fungi staining with calcofluor white stain?

- ❏ (A) Chitin
- ❏ (B) DNA
- ❏ (C) Ergosterol
- ❏ (D) Glucan
- ❏ (E) Peptidoglycan

31 A 56-year-old man goes to his physician with a complaint of hypopigmented macular lesions on his chest and neck. Although they are not painful, they are unattractive, and he feels embarrassed when he is at the beach. His doctor takes some scrapings of the lesions, and a microscopic examination reveals the presence of organisms (see figure). His doctor also wants to culture the organism. Which supplement should be added to the culture medium to optimize recovery of this organism?

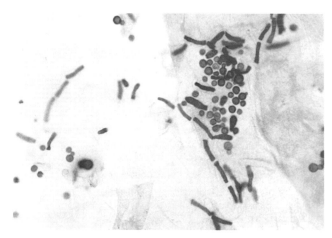

From Connor DH, et al: *Pathology of infectious diseases,* Stanford, 1997, Appleton & Lange.

☐ (A) Albumin
☐ (B) Bovine serum
☐ (C) Cysteine
☐ (D) Hemin
☐ (E) Olive oil

1 **(E) Pentamidine.** Pneumocystis, formerly classified as a parasite but now recognized to be a fungus, is susceptible to pentamidine. Pentamidine is also used in the treatment of leishmaniasis and African trypanosomiasis.
MM5 798-800

2 **(A) Ergosterol.** Fungi are eukaryotic organisms. As such, they do not have many of the components found in prokaryotic organisms, such as lipid A (endotoxin), peptidoglycan (in the cell wall of most bacteria), teichoic acid (in the cell wall of *Staphylococcus*), or 70S ribosome (consisting of 30S and 50S subunits). A prominent component of the fungal cell wall is ergosterol.
MM5 67-71, 719-723

3 **(E) *Trichophyton*.** This patient has a dermatophyte infection caused by *Trichophyton tonsurans*. The negative Wood's light examination is consistent with the characteristics of this organism. Microsporum infections typically fluoresce under the Wood's lamp. The presence of abundant microconidia but few or no macroconidia is also consistent with *T. tonsurans*. *Epidermophyton* infections are characterized by abundant macroconidia but not microconidia. *Malassezia* grows as a yeast and not as a mold. *Trichosporon* causes infections of the hair, forming adherent nodules on the hair shaft. Conidia are not observed in culture.
MM5 748-754

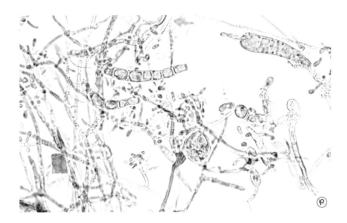

From Marler LM, Siders JA, et al: *Mycology* CD-ROM, Indiana Pathology Images, 2004.

4 **(C) Enzyme-linked immunosorbent assay (ELISA) test for *Cryptococcus* antigen in CSF.** Although *C. neoformans* is gram-positive, the fungi stain weakly and may be missed by an inexperienced microscopist. A gram stain is certainly less sensitive compared to the antigen tests. Detection of the polysaccharide antigen from the capsule of *C. neoformans* in the CSF is a sensitive and specific method for the rapid diagnosis of infections with this organism. This can be done by either an ELISA test or a latex agglutination test. Virtually all patients with an infection will have a positive antigen test. In some patients, particularly HIV-infected patients, the titers of antigen will be extremely high, which persists for months to years. The ELISA and latex agglutination tests have replaced the India ink stain and are the tests of choice for early diagnosis. The India ink stain (used to highlight the encapsulated cell) is less sensitive compared to the antigen tests. In contrast with some other pathogens, cryptococcal antigen is not detected in urine. Most patients with cryptococcosis are immunocompromised and produce a poor antibody response to infection.
MM5 787-789

5 **(A) Calcofluor white stain.** Calcofluor white is used for the detection of fungi and parasites. This is a nonspecific fluorochrome that binds to cellulose and chitin. Chitin is present in the cell wall of fungi. *C. neoformans* can stain with the Gram stain, but this result is not specific for this organism. The Kinyoun stain is an acid-fast stain and will not stain *C. neoformans*. The trichrome stain is used to detect parasites, particularly protozoa. The Wright-Giemsa stain is used to detect blood-borne pathogens (e.g., *Borrelia*, *Ehrlichia*, *Anaplasma*, *Rickettsia*, *Plasmodium*, *Babesia*, microfilaria).
MM5 734-738

6 **(B) *Aspergillus fumigatus*.** *A. fumigatus* is the most common *Aspergillus* species associated with opportunistic infections in immunocompromised patients. The genus *Aspergillus* is a member of the group of fungi with septated, hyaline (colorless) hyphae. Identification of the specific species is based on their morphologic appearance: macroscopic and microscopic. *A. fumigatus* typically has a green pigment on the surface of the colonies, club-shaped head with conidia (spores) radiating from the upper two thirds of the head.
MM5 791-793

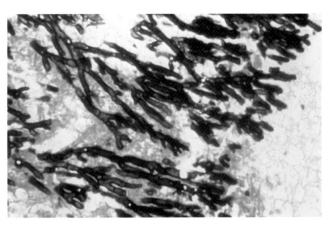

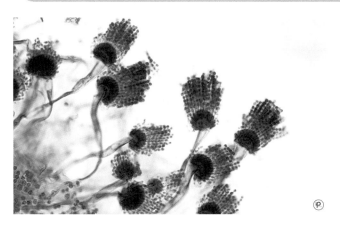

From Marler LM, Siders JA, et al: *Mycology* CD-ROM, Indiana Pathology Images, 2004.

7 **(E) *Sporothrix schenckii*.** This patient has chronic arthritis caused by *Sporothrix*. Her course was complicated by the failure to identify this dimorphic fungus when she initially complained of her symptoms. Microscopy is generally insensitive for making the diagnosis because the yeast cells are generally not abundant. If seen, they are described as looking "cigar-like." The mold grows relatively rapidly for a dimorphic fungus. The colonies will initially appear waxy and then turn more filamentous with extended incubation. The surface will also turn a brown-black color with time. This is a dermatiaceous mold (pigmented hyphae) that has characteristics of a fruiting structure resembling flowers that develop off the hyphae. The other fungi listed in the answers to this question all have hyaline hyphae and do not produce a dark mold.
MM5 755-757

8 **(B) Chlorine.** Most disinfectants have some activity against fungi and enveloped viruses; however, of the agents listed in the answers to this question, only chlorine compounds (e.g., elemental chlorine, hypochlorous acid, hypochlorite ion) have uniform activity against all fungi and viruses. Alcohol and phenolics have good activity against fungi but not against some viruses. Iodophors and quaternary ammonium compounds have poor activity against some fungi; some iodophors have some activity against viruses, and quarternary ammonium compounds have activity against all viruses.
MM5 92-94

9 **(E) *Rhizopus*.** The organism in the figure is a nonseptated mold (a zygomycetes). The only mold listed in this question that is nonseptated is *Rhizopus*. Other zygomycetes that cause human disease include *Absidia, Cunninghamella, Mucor, Rhizomucor,* and *Saksenaea*. These molds are ubiquitous, and exposure for most people is inconsequential. Some individuals, such as patients with uncontrolled diabetes mellitus, are at increased risk for infections. Rhinocerebral mucormycosis (invasion of a zygomycetes into the sinuses and then to the orbit or brain) is a

particular concern in diabetic patients in acidosis. This disease is fatal unless promptly treated.
MM5 793-795

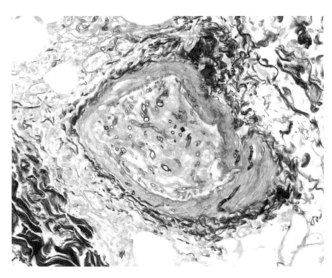

10 **(D) Potassium iodide.** Sporotrichosis is most effectively treated with potassium iodide administered orally. For patients who cannot tolerate this treatment, itraconazole has been successful. Amphotericin B is considered too toxic for treating lymphocutaneous sporotrichosis. The other agents listed in the answers to this question are ineffective against *S. schenckii*.
MM5 755-757

11 **(C) *Histoplasma capsulatum*.** *B. dermatitidis, C. immitis, H. capsulatum,* and *S. schenckii* are dimorphic fungi—they grow as filamentous molds at room temperature and as unicellular cells when infecting humans and grow at 37°C. Each fungus grows slowly, requiring up to 2 to 4 weeks incubation before growth is detected. Identification of the fungi is based on their morphological appearance at both temperatures. The yeast phase of *H. capsulatum* appears as budding cells 3 to 4 μm in diameter. The mold form of *H. capsulatum* appears as thin mycelia with both macroconidia and microconidia. The macroconidia are described as tuberculate or cells with knobby projections. *H. capsulatum* typically infects humans by the respiratory route, where an asymptomatic infection most commonly occurs. Symptomatic disease may present as a mild flu-like illness or progress to cavitary disease. Disseminated disease can involve multiple organs, including the central nervous system, liver, spleen, and bones. In this case, the active disseminated disease weakened the girl's humerus and then spread to the overlying tissues following the break. *S. aureus* is the most common bacterium that produces a similar disease; however, the culture results are inconsistent with *S. aureus*.
MM5 772-775

12 **(A) Amphotericin B.** Amphotericin B binds to ergosterol, a sterol present in the fungal cell membrane. Although this drug is relatively toxic, it is a mainstay in the treatment of disseminated fungal infections. The other agents listed in the answers to this question are ineffective against *C. glabrata*.
MM5 719-723

13 **(E) Sporothrix.** This woman has an infection with the dimorphic fungus *Sporothrix schenckii.* The mold lives in soil rich in organic material. Most infections are acquired when the fungus is introduced into the cutaneous tissues by mild trauma, usually associated with gardening. At body temperature, the fungus replicates as a yeast and has been referred to as "cigar-shaped." At 25° to 30°C, the fungus grows as a dematiaceous mold. The delicate "rosette" arrangement of the conidia on the conidophores is characteristic of *Sporothrix* (suggesting the dangers of rose gardening). *Candida* exists only in the yeast form and *Microsporum* only as a mold. *Blastomyces* and *Histoplasma* are both dimorphic fungi (have both a yeast and a mold phase) and can cause skin lesions (much more common with *Blastomyces*). The yeast and mold phases, however, do not resemble those of *Sporothrix*.
MM5 755-757

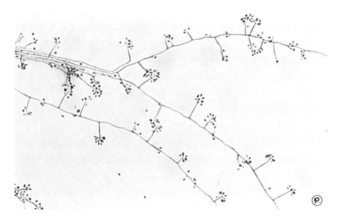

From Marler LM, Siders JA, et al: *Mycology* CD-ROM, Indiana Pathology Images, 2004.

14 **(D) Trichophyton rubrum.** This man has a dermatophyte infection of his feet. Each of the fungi listed in the answers to this question are dermatophytes, so the specific diagnosis of the causal agent requires examination of the macroscopic and microscopic morphology of the isolate. Colonies of *T. rubrum* are white to buff-colored on the surface and red to purple on the reverse side (observed because media used for the isolation of dermatophytes is clear). Microscopically, all dermatophytes have hyaline, septated hyphae. Differentiation of the different genera and species is determined by the presence and shape of microconidia and macroconidia. *Trichophyton* species have numerous microconidia and rare, thin-walled, smooth macroconidia. *M. canis* has microconidia and numerous, thick-walled, rough

macroconidia. *E. floccosum*, the third dermatophyte genus, does not form microconidia and has numerous, thin- and thick-walled macroconidia. The microscopic appearance of this patient's mold is consistent with a *Trichophyton* species. The microconidia of *T. rubrum* are typically singly arranged compared with microconidia clusters of *T. mentagrophytes*. In addition, the bottom of *T. mentagrophytes* colonies is typically tan in color. Because *T. mentagrophytes* is a common cause of "athlete's foot," differentation from *T. rubrum* is important. *T. tonsurans*, a cause of scalp infections and infections of nails, has variably shaped microconidia and enlarged balloon forms. *M. canis* causes infections of the scalp and skin, particularly in children exposed to infected dogs or cats. *E. floccosum* causes infections in skin and nails.
MM5 748-754

15 **(D) Malassezia.** *Malassezia* is a lipophilic fungus that is found in areas of the body that are rich in sebaceous glands. This fungus is part of the normal flora of the human skin. *Bacteroides* species and *Escherichia* species are primarily restricted to the intestines; *Lactobacillus* species infect acidic areas such as the stomach, upper small intestine, and genitourinary tract; and *Streptococcus* is found primarily in the upper respiratory tract.
MM5 745-746

16 **(C) Miconazole.** All but the most severe dermatophyte infections are treated with a topical azole, such as miconazole. These agents are uniformly active and, if used for a sufficient duration, effect cure. The other agents listed in the answers to this question are ineffective against *T. mentagrophyte* and other dermatophytes.
MM5 723-725

17 **(C) Coccidioides immitis.** This man has coccidioidomycosis. This fungus is endemic in the southwestern states of the United States, with infections common in Arizona. Most exposures result in an asymptomatic infection; however, progressive pulmonary disease and meningitis can occur. The mold form of this dimorphic fungus grows in nature and is highly contagious. The arthroconidia (barrel-shaped spores seen in the figure) can be readily dispersed in winds and drift for many miles. Inhalation of these spores can initiate infection. The form of the fungus that is seen in patients is that of an endospore-filled, thick-walled spherule. None of the other fungi listed in the answers to this question can produce arthroconidia.
MM5 769-772

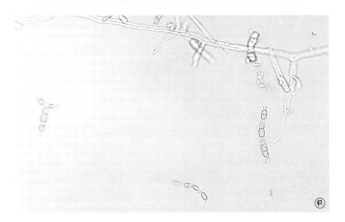

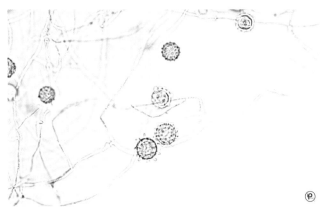

From Marler LM, Siders JA, et al: *Mycology* CD-ROM, Indiana Pathology Images, 2004.

From Marler LM, Siders JA, et al: *Mycology* CD-ROM, Indiana Pathology Images, 2004

18 **(B) DNA.** Acridine orange is a fluorochrome that intercalates nucleic acid. Bacterial and fungal DNA fluoresce as an orange color, and mammalian DNA fluoresces as a green color with ultraviolet (UV) excitation using a fluorescent microscope. Acridine orange will not bind to other components, such as chitin, ergosterol, and glucan present in the fungal cell wall and peptidoglycan found in bacterial cell walls.
MM5 734-738

19 **(A) *Candida albicans.*** This patient has a line infection with *C. albicans*. The key identification test for this fungus is the germ tube. *C. albicans* can be identified if the 2-h test is positive. If it is negative, additional tests, such as carbohydrate utilization tests, must be performed. *C. glabrata* is a common pathogen, particularly associated with urinary tract infections. *C. parapsilosis* has a predilection for infections associated with hyperalimentation lines. *C. tropicalis* is associated with infections of immunocompromised patients. *C. neoformans* (positive for both urease and phenol oxidase) is also an important pathogen in immunocompromised patients.
MM5 779-787

20 **(E) *Histoplasma capsulatum.*** This man has pulmonary histoplasmosis. Characteristically, this dimorphic fungus grows as small, oval yeast cells in patients and as a mold when cultures are incubated at room temperature. The characteristic structure that allows identification of this slow-growing mold is the presence of thin, septated, hyaline hyphae with large, thick-walled tuberculated or knobby macroconidia and small, pear-shaped microconidia. The mold phases of *B. dermatitidis* and *C. immitis* do not resemble the phase of *H. capsulatum*, and C. *albicans* and C. *neoformans* only are observed as yeasts.
MM5 772-775

21 **(A) Amphotericin B.** Amphotericin B binds to ergosterol, a sterol present in the fungal cell membrane. Although this drug is relatively toxic, it is a mainstay in the treatment of disseminated fungal infections. The other agents listed in the answers to this question are ineffective against *H. capsulatum*.
MM5 719-723

22 **(A) *Blastomyces dermatitidis.*** This patient has pulmonary blastomycosis with dissemination to the skin. This is a dimorphic fungus. The mold phase (at 25° to 30°C) grows slowly, first forming yeast-like colonies and then turning "cottony" with a white surface and tan bottom. Small, pear-shaped conidia grow on the septated hyphae (resembling lollipops). The yeast cells seen in the patient's specimens are large (8 to 15 μm in diameter) with a thick wall and are connected at a broad base. Yeast forms of *C. albicans*, *C. neoformans*, and *H. capsulatum* are smaller and more delicate. *C. immitis* does not form yeast cells; rather, spherules are seen in patient specimens.
MM5 765-769

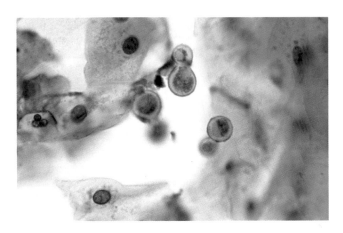

23 **(A)** *Candida albicans.* This woman has fungal peritonitis. The diagnostic test described in this question is the germ tube test. *C. albicans* has the unique ability to form germ tubes (hyphal extensions from the yeast cells) when incubated in serum for 2 h. If the incubation period is extended, other yeast can also form germ tubes. Care must be taken to differentiate germ tubes from pseudohyphae, which are found in many yeasts. Although *E. faecalis* can produce peritonitis, the lack of response to broad-spectrum antibiotics would tend to exclude this organism from the diagnosis. In addition, enterococci and most bacteria are significantly smaller than yeast cells, and enterococci do not form hyphal extensions.
MM5 779-787

24 **(B)** *Candida albicans.* This man has oral thrush. This infection is most commonly caused by *C. albicans*, although other *Candida* species (e.g., *C. tropicalis*, *C. glabrata*, *C. krusei*) can also cause these symptoms. Mucosal *Candida* infections are typically associated with impaired cellular immunity, with the incidence of disease greatest when the CD4+ cell counts fall below 200/mm^3. The other fungi listed in the answers to this question do not produce mucosal infections as described here.
MM5 779-787

25 **(C)** *Coccidioides immitis.* The structure in the figure is a spherule, characteristic of *Coccidioides*. Spherules are produced by *C. immitis* when it grows in a human. When the organism is cultured in the laboratory, it grows as a filamentous mold. The characteristic structure of the mold is barrel-shaped arthroconidia. These can be easily dispensed in the air and are highly infectious. None of the other fungi listed in the answers to this question can form spherules.
MM5 769-772

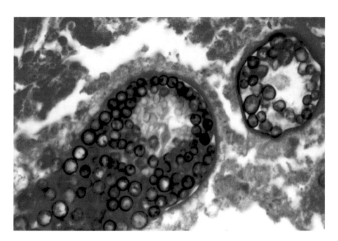

From Chandler FW, Watts JC: *Pathologic diagnosis of fungal infections*, Chicago, 1987, ASCP Press.

26 **(D) Glucan.** The periodic acid-Schiff stain (PAS) stains cell wall carbohydrates in fungi (e.g., glucan). It is a time-consuming stain and primarily used in anatomic pathology labs. The stain is used most commonly to detect *Cryptococcus neoformans* in tissue specimens. The capsule surrounding *Cryptococcus* will stain intensely pink with the PAS stain. PAS does not bind to chitin, DNA, ergosterol, or peptidoglycan.
MM5 734-738

27 **(E)** *Pneumocystis (carinii) jiroveci.* This patient has *Pneumocystis* pneumonia. *P. jiroveci*, like all yeasts, will stain with silver stains. This fungus must be distinguished from *C. albicans* and the yeast forms of other fungi. *C. albicans* rarely causes pulmonary infections, so this organism is less likely than *P. jiroveci* to be responsible for the patient's infection. *A. fumigatus* does not form yeast-like cells. *C. neoformans* causes pulmonary infections, particularly in immunocompromised patients; however, the cells are slightly larger (4 to 8 μm) and are typically surrounded by a capsule. The yeast form of *Histoplasma* is smaller (2 to 3 μm by 4 to 5 μm) and is typically intracellular.
MM5 798-800

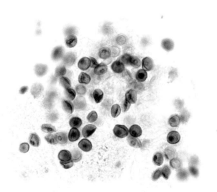

28 **(E) Selenium sulfide.** *Malassezia furfur* infections (tinea versicolor) are treated with the topical application of selenium sulfide, an over-the-counter solution that can be purchased at any drug store. Amphotericin B can be used for systemic infections, but the other organisms listed in the answers to this question are ineffective.
MM5 745-746

29 **(C) Fluorescent antibody test.** This patient most likely has an infection with *Pneumocystis (carinii) jiroveci*. This fungus (formerly thought to be a protozoa) is a significant cause of pulmonary disease in patients with AIDS. The chest radiograph is typical of this infection. A number of different methods have been used to detect this organism, including use of calcofluor white, Giemsa, and silver stains. The calcofluor white stain will stain all fungi, and these may be difficult to distinguish from *P.*

jiroveci. The Giemsa stain is a reliable procedure, but *P. jiroveci* may be difficult to detect for inexperienced microscopists. Silver stains will stain all fungi, which may also cause a problem. Fluorescent antibody tests have been developed that specifically stain *Pneumocystis* species, and these are the microscopic tests of choice. Specific polymerase chain reaction (PCR) tests are also available in some laboratories and are the most sensitive and specific tests. The organism does not stain with the acid-fast stain or trichrome stain and stains weakly with the Gram stain. The organism cannot be cultured.

MM5 798-800

30 **(A) Chitin.** Calcofluor white is a nonspecific fluorochrome that binds to β1,3- and β1,4-polysaccharides, specifically, cellulose and chitin in the cell walls of fungi. Fungal elements appear bluish white against a dark background when chitin is used to stain a fungal preparation and when the preparation is examined using a fluorescent microscope.

MM5 734-738

31 **(E) Olive oil.** This man's infection is pityriasis (tinea) versicolor caused by *Malessezia furfur.* The organism can also cause catheter-related systemic infection in infants and adults receiving intravenous lipids. The organism can grow rapidly in culture if a source of lipids is provided. This is most conveniently done by adding a few drops of olive oil to the surface of a blood agar plate. None of the other supplements listed in the answers to this question, although commonly used as media supplements, would affect the growth of this organism. Morphologically, the organism grows as yeast-like cells (1.5 to 4.5 μm by 2.0 to 6.5 μm in size). A small collar is seen encircling the upper third of the cell.

MM5 745-746

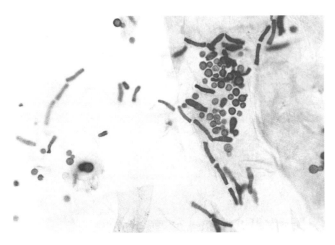

From Connor DH, et al: *Pathology of infectious diseases,* Stanford, 1997, Appleton & Lange.

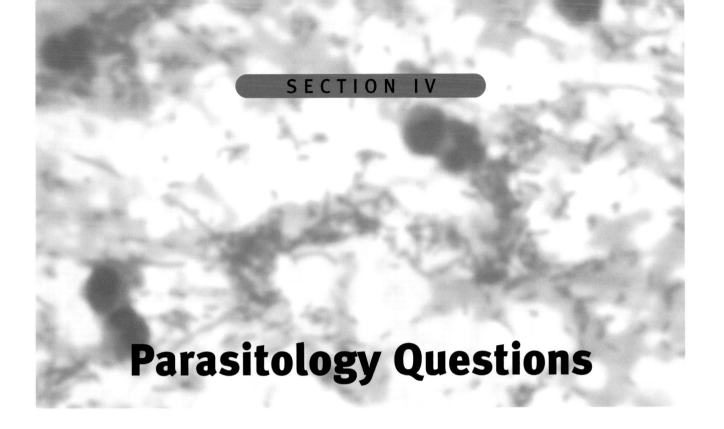

Parasitology Questions

1 Which antimicrobial would be used to treat infections with *Naegleria?*

- ❐ (A) Amphotericin B
- ❐ (B) Albendazole
- ❐ (C) Chloroquine
- ❐ (D) Metronidazole
- ❐ (E) Pentamidine

2 Which route of infection is common for *Strongyloides stercoralis?*

- ❐ (A) Direct inoculation
- ❐ (B) Direct skin penetration
- ❐ (C) Fecal-oral
- ❐ (D) Inhalation
- ❐ (E) Mosquito bite

3 Which microscopic staining method should be used to detect *Babesia?*

- ❐ (A) Calcofluor white
- ❐ (B) Giemsa
- ❐ (C) Gram
- ❐ (D) Kinyoun
- ❐ (E) Trichrome

4 Approximately 3 days after attending a wedding reception in St. Louis, Missouri, 32 guests become ill with symptoms that include diarrhea, anorexia, abdominal cramping, and a low-grade fever. Cultures for bacteria and viral pathogens are negative. Coccoid forms, 8 to 10 μm in diameter that stain acid-fast are seen on ova and parasite (O&P) examination (see figure). Which organism is most likely responsible for these infections?

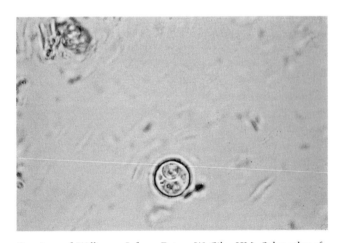

Courtesy of Williams, J; from Peters W, Giles HM: *Color atlas of tropical medicine and parasitology*, ed 4, London, 1995, Mosby-Wolfe.

- ❐ (A) *Candida*
- ❐ (B) *Cryptosporidium*
- ❐ (C) *Cyclospora*
- ❐ (D) *Isospora*
- ❐ (E) Microsporidia

5 Which vector is associated with disease caused by *Onchocerca volvulus?*

- ❐ (A) Chrysops fly
- ❐ (B) Reduviid bug
- ❐ (C) Sandfly
- ❐ (D) Simulium black fly
- ❐ (E) Tsetse fly

6 A 23-year old man returns from a camping trip in Mexico. He presents to the emergency department suffering from abdominal pain, nausea, fever, and bloody diarrhea. Stool specimens are collected and submitted to the laboratory for bacterial cultures and (O&P) examination. Bacterial cultures are negative for enteric pathogens, but the (O&P) examination reveals an organism (see figure). Which host is a primary reservoir for this parasite?

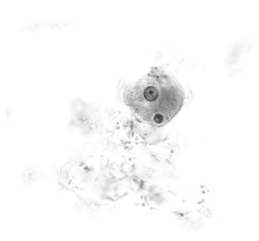

From Marler LM, Siders JA, et al: *Parasitology* CD-ROM, Indiana Patholgy Images, 2003.

☐ (A) Cockroach
☐ (B) Dog
☐ (C) Fly
☐ (D) Human
☐ (E) Mosquito

7 Which disease is transmitted by fleas?

☐ (A) African trypanosomiasis
☐ (B) Plague
☐ (C) Epidemic relapsing fever
☐ (D) Rickettsial pox
☐ (E) Tularemia

8 Which route of infection is most common for *Ascaris lumbricoides?*

☐ (A) Direct inoculation
☐ (B) Direct skin penetration
☐ (C) Fecal-oral route
☐ (D) Inhalation
☐ (E) Mosquito bite

9 Which disease is transmitted by ticks?

☐ (A) African trypanosomiasis
☐ (B) Babesiosis
☐ (C) Epidemic relapsing fever
☐ (D) Rickettsial pox
☐ (E) Toxoplasmosis

10 A 36-year-old man returns from a fishing trip in Colorado. He presents to the emergency department of a local hospital with complaints of 4 days of watery diarrhea, crampy epigastric pain, and foul-smelling flatulence. A stool specimen submitted for (O&P) examination is positive for a parasite (see figure). Which host is the most common reservoir?

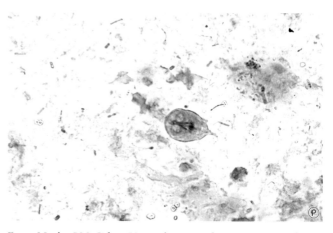

From Marler LM, Siders JA, et al: *Parasitology* CD-ROM, Indiana Patholgy Images, 2003.

☐ (A) Beaver
☐ (B) Dog
☐ (C) Rabbit
☐ (D) Snake
☐ (E) Trout

11 Which disease is transmitted by ticks?

☐ (A) African trypanosomiasis
☐ (B) Plague
☐ (C) Epidemic relapsing fever
☐ (D) Rickettsial pox
☐ (E) Tularemia

12 Which parasitic disease is distributed worldwide?

☐ (A) *Babesia microti*
☐ (B) *Cryptosporidium parvum*
☐ (C) *Plasmodium falciparum*
☐ (D) *Strongyloides stercoralis*
☐ (E) *Trypanosoma cruzi*

13 A previously healthy 45-year-old man sees his physician with a history of 10 days of diarrhea alternating with constipation, abdominal discomfort, vomiting, anorexia, intense fatigue, and myalgia. He tells the physician that his wife and four other friends are suffering from similar symptoms. Approximately 5 days before his symptoms began, he and his wife and friends had eaten at a local restaurant. An organism is observed when an acid-fast stain of the patient's stool specimen is performed. The organism is approximately 10 μm in diameter. What is this organism?

❏ (A) *Cryptosporidium parvum*

❏ (B) *Cyclospora cayetanensis*

❏ (C) *Entamoeba histolytica*

❏ (D) *Mycobacterium avium*

❏ (E) *Rhodococcus equi*

14 Which route of infection is most common for *Acanthamoeba?*

❏ (A) Direct inoculation

❏ (B) Direct skin penetration

❏ (C) Fecal-oral

❏ (D) Inhalation

❏ (E) Mosquito bite

15 Which antimicrobial drug would be used to treat infections with *Trichinella?*

❏ (A) Amphotericin B

❏ (B) Albendazole

❏ (C) Chloroquine

❏ (D) Metronidazole

❏ (E) Pentamidine

16 A 36-year-old Peace Corps worker in West Africa returns to the United States for an extended family visit. While at home, he complains of not feeling well. During the course of 1 week, he develops symptoms of severe myalgia, abdominal discomfort, vomiting, diarrhea, fever, chills, and sweats. Because his symptoms are not improving, he goes to the local university hospital. Upon physical examination, the physician notes enlarged cervical lymph nodes. Blood is drawn for culture, and thick and thin smears are prepared and stained by the Giemsa method. The lymph node is also aspirated and Gram stained and cultured for bacteria; a Giemsa stain is prepared. The bacterial stains and cultures of blood and lymph nodes are negative. Slender protozoa with long, free flagella, however, are observed in the blood and lymph nodes. Which organism is most likely responsible for this patient's infection?

❏ (A) *Leishmania donovani*

❏ (B) *Plasmodium falciparum*

❏ (C) *Toxoplasma gondii*

❏ (D) *Trypanosoma cruzi*

❏ (E) *Trypanosoma brucei*

17 The public health department notifies owners of an aquatic park that eight children have developed diarrheal disease in the week following their visit to the park. The children have profuse, watery diarrhea; abdominal cramping; and low-grade fevers. Parasitology examination of their stool specimens is positive with acid-fast cocci that are 4 to 6 μm in diameter. The public health department closes the park and collects specimens from the food service and water pools. Which source is the most likely cause of these infections?

❏ (A) Basil in salad

❏ (B) Chicken

❏ (C) Contaminated water

❏ (D) Seafood appetizer

❏ (E) Cake

18 A 32-year-old woman infected with human immunodeficiency virus (HIV) presents to her primary care physician with a 1-month history of chronic, nonbloody, watery diarrhea and a 15-lb weight loss. Her CD4 lymphocyte count is less than 50/mm^3. A stool examination for bacterial pathogens and routine (O&P) examination are negative. A jejunal biopsy is then performed, which reveals parasites that are 1 to 2 μm (see figure) Which parasite is most likely responsible for this infection?

From Marler LM, Siders JA, et al: *Parasitology* CD-ROM, Indiana Patholgy Images, 2003.

❏ (A) *Cryptosporidium*

❏ (B) *Cyclospora*

❏ (C) *Giardia*

❏ (D) *Isospora*

❏ (E) *Microsporidium*

19 Which disease is transmitted by lice?

❏ (A) African trypanosomiasis

❏ (B) Plague

❏ (C) Epidemic relapsing fever

❏ (D) Rickettsial pox

❏ (E) Tularemia

20 A 25-year-old man infected with HIV presents to his physician with a 10-week history of profuse, nonbloody, watery diarrhea and an 18-lb weight loss. A stool examination for ova and parasites demonstrates an organism (see figure). The parasite measures 25 μm long and 15 μm in width with tapering ends. The parasites are also observed when the stool specimen is stained with an acid-fast stain. Which organism is most likely responsible for this patient's disease?

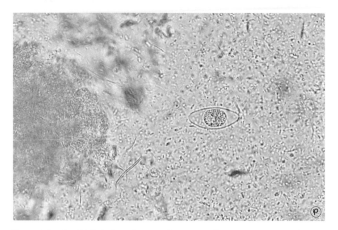

From Marler LM, Siders JA, et al: *Parasitology* CD-ROM, Indiana Patholgy Images, 2003.

□ (A) *Cryptosporidium*
□ (B) *Cyclospora*
□ (C) *Entamoeba*
□ (D) *Giardia*
□ (E) *Isospora*

21 Disease caused by which parasite is associated with consumption of contaminated fish?

□ (A) *Diphyllobothrium latum*
□ (B) *Echinococcus multilocularis*
□ (C) *Fasciola hepatica*
□ (D) *Hymenolepis diminuta*
□ (E) *Paragonimus westermani*

22 Which disease is transmitted by flies?

□ (A) African trypanosomiasis
□ (B) Plague
□ (C) Epidemic relapsing fever
□ (D) Rickettsial pox
□ (E) Tularemia

23 A 24-year-old marine returns to the United States after spending 15 months in Iraq. When he returns to his base, he notices a small raised erythematous area next to his eye. During the next 5 weeks, the area enlarges to the size of a quarter and develops into an ulcer with a serous exudate. The lesion is itchy but not painful. Upon examination, enlarged axillary and cervical lymph nodes are also noted. One of the enlarged nodes is aspirated, and an organism is observed on a stained impression smear (see figure). Which organism is most likely responsible for this patient's infection?

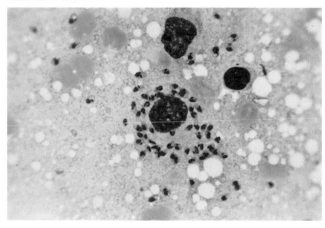

From Cohen J, Powderly WG: *Infectious diseases*, ed 2, St Louis, 2004, Mosby.

□ (A) *Babesia microti*
□ (B) *Leishmania braziliensis*
□ (C) *Plasmodium vivax*
□ (D) *Toxoplasma gondii*
□ (E) *Trypanosoma cruzi*

24 Which route of infection is most common for *Enterobius vermicularis?*

□ (A) Direct inoculation
□ (B) Direct skin penetration
□ (C) Fecal-oral
□ (D) Inhalation
□ (E) Mosquito bite

25 A 56-year-old woman returns from a 2-week vacation in Kenya. While in Africa, she traveled extensively throughout both urban and rural areas. During her trip, she ate local foods prepared in restaurants and by street vendors. She drank local water when she did not have bottled water. Upon her return to the United States, she develops diarrhea and a low-grade fever. She takes ciprofloxacin for her illness (self-prescribed) and, within 3 days, begins to feel better. Her fever, however, persists, and she develops night sweats. Because of these symptoms, she goes to her physician. He orders blood cultures and a thick and thin smear of her blood. The tests reveal organisms in her blood (see figure). Which organism is most likely responsible for her infection?

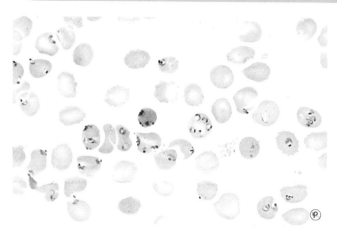

From Marler LM, Siders JA, et al: *Parasitology* CD-ROM, Indiana Pathology Images, 2003.

- ❐ (A) *Babesia microti*
- ❐ (B) *Plasmodium falciparum*
- ❐ (C) *Plasmodium malariae*
- ❐ (D) *Plasmodium vivax*
- ❐ (E) *Trypanosoma cruzi*

26 *Toxoplasma gondii* is able to avoid the host immune response by which mechanism?

- ❐ (A) Acquisition of host antigens
- ❐ (B) Encystment in muscle
- ❐ (C) Formation of thick extracellular cuticle
- ❐ (D) Inhibition of phagosome/lysosome fusion
- ❐ (E) Intracellular replication

27 Which organism can be stained with a modified acid-fast stain?

- ❐ (A) *Actinomyces*
- ❐ (B) *Corynebacterium*
- ❐ (C) *Cryptosporidium*
- ❐ (D) *Giardia*
- ❐ (E) *Streptomyces*

28 A 22-year-old man presents to the emergency department with complaints of eye pain and blurred vision during the preceding day. He does not remember an eye injury but has been wearing contact lenses for an extended period when the eye pain started. The patient also admits to cleaning his contacts with nonsterile water. Examination of the eye reveals ulceration of the cornea. Cultures for bacteria, including *Neisseria gonorrhoeae* and *Chlamydia trachomatis*, are negative. However, Giemsa stain of the eye scrapings reveal an organism (see figure). Which organism is most likely responsible for this infection?

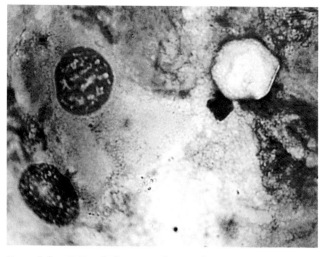

From Cohen J, Powderly WG: *Infectious diseases*, ed 2, St Louis, 2004, Mosby.

- ❐ (A) *Acanthamoeba*
- ❐ (B) *Dientamoeba*
- ❐ (C) *Entamoeba*
- ❐ (D) *Isospora*
- ❐ (E) Microsporidia

29 A 24-year-old woman presents to the emergency department with profuse, nonbloody, watery diarrhea. The diarrhea developed over the preceding 5 days. She has a history of HIV infection, has not taken her antiviral drugs, and has a low CD4 lymphocyte count (less than 50/mm^3) when she arrives at the hospital. Stool samples are collected for bacterial and parasitic examinations. The bacterial cultures are negative for common pathogens, and the *Clostridium difficile* assay is negative. The parasitic examine is positive for organisms (see figure). The organisms are small (between 1 to 2 μm in diameter) and observed with a special stain. Which organism are most likely responsible for this patient's chronic diarrhea?

From Cohen J, Powderly WG: *Infectious diseases*, ed 2, St Louis, 2004, Mosby.

- ❐ (A) *Cryptosporidium*
- ❐ (B) *Cyclospora*
- ❐ (C) *Entamoeba*
- ❐ (D) *Giardia*
- ❐ (E) Microsporidia

30 Which antimicrobial drug would be used to treat infections with *Trichomonas vaginalis?*

- ❐ (A) Amphotericin B
- ❐ (B) Albendazole
- ❐ (C) Chloroquine
- ❐ (D) Metronidazole
- ❐ (E) Pentamidine

31 A family with 25 members meets for an annual picnic. In the week following the picnic, 15 children and adults develop a diarrheal disease with 5 to 10 bowel movements a day, anorexia, abdominal cramping, and a low-grade fever. Stool specimens are submitted for culture and (O&P) examination. The parasitology tests are reported to be positive for acid-fast cocci, 8 to 10 μm in diameter. Which source most likely led to these infections?

- ❐ (A) Basil in salad
- ❐ (B) Chicken
- ❐ (C) Contaminated water
- ❐ (D) Seafood appetizer
- ❐ (E) Cake

32 A mother notices that her 4-year-old boy is persistently scratching his anus. The boy is taken to his pediatrician for an evaluation. A parasitic examination reveals the presence of eggs (see figure). Which organism is responsible for this patient's symptoms?

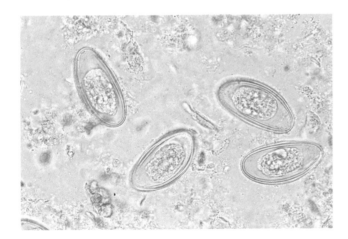

- ❐ (A) *Ascaris*
- ❐ (B) *Enterobius*
- ❐ (C) *Necator*
- ❐ (D) *Toxocara*
- ❐ (E) *Trichuris*

33 Which vector is associated with disease caused by Loa loa?

- ❐ (A) Chrysops fly
- ❐ (B) Reduviid bug
- ❐ (C) Sandfly
- ❐ (D) Simulium black fly
- ❐ (E) Tsetse fly

34 A 56-year-old businessman returns from China after a 1-year stay; he develops diarrhea and abdominal pain in the right upper quadrant. Examination in the hospital reveals a palpable liver, and laboratory tests document an elevation in liver enzymes. When questioned about his diet, he states he enjoyed eating many of the local delicacies, including raw fish and uncooked watercress. Eggs are observed when the stool is examined for parasites (see figure). Which organism is responsible for this patient's illness?

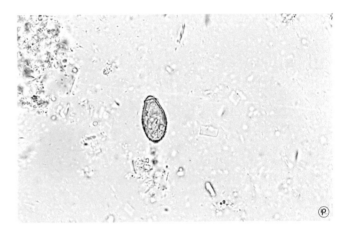

- ❐ (A) *Ancyclostoma duodenale*
- ❐ (B) *Fasciola hepatica*
- ❐ (C) *Opisthorchis sinensis*
- ❐ (D) *Paragonimus westermani*
- ❐ (E) *Schistosoma mansoni*

35 Disease caused by which parasite is associated with consumption of contaminated meat?

- ❐ (A) *Diphyllobothrium latum*
- ❐ (B) *Echniococcus multilocularis*
- ❐ (C) *Fasciola hepatica*
- ❐ (D) *Giardia lamblia*
- ❐ (E) *Taenia saginata*

36 A previously healthy 18-year-old boy is brought to the emergency department suffering from a 40.2°C fever, a severe headache, and vomiting. Because the weather is warm, he has spent the last several weeks swimming in a local pond. The physician notes the patient has a stiff neck and performs a lumbar puncture. The laboratory reports a cell count of 20,000/mm^3 with a predominance of neutrophils. The glucose level is low, and the protein level is markedly elevated. No bacteria are observed on Gram stain, and the culture is negative. Which test of the cerebrospinal fluid (CSF) should be considered?

- ❐ (A) Acid-fast stain
- ❐ (B) Bacterial antigen test
- ❐ (C) Cryptococcal antigen test
- ❐ (D) Enzyme-linked immunosorbent assay (ELISA) test for *Borrelia*
- ❐ (E) Trichrome stain

37 A 23-year-old Peace Corps worker living in Africa for the previous year develops symptoms of nausea, vomiting, and diarrhea while visiting family in New York. Stool specimens are collected for bacterial culture and O&P examination. The bacterial cultures are negative, but the O&P examination is positive for an organism (see figure). What is the most likely source of this woman's infection?

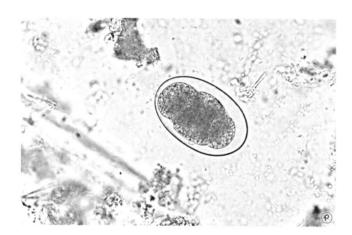

- ❐ (A) Consumption of uncooked pork
- ❐ (B) Consumption of contaminated raw vegetables
- ❐ (C) Direct skin penetration by infectious larvae
- ❐ (D) Oral exposure to the feces of an infected dog
- ❐ (E) Oral exposure to the feces of an infected human

38 *Trichinella spiralis* is able to avoid the host's immune response by which mechanism?

- ❐ (A) Acquisition of host antigens
- ❐ (B) Encystment in muscle
- ❐ (C) Formation of thick extracellular cuticle
- ❐ (D) Inhibition of phagosome/lysosome fusion
- ❐ (E) Intracellular replication

39 A 20-year-old woman returns from a 1-month vacation in Puerto Rico suffering from crampy abdominal pain and diarrhea. She spent most of her vacation in rural areas and took no precautions with the food or water she consumed. Her physician is concerned about a parasitic infection, so stool specimens are collected for O&P examination; an organism is found in her stool specimens (see figure). Which organism is responsible for her infection?

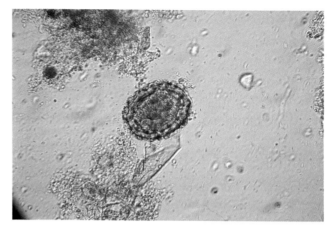

From Cohen J, Powderly WG: *Infectious diseases*, ed 2, St Louis, 2004, Mosby.

- ❐ (A) *Ascaris lumbricoides*
- ❐ (B) *Enterobius vermicularis*
- ❐ (C) *Necator americanus*
- ❐ (D) *Strongyloides stercoralis*
- ❐ (E) *Trichuris trichiura*

40 Which microscopic staining method should be used to detect *Entamoeba histolytica*?

- ❐ (A) Calcofluor white stain
- ❐ (B) Gram stain
- ❐ (C) Kinyoun stain
- ❐ (D) Trichrome stain
- ❐ (E) Wright-Giemsa stain

41 Which route of infection is common for *Entamoeba histolytica*?

- ❐ (A) Direct inoculation
- ❐ (B) Direct skin penetration
- ❐ (C) Fecal-oral
- ❐ (D) Inhalation
- ❐ (E) Mosquito bite

42 A 36-year-old woman presents to her primary care physician with complaints of pain on urination and hematuria. Her relevant medical history is that 3 months before her symptoms developed, she lived in Egypt for 5 years. Urinalysis is performed, and normal levels of glucose and protein are found. Bacteria are not observed on microscopy, but eggs are present (see figure). Which organism is most likely responsible for this woman's infection?

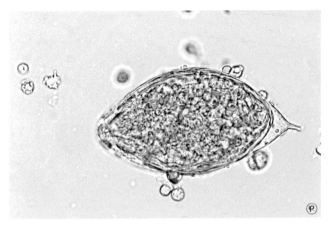

From Marler LM, Siders JA, et al: *Parasitology* CD-ROM, Indiana Patholgy Images, 2003.

☐   (A)   *Fasciolopsis buski*
☐   (B)   *Paragonimus westermani*
☐   (C)   *Schistosoma haematobium*
☐   (D)   *Schistosoma japonicum*
☐   (E)   *Schistosoma mansoni*

43   An HIV-infected patient develops profuse, watery diarrhea. His physician collects stool specimens for bacterial, fungal, mycobacterial, and parasitology examination. Later that day, the clinical laboratory telephones the physician and informs her that acid-fast cocci, 4 to 6 μm in diameter, are observed on parasitology examination. Which organism most likely responsible for these infections?

☐   (A)   *Candida*
☐   (B)   *Cryptosporidium*
☐   (C)   *Cyclospora*
☐   (D)   *Isospora*
☐   (E)   Microsporidia

44   *Schistosoma mansoni* is able to avoid the host immune response by which mechanism?

☐   (A)   Acquisition of host antigens
☐   (B)   Encystment in muscle
☐   (C)   Formation of thick extracellular cuticle
☐   (D)   Inhibition of phagosome/lysosome fusion
☐   (E)   Intracellular replication

45   A 61-year-old-man presents to his physician with diarrhea, abdominal pain, and a nonproductive cough. The diagnosis of multiple myeloma was made 2 years prior to this visit, and 1 month before his current illness began, he underwent a bone marrow transplant. An induced sputum and blood are collected for bacterial culture, and stool specimens are collected for bacterial culture and O&P examination. The sputum and stool cultures are negative, but the blood culture is positive for *Escherichia coli*. The O&P examination is also positive for an organism (see figure). Which parasite is most likely responsible for this patient's illness?

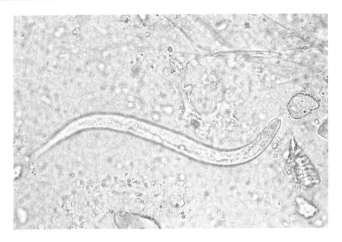

☐   (A)   *Ancyclostoma*
☐   (B)   *Ascaris*
☐   (C)   *Necator*
☐   (D)   *Strongyloides*
☐   (E)   *Trichinella*

46   A 56-year-old man with acquired immune deficiency virus (AIDS) is brought to the local hospital by his companion. The patient has been suffering from a headache, fever, and fatigue for several weeks and appears to be disoriented. The patient's CD4 T lymphocyte count is $25/mm^3$. The physician who examines the patient considers toxoplasmosis in his differential. Which test would be most useful in confirming this diagnosis?

☐   (A)   Detection of *Toxoplasma*-specific antibodies in blood
☐   (B)   Detection of *Toxoplasma*-specific antibodies in CSF
☐   (C)   Culture CSF in tissue culture cells
☐   (D)   Immunoperoxidase staining of brain biopsy
☐   (E)   *Toxoplasma*-specific polymerase chain reaction (PCR) using CSF

47   Which route of infection is most common for *Opisthorchis (Clonorchis) sinensis?*

☐   (A)   Direct inoculation
☐   (B)   Direct skin penetration
☐   (C)   Fecal-oral
☐   (D)   Ingestion
☐   (E)   Mosquito bite

48   A 7-year-old girl living in El Paso, Texas, develops bloody diarrhea, abdominal pain, and nausea. Bacterial culture of a stool specimen is negative, but O&P examination is positive for an organism (see figure). Which organism is responsible for her infection?

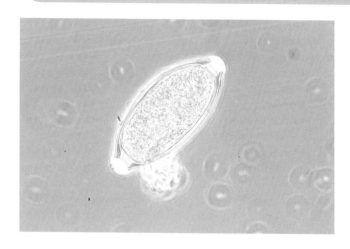

49 Which vector is associated with disease caused by *Babesia microti?*

❐   (A)   Mosquito
❐   (B)   Reduviid bug
❐   (C)   Sandfly
❐   (D)   Tick
❐   (E)   Tsetse fly

❐   (A)   *Ascaris lumbricoides*
❐   (B)   *Enterobius vermicularis*
❐   (C)   *Necator americanus*
❐   (D)   *Toxocara canis*
❐   (E)   *Trichuris trichuria*

1 **(A) Amphotericin B.** Amphotericin B is thought of as an antifungal agent; however, it also has activity against the free-living protozoa, *Naegleria fowleri*. *N. fowleri* is exquisitely susceptible to amphotericin B. Unfortunately, the other free-living protozoa associated with amebic encephalitis, *Acanthamoeba*, is resistant to this antimicrobial. The other agents listed in the answers to this question are ineffective against *Naegleria*.
MM5 869-870

2 **(B) Direct skin penetration.** The filariform larva of *S. stercoralis* is infectious and can infect humans by directly penetrating the skin. Autoinfections can also occur in patients with severe disease. In this case, the noninfectious rhabditiform larva is able to develop into the infectious filariform larva and penetrate the intestine or perianal skin and initiate a new cycle of infection. Sexual transmission can also occur.
MM5 885-887

3 **(E) Giemsa.** Giemsa stain is used to detect blood-borne pathogens (e.g., *Borrelia*, *Ehrlichia*, *Anaplasma*, *Rickettsia*, *Plasmodium*, *Babesia*, microfilaria). Calcofluor white is a nonspecific fluorochrome that binds to cellulose and chitin. Chitin is present in the cell wall of fungi. Gram stain is used primarily to stain bacteria and will not stain *Babesia*. Kinyoun stain is an acid-fast stain and will not stain *Babesia*. Trichrome stain is used to detect intestinal and urogenital protozoa.
MM5 866-867

4 **(C) *Cyclospora*.** Of the organisms listed in the answers to this question, all are acid-fast except *Candida*. The easiest way to differentiate the acid-fast parasites is by their size: microsporidia are 1 to 2 μm in diameter; *Cryptosporidium* is 4 to 6 μm; *Cyclospora* is 8 to 10 μm; and *Isospora* is 10 to 19 μm wide and 20 to 30 μm long.
MM5 856-858

5 **(D) Simulium black fly.** The Simulium black fly is the vector of *O. volvulus* infections (onchocerciasis). The black fly becomes infected when it bites the skin of a person with onchocerciasis. The fly ingests the microfilaria in the skin of the infected individual, and then the microfilaria (or embryo) penetrates through the stomach wall of this fly and localizes in the thoracic muscles, where it mature to a first stage larva. The larva then migrates to the head and proboscis and matures to the second- and then third-stage larval forms. During this third stage, the larva is infectious and, when transmitted to a new human host during a bite, establishes disease in humans. *Onchocerca* larvae mature to adults in the subcutaneous tissues of humans and produce microfilariae that migrate in the skin.
MM5 891-893, 929-930

6 **(D) Human.** The parasite observed in the figure is the trophozoite form of *Entamoeba histolytica*, the etiologic agent of amebiasis. Characteristically, the trophozoites are motile and vary in average size from 15 to 30 μm. The single nucleus is round with a central karyosome and an even distribution of chromatin granules around the nuclear membrane. Ingested erythrocytes may be in the cytoplasm. The cysts are smaller (15 to 20 μm) and contain one to four nuclei (usually four). Round chromatoidal bars may be in the cytoplasm. Patients infected with *E. histolytica* pass noninfectious trophozoites and the infectious cysts in their stools. The trophozoites cannot survive in the external environment or when transported through the stomach. Therefore the main source of water and food contamination is the asymptomatic carrier who passes cysts. Cockroaches and flies can serve as vectors of this parasite by transferring the cysts from human feces to food or water. Dogs do not serve as reservoirs, and mosquitoes have not been implicated as vectors.
MM5 847-849

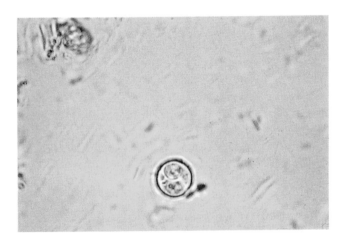

Courtesy of Williams, J; from Peters W, Giles HM: *Color atlas of tropical medicine and parasitology*, ed 4, London, 1995, Mosby-Wolfe.

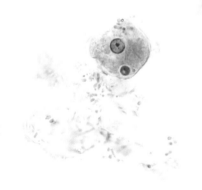

From Marler LM, Siders JA, et al: *Parasitology* CD-ROM, Indiana Patholgy Images, 2003.

7 **(B) Plague.** *Yersinia pestis* is the etiologic agent of the plague. This is a zoonotic infection, with rats as the natural reservoir in urban plague, and squirrels, rabbits, field rats, and domestic cats as the reservoirs in sylvan plague. Urban plague is maintained in rat populations and is spread among rats or between rats and among humans by infected fleas. The fleas become infected during a blood meal from a bacteremic rat. After the bacteria replicate in the flea gut, the organisms are transferred to another rodent or to humans during feeding. Sylvan plague is maintained in mammalian reservoirs and is spread among animals and occasional humans also by infected fleas.
MM5 932-933

8 **(C) Fecal-oral route.** *A. lumbricoides* is commonly known as a roundworm because the adult can resemble an albino earthworm. *A. lumbricoides* is prevalent where sanitation is poor and food and water can become contaminated with human feces. Disease is primarily acquired by ingestion of fecally contaminated products. The parasite is not transmitted by direct inoculation, direct skin penetration, inhalation, or insect bites.
MM5 881-882

9 **(B) Babesiosis.** *Babesia microti* is the most common species responsible for babesiosis in the United States. This is a zoonotic disease with a variety of animals serving as reservoir hosts, including deer, cattle, and rodents, and humans serving as accidental hosts. Human infection follows contact with an infected tick. The infectious pyriform bodies are introduced into the blood and infect erythrocytes. The intraerythrocytic trophozoites multiply by binary fission, forming tetrads, and then lyse the erythrocytes, releasing the merozoites. The merozoites can reinfect other cells to maintain the infection. Infected cells can also be ingested by feeding ticks, in which additional replication can take place. Infection in the tick population can also be maintained by transovarian transmission.
MM5 866-867

10 **(A) Beaver.** The organism in the figure is *Giardia lamblia*. *Giardia* trophozoites are 9 to 12 μm long and 5 to 15 μm wide. Flagella are present, as are two nuclei with large central karyosomes, a large ventral sucking disk for attachment to the intestinal villi, and two oblong parabasal bodies below the nuclei. Cysts are smaller at 8 to 12 μm long and 7 to 10 μm wide. Four nuclei and four parabasal bodies are present. *Giardia* has a worldwide distribution with streams and lakes contaminated in mountainous areas. The sylvan distribution is maintained in reservoir animals such as beavers and muskrats. In this setting, giardiasis is acquired through the consumption of inadequately treated contaminated water. The other animals listed in the answers to this question (i.e., dog, rabbit, snake, trout) have not been implicated in disease caused by this parasite.
MM5 850-852

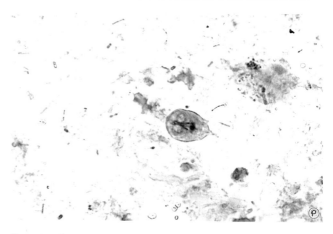

From Marler LM, Siders JA, et al: *Parasitology* CD-ROM, Indiana Patholgy Images, 2003.

11 **(E) Tularemia.** *Francisella tularensis* is the etiologic agent of tularemia. The organism is found in many wild mammals, domestic animals, birds, fish, and blood-sucking arthropods. The most common reservoirs of *F. tularensis* in the United States are rabbits, muskrats, and ticks. Infections can be maintained in the tick population with transovarian transmission. Human tularemia is acquired most often from the bite of an infected tick or contact with an infected animal.
MM5 926-927

12 **(B) *Cryptosporidium parvum.*** *C. parvum* has worldwide distribution, producing infection in a wide variety of animals, including mammals, reptiles, and fish. Specific *Cryptosporidium* species are associated with specific animal hosts, with *C. parvum* and *C. hominis* most commonly responsible for human disease. More than 70 species of *Babesia* are found in Africa, Asia, Europe, and North America, with *B. microti* responsible for disease along the northeastern seaboard of the United States. *P. falciparum* occurs almost exclusively in tropical and subtropical regions. *S. stercoralis* is present in the northern United States and Canada. *T. cruzi* disease in humans occurs most commonly in South and Central America.
MM5 855-856

13 **(B) *Cyclospora cayetanensis.*** *Cyclospora* is a coccidian parasite that can infect the small intestine and cause a chronic diarrheal disease. This organism, like *C. parvum*, *M. avium*, and *R. equi*, is acid-fast. It is distinguished from *C. parvum* by its size: *C. parvum* is 5 to 7 μm in diameter, and *C. cayetanensis* is 8 to 10 μm in diameter. *M. avium* is a small rod-shaped bacterium, 2 to 3 μm long. *R. equi* will initially appear rod-like, but within 24 h of growth, it will form 2 to 5 μm coccoid cells. *E. histolytica* is not acid-fast and is much larger that the other organisms listed in the answers to this question.
MM5 856-858

14   (A) Direct inoculation. *Acanthamoeba* are free-living amoebae that are primarily associated with infections of the eyes (keratitis) and central nervous system (encephalitis). The most common route of exposure to this organism is direct exposure to contaminated water (e.g., contaminated solutions used to clean contact lenses), soil, or air. Most infections follow direct inoculation into the eye (e.g., previously abraded cornea from the use of dirty contact lenses) or inhalation. The organism does not directly penetrate into the skin like some other parasites do (e.g., hookworm, *Strongyloides*). There is no evidence of person-to-person spread (e.g., by the fecal-oral route), of infections following ingestion of water or foods contaminated with *Acanthamoeba*, or of mosquitoes serving as carriers of the parasite.
MM5 869-870

15   (B) Albendazole. The benzimidazoles are broad-spectrum antihelminthic agents that include mebendazole, thiabendazole, and albendazole. The agents disrupt microtubular function, thus reducing the motility of the worms. Albendazole is active against *Trichinella*, as well as against other helminthes, including *Enterobius* (pinworm), hookworm, *Toxocara*, and *Trichuris*. The cestodes *Cysticercus* and *Echinococcus* are also susceptible.
MM5 834

16   (E) *Trypanosoma brucei*. *T. brucei*, which is the etiologic agent of sleeping sickness, is endemic from central West Africa (*T. brucei gambiense*) to central East Africa (*T. brucei rhodesiense*). The infectious stage of the parasite is the trypomastigote. This develops in the salivary glands of the tsetse fly and is transmitted during a bite. The trypomastigote enters the bite wound and then eventually the patient's blood, lymph nodes, and cerebrospinal fluid, where it replicates. Diagnosis is made by examining thick and thin blood films and aspirations from lymph nodes and concentrated cerebrospinal fluid. *T. cruzi* infections (American trypanosomiasis) occur in the Western Hemisphere from southern California to Argentina. *L. donovani* (visceral leishmaniasis) is present in China, India, the Middle East, and Africa. The amastigote stage (small ovoid cell) is diagnostic for leishmaniasis. *P. falciparum* is present in Africa but does not resemble the flagellated organism described in this question. *T. gondii* would also not be mistaken for *T. brucei*.
MM5 873-875

17   (C) Contaminated water. This outbreak is caused by *Cryptosporidium*, the only acid-fast parasite that is 4 to 6 μm in diameter. The most common source for *Cryptosporidium* infections in the United States has been contaminated water.
MM5 855-856

18   (E) *Microsporidium*. All of the parasites listed in the answers to this question can cause chronic diarrhea in HIV-infected patients. The characteristic that separates these parasites is their size. *Cryptosporidium* is 5 to 7 μm in diameter; *Cyclospora* is 8 to 10 μm in diameter; and *Giardia* and *Isospora* are much larger. Microsporidia are a large group of intracellular parasites in the phylum Microspora. Six genera of microsporidia have been reported in humans: *Encephalitozoon*, *Enterocytozoon*, *Nosema*, *Pleistophora*, *Trachipeleistophora*, and *Vittaforma*. The spores of microsporidia can stain with the tissue Gram stain, acid-fast stain, Giemsa stain, and a special chromotrope-based stain developed to detect the parasites. Infections in immuno-compromised patients are generally chronic because effective treatment of microsporidian infections has not been found.
MM5 858-859

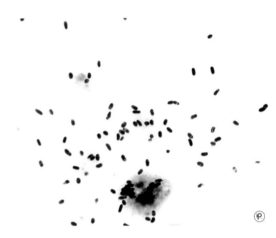

From Marler LM, Siders JA, et al: *Parasitology* CD-ROM, Indiana Patholgy Images, 2003.

19   (C) Epidemic relapsing fever. Two forms of relapsing fever are caused by *Borrelia* species: epidemic or louse-borne relapsing fever and endemic relapsing fever caused by exposure to soft ticks of the genus *Ornithodorus*. The human body louse, *Pediculus humanus*, spreads epidemic relapsing fever. Lice become infected after feeding on an infected person. The organisms are ingested, pass through the wall of the gut, and multiply in hemolymph. Human infection occurs when the lice are crushed during feeding. Because lice do not survive for more than a few months, maintenance of disease in a population requires crowded, unsanitary conditions (e.g., wars, natural disasters).
MM5 931-932

20   (E) *Isospora*. *Isospora* is the largest acid-fast parasite responsible for human disease. *Cryptosporidia* are 5 to 7 μm in diameter, and *Cyclospora* are 8 to 10 μm in diameter. *Entamoeba* and *Giardia* are not acid-fast. Each of the parasites causes diarrheal disease, with *Entamoeba histolytica* responsible for a hemorrhagic colitis and the other parasites causing a watery diarrhea.
MM5 854-855

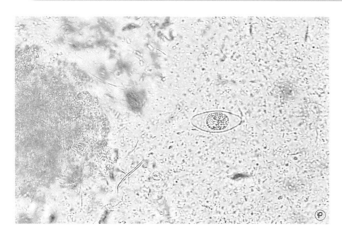

From Marler LM, Siders JA, et al: *Parasitology* CD-ROM, Indiana Patholgy Images, 2003.

21 **(A)** *Diphyllobothrium latum.* D. latum, the fish tapeworm, has a complex life cycle involving freshwater crustacean and fish as intermediate hosts and humans as the primary host. Ingestion of inadequately cooked fish exposes the human host to the larval worm (sparganum). Within 1 month, the larval worm will mature to the adult stage in the small intestine and begin to produce eggs that can continue for months to years. Human infection with *E. multilocularis* follows the accidental exposur to the parasite's eggs present in the feces of infected foxes, wolves, dogs, or cats. Infection with *F. hepatica* follows ingestion of the encysted larval stage (metacercaria) present in aquatic vegetation, such as water chestnuts. Infection with *H. diminuta* follows ingestion of grain products contaminated with infected larval insects. Infection with *P. westermani* follows ingestion of uncooked freshwater crabs and crayfish infected with the parasite.
MM5 910-911

22 **(A)** African trypanosomiasis. *Trypanosoma brucei* is the etiologic agent of African trypanosomiasis or sleeping sickness. Human disease is acquired by the bite of an infected tsetse fly. Tsetse flies become infected by biting an infected host and ingesting the trypomastigotes in the blood. The organisms replicate in the midgut and then migrate to the salivary glands, where an epimastigote form continues reproduction to the infective trypomastigote stage. The trypomastigotes are then transferred to the next host during a bite.
MM5 873-875

23 **(B)** *Leishmania braziliensis.* L. braziliensis is one of the *Leishmania* species that causes cutaneous and mucocutaneous leishmaniasis. Infections have been particularly common in soldiers in the Middle East. Diagnosis is made by detecting the amastigote stage in tissue or lymph nodes. Amastigotes are spherical-shaped cells, 1 to 5 μm long and 1 to 2 μm wide, with a large nucleus and prominent kinetoplast. The other organisms

listed in the answers to this question (i.e., *B. microti*, *P. vivax*, *T. gondii*, and *T. cruzi*) would not be mistaken for *L. braziliensis*.
MM5 872-873

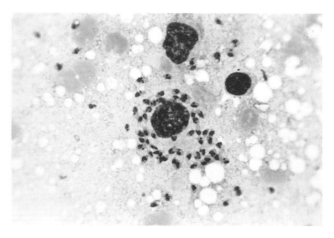

From Marler LM, Siders JA, et al: *Parasitology* CD-ROM, Indiana Patholgy Images, 2003.

24 **(C)** Fecal-oral. *Enterobius vermicularis* is commonly known as the pinworm. It causes gastrointestinal disease in humans, particularly in children. The adult worm lays her eggs in the perianal area, and person-to-person spread occurs most commonly by the fecal-oral route. The organism is unable to cause disease by direct inoculation, direct skin penetration, inhalation, or mosquito bites.
MM5 879-881

25 **(B)** *Plasmodium falciparum.* The question does not state whether the woman took any prophylaxis for malaria; however, because she did not take other precautions, malaria is certainly a disease to consider. *P. falciparum* is present in tropical and subtropical regions. Diagnosis of malaria is made by examination of thick and thin blood smears. *P. falciparum* can be identified by the presence of small, delicate ring forms to the exclusion of other forms (e.g., trophozoites, schizonts) in infected erythrocytes. Cells may be infected with multiple organisms, stippling (dots) is uncommon, and the rings may be arranged at the edge of the cell (appliqué form). Crescent-shaped gametocytes may also be observed. The other *Plasmodium* species listed in the answers to this question should not be confused with *P. falciparum*. Ring forms, as well as trophozoites and schizonts, should be observed in the blood. Trophozoites of *B. microti* can be mistaken for *Plasmodium* ring forms unless carefully examined. The travel history is inconsistent with babesiosis. *T. cruzi* would not be confused with *P. falciparum*.
MM5 861-869

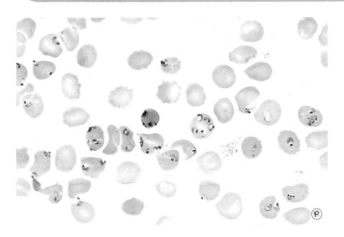

From Marler LM, Siders JA, et al. *Parasitology* CD-ROM, Indiana Patholgy Images, 2003.

26 **(D) Inhibition of phagosome/lysosome fusion.** Toxoplasma is an intracellular parasite that exists in two forms in humans: the actively proliferating trophozoites and the resting form or cysts. If the parasite is phagocytosed by macrophages, intracellular killing is avoided by the parasite's inhibition of fusion of the phagosome and the lysosome.
MM5 867-869

27 **(C) *Cryptosporidium.*** Acid-fast organisms include *Mycobacterium, Nocardia, Rhodococcus, Tsukamurella, Gordonia,* microsporidia, *Cryptosporidium, Cyclospora,* and *Isospora.* *Actinomyces, Corynebacterium, Giardia,* and *Streptomyces* will not stain with acid-fast stains. *Corynebacterium* species that were previously reported as acid-fast have now been reclassified in other genera (i.e., *Rhodococcus, Tsukamurella, Gordonia*).
MM5 855-856

28 **(A) *Acanthamoeba.*** *Acanthamoeba* species can produce a devastating keratitis that is difficult to treat and frequently leads to enucleation of the eye. The keratitis is usually associated with eye trauma that occurred before contact with contaminated soil, dust, or water. In this patient's situation, the eye trauma is likely related to contact wear that can abrade the surface of the cornea. The use of contaminated water to clean the contacts can introduce the amoeba on the contacts. The other parasites listed in the answers to this question are not associated with eye infections.
MM5 869-870

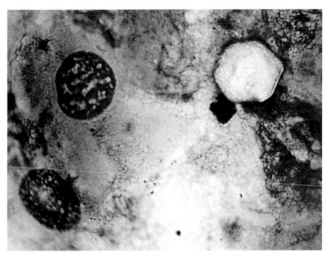

From Cohen J, Powderly WG: *Infectious diseases,* ed 2, St Louis, 2004, Mosby.

29 **(E) Microsporidia.** Microsporidia are obligate intracellular pathogens belonging to the phylum Microspora. Infection is acquired by ingestion of the spores. The spores multiply in the cells lining the small intestine. Immunocompetent patients generally do not have symptoms from ingestion of the spores, but immunocompromised patients, such as this patient, can develop persistent and debilitating diarrhea similar to patients with cryptosporidiosis, cyclosporiasis, and isosporiasis. The parasites are most easily distinguished by size, with microsporidia being the smallest. *Entamoeba* and *Giardia* are much larger than microsporidia and would not be confused with these parasites.
MM5 858-859

From Cohen J, Powderly WG: *Infectious diseases,* ed 2, St Louis, 2004, Mosby.

30 (D) Metronidazole. Metronidazole is a nitroimidazole agent that is believed to inhibit DNA and RNA synthesis, as well as the metabolism of glucose and mitochondrial function. Metronidazole is the drug of choice for trichomoniasis and giardiasis. It is also active against strict anaerobic bacteria.
MM5 833-844

31 (A) Basil in salad. This infection is caused by *Cyclospora*, the only acid-fast parasite that is 8 to 10 µm in diameter. In developing countries, *Cyclospora* is frequently found in contaminated water, and this is a likely source of infection for travelers. In the United States, however, most outbreaks of *Cyclospora* infections have been associated with imported berries and basil.
MM5 856-858

32 (B) *Enterobius*. Eggs of *Enterobius vermicularis*, the pinworm, are seen in the figure. Infection is most common in children who become infected when they ingest the eggs. The larvae hatch in the small intestine and migrate to the large intestine, where they mature into adults. The females are fertilized by male worms, and then egg laying commences. The eggs are laid in the perianal folds by the migrating female. The eggs are characteristically flattened on one side, 50 to 60 µm long and 20 to 30 µm wide. These eggs would not be confused with eggs produced by the other nematodes listed in the answers to this question.
MM5 879-881

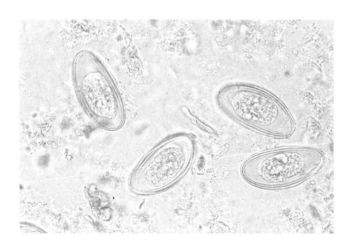

33 (A) Chrysops fly. The vector of Loa loa is the biting fly Chrysops or the mango fly. Microfilariae, present in the blood of humans, are ingested by the mango fly during the initial bite. The microfilariae then penetrate the stomach wall of the insect, localize in the thoracic muscles, and undergo two stages of larval development. The larvae migrate to the head and proboscis of the fly and infect a new human host when the fly bites. The microfilariae mature to adults in the lymphatic system and produce microfilariae that are observed in the patient's blood.
MM5 890-891

34 (C) *Opisthorchis sinensis*. *O. sinensis* is the Chinese liver fluke. This patient's travel history and diet indicate that he could have been infected with this organism or *F. hepatica*, the sheep liver fluke. *O. sinensis* is associated with consumption of infected raw fish and *F. hepatica* with uncooked watercress. The diagnosis is made by examination of the stool for characteristic eggs. *O. sinensis* eggs are 27 to 35 µm long and 12 to 19 µm wide. An opening or operculum with a prominent ridge or shoulders is at one end, and a small button is at the other end. *F. hepatica* eggs are significantly larger, 130 to 150 µm long and 63 to 90 µm wide with a small and indistinct operculum. The other parasites listed in the answers to this question are not associated with hepatitis, and their eggs would not be confused with *O. sinensis*.
MM5 899-900

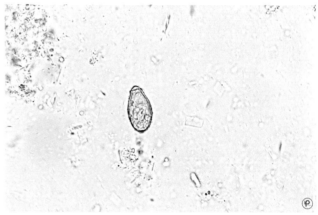

35 (E) *Taenia saginata*. Human infection with *T. saginata*, the beef tapeworm, follows ingestion of insufficiently cooked beef. The cysticerci in cattle mature in 1 month to the adult stage in the human small intestine, and egg laying may persist for up to 25 years. Ingestion of inadequately cooked freshwater fish exposes the human host to the larval worm (sparganum) of *D. latum*. Human infection with *E. multilocularis* follows the accidental exposure to the parasite's eggs present in the feces of infected foxes, wolves, dogs, or cats. Infection with *F. hepatica* follows ingestion of the encysted larval stage (metacercaria) present in aquatic vegetation, such as in water chestnuts. *G. lamblia* infections follow ingestion of the cyst form of the flagellate.
MM5 909-910

36 (E) Trichrome stain. This boy has meningoencephalitis caused by a free-living amoeba, most likely *Naegleria fowleri*. Infections are acquired by exposure to contaminated water. Acute infections are characterized by a fulminant, rapidly fatal meningoencephalitis. This infection commonly occurs in patients with no underlying diseases. An acid-fast stain can be used to diagnose infections with mycobacteria or *Nocardia*, but there is nothing in the clinical history to suggest infections with these organisms. A cryptococcal infection in a previously healthy patient is very uncommon, and the cerebrospinal fluid (CSF) profile is inconsistent with this pathogen. Late-stage Lyme

disease would not present with this fulminant course and without a prior history of a rash, carditis, or arthritis.
MM5 869-870

37 **(C) Direct skin penetration by infectious larvae.** This woman is infected with a hookworm, either *Ancyclostoma duodenale* or *Necator americanus*. The eggs of these two parasites are indistinguishable, having a thin outer shell and measuring 60 to 75 µm long and 35 to 40 µm wide. Eggs are shed in the feces of an infected patient; if the eggs are deposited on shady, well-drained soil, they can hatch and mature into infectious larvae. The larvae then penetrate unbroken skin, migrate to the lungs, and find their way to the small intestine. *Strongyloides* is the other important nematode that initiates infections in humans by penetrating the skin.
MM5 844-845

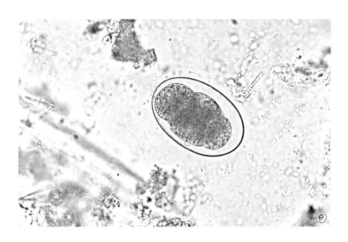

38 **(B) Encystment in muscle.** Trichinosis infection in humans is initiated when meat with encysted larvae of *Trichinella spiralis* is ingested. The larvae rapidly develop into adults in the small intestine and begin production of larval worms. These larvae move from the intestinal mucosa into the blood and are carried to striated muscle where they encyst.
MM5 887-888

39 **(A) *Ascaris lumbricoides*.** This woman has an *Ascaris* infection. Diagnosis is made by detection of the characteristic thick-walled eggs in her stool specimens. Eggs are typically 55 to 75 µm long and 35 to 50 µm wide. Both fertilized and infertile eggs may be seen. Although other parasites listed in the answers to the question may cause gastrointestinal symptoms, the eggs of *A. lumbricoides* (the roundworm) are readily distinguished from these other parasites.
MM5 881-882

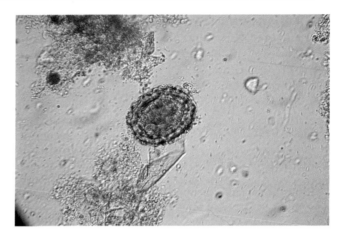

From Cohen J, Powderly WG: *Infectious diseases*, ed 2, St Louis, 2004, Mosby.

40 **(D) Trichrome stain.** Trichrome stain is used to detect intestinal and urogenital protozoa, including *Entamoeba histolytica*. Calcofluor white is a nonspecific fluorochrome that binds to cellulose and chitin. Chitin is present in the cell wall of fungi. Gram stain is used primarily to stain bacteria; Kinyoun stain is an acid-fast stain. The only parasites that are acid-fast are microsporidia, *Cryptosporidium*, *Cyclospora*, and *Isospora*. The Wright-Giemsa stain is used to detect blood-borne pathogens (e.g., *Borrelia*, *Ehrlichia*, *Anaplasma*, *Rickettsia*, *Plasmodium*, *Babesia*, microfilariae).
MM5 847-849

41 **(C) Fecal-oral.** *E. histolytica* is responsible for amebiasis, a disease that is primarily restricted to the intestine although direct spread to the liver can occur in severe infections. Most infections are acquired by ingestion of fecally contaminated food products or water. Symptomatic or asymptomatic carriers pass the amoeba in their stools. The infectious cyst form can survive in the environment for long periods. Infections can also be transmitted by oral-anal sexual practice, and disease is prevalent in homosexual populations.
MM5 847-849

42 **(C) *Schistosoma haematobium*.** This patient has schistosomiasis caused by the blood fluke, *S. haematobium*. Infection occurs when an individual comes into contact with the free-swimming cercaria that can penetrate unbroken skin. The cercaria enter the circulation and move to the vesical, prostatic, rectal, and uterine plexuses and veins, where they mature into adult worms. Adult *S. haematobium* worms reside in the veins around the urinary bladder, where they proceed with egg laying. The eggs elicit an intense inflammatory reaction and stimulate microabscess formation. In addition, the larvae inside the eggs produce enzymes that aid in tissue destruction and allow the eggs to pass through the mucosa and into the lumen of the bowel and bladder, where they are passed in feces and urine. *S. haematobium* eggs are 112 to 170 µm long and 40 to 70 µm

wide, with a prominent terminal spine. *S. mansoni* has a lateral spine, and *S. japonicum* has smaller eggs with no prominent spine. *Fasciolopsis buski* eggs are larger than *S. haematobium* eggs, oval without a terminal spine, and with an operculum. *Paragonimus westermani* eggs are smaller than *S. haematobium* eggs, oval, and with an operculum. *F. buski* is the giant intestinal fluke and *P. westermani* is the lung fluke.
MM5 902-905

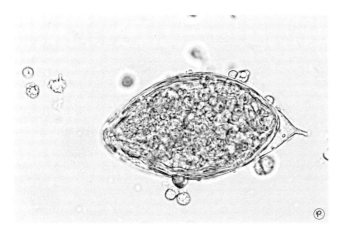

From Marler LM, Siders JA, et al. *Parasitology* CD-ROM, Indiana Pathology Images, 2003.

43 **(B) *Cryptosporidium*.** This infection is caused by *Cryptosporidium*, the only acid-fast parasite that is 4 to 6 μm in diameter. *Candida* is not acid-fast, whereas the other parasites listed in the answers to this question are weakly acid-fast. Microsporidia are 1 to 2 μm; *Cyclospora* are 8 to 10 μm; and *Isospora* are 10 to 19 μm wide and 20 to 30 μm long.
MM5 855-856

44 **(A) Acquisition of host antigens.** Human infection with *S. mansoni* is initiated when infected, free-swimming cercaria penetrate the skin. The cercaria are carried in the blood to the intrahepatic portal circulation where the worms will mature to adults. As the worms develop, they coat themselves with host antigens, thus protecting them from the host immune response. In contrast with the adult worms, the released eggs elicit an intense inflammatory reaction with mononuclear and polymorphonuclear cellular infiltrates, resulting in the formation of microabscesses.
MM5 902-905

45 **(D) *Strongyloides*.** This patient has an infection with *Strongyloides stercoralis*. The larvae of the parasite are able to penetrate skin, enter the circulatory system, and pass through the lungs. The worms are coughed up, swallowed, and then develop into adults in the small intestine. Eggs are deposited in the intestinal mucosa, where they hatch, releasing the larvae. Larvae and not eggs are detected in the stool specimens. Autoinfections can occur in immunocompromised patients. In this situation, the larvae in the stool develop into the infectious filariform larvae and repenetrate the intestines, initiating their migratory path from the circulatory system to the lungs and then to the small intestine. Autoinfections (hyperinfections) are characterized by perforation of the intestines when the larvae penetrate the intestinal wall to the circulatory system and pneumonitis when the worms migrate through the lungs. *Ancyclostoma* and *Necator* (hookworms) have a similar developmental cycle, but eggs and not larvae are found in stool specimens. Larvae for *Ascaris* or *Trichinella* would not be observed in clinical specimens.
MM5 885-887

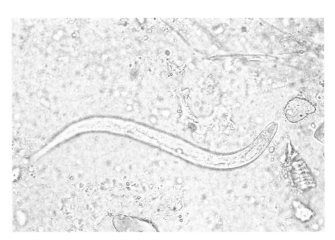

46 **(D) Immunoperoxidase staining of brain biopsy.** This test is sensitive and specific. The biopsy material could also be stained with the Giemsa stain, but this test is less sensitive. The detection of antibodies in blood does not discriminate between a current infection and a past infection. Detection of antibodies in CSF is insensitve. Isolation of *Toxoplasma* in tissue culture cells is a specific but insensitve test. PCR testing is used commonly in clinical laboratories but is less sensitive compared with immunoperoxidase staining.
MM5 867-869

47 **(D) Ingestion.** *Opisthorchis sinensis* is commonly called the Chinese liver fluke. This parasite has a complex life cycle, maturing first in snails and then in water plants (i.e., water chestnuts). Ingestion of the water chestnuts by humans leads to human disease. The organism is unable to infect humans by other routes (e.g., inoculation, skin penetration, fecal-oral, or mosquito bites).
MM5 899-900

48 **(E) *Trichuris trichuria*.** This patient is infected with *T. trichuria*, the whipworm. Infection is initiated by ingestion of infectious, embryonated eggs. After passing through the stomach, the egg hatches, releasing the larvae that migrate to the large intestine. The adult worm attaches to the cecum and begins egg laying. The eggs have a characteristic morphology: 50

to 55 µm long, 22 to 24 µm wide, and barrel-shaped with a thick shell and clear plugs at each end.

MM5 883-884

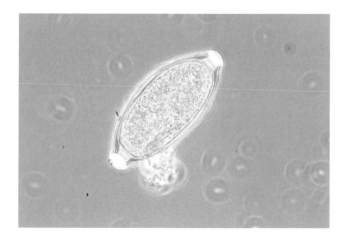

49 **(D) Tick.** *Babesia microti* is the etiologic agent of babesiosis, a zoonotic disease affecting a variety of animals with humans as an accidental host. This blood-borne infection is transmitted by the ixodid tick. Other biting insects (e.g., mosquito, reduviid bug, sandfly, or tsetse fly) have not been associated with this infection.

MM5 866-867